D0844681

WINDOWS TO THE BRAIN

Insights From Neuroimaging

WINDOWS TO THE BRAIN

Insights From Neuroimaging

Edited by

Robin A. Hurley, M.D.
W.G. "Bill" Hefner VAMC
Salisbury, North Carolina

Katherine H. Taber, Ph.D.
W.G. "Bill" Hefner VAMC
Salisbury, North Carolina

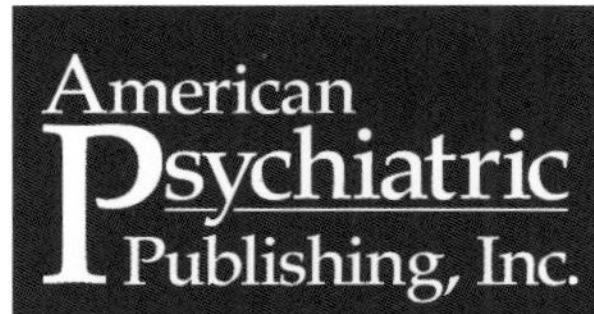

Washington, DC
London, England

Note: The authors have worked to ensure that all information in this book is accurate at the time of publication and consistent with general psychiatric and medical standards, and that information concerning drug dosages, schedules, and routes of administration is accurate at the time of publication and consistent with standards set by the U.S. Food and Drug Administration and the general medical community. As medical research and practice continue to advance, however, therapeutic standards may change. Moreover, specific situations may require a specific therapeutic response not included in this book. For these reasons and because human and mechanical errors sometimes occur, we recommend that readers follow the advice of physicians directly involved in their care or the care of a member of their family.

Books published by American Psychiatric Publishing, Inc., represent the views and opinions of the individual authors and do not necessarily represent the policies and opinions of APPI or the American Psychiatric Association.

If you would like to buy between 25 and 99 copies of this or any other APPI title, you are eligible for a 20% discount; please contact APPI Customer Service at appi@psych.org or 800–368–5777. If you wish to buy 100 or more copies of the same title, please e-mail us at bulksales@psych.org for a price quote.

Drs. Hurley and Taber have no competing interests to disclose.

Manufactured in China on acid-free paper
11 10 09 08 07 5 4 3 2 1
First Edition

Typeset in Adobe's Berkeley and Formata

American Psychiatric Publishing, Inc.
1000 Wilson Boulevard
Arlington, VA 22209–3901
www.appi.org

Library of Congress Cataloging-in-Publication Data
Windows to the brain : insights from neuroimaging / edited by Robin A. Hurley, Katherine H. Taber.—1st ed.
p. ; cm.
Includes bibliographical references and index.
ISBN 978-1-58562-302-0 (hardcover : alk. paper)
1. Brain—Imaging. 2. Nervous system—Imaging. 3. Mental illness—Diagnosis. I. Hurley, Robin A. II. Taber, Katherine H.
[DNLM: 1. Brain Diseases—diagnosis. 2. Diagnostic Imaging. 3. Diagnostic Techniques, Neurological. 4. Mental Disorders—diagnosis. WL 141 W7655 2008]
RC473.B7W56 2008
616.8′04754—dc22

2007038071

British Library Cataloguing in Publication Data
A CIP record is available from the British Library.

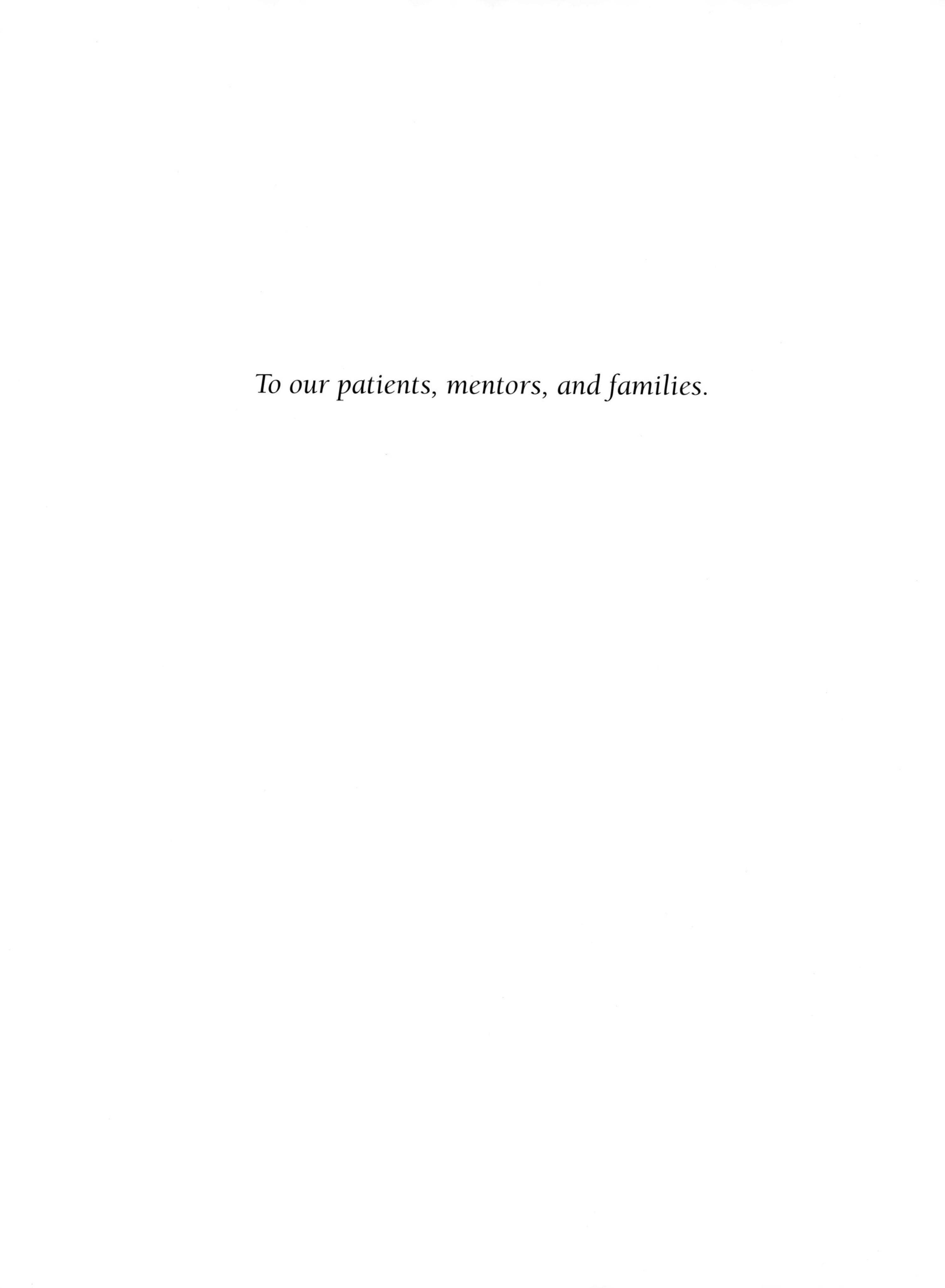

To our patients, mentors, and families.

CONTENTS

Part 1
IMAGING TECHNIQUES

Part 2
SPECIFIC DISEASES

Contributors

Anissa Abi-Dargham, M.D.
Department of Clinical Psychobiology, New York State Psychiatric Institute, New York, New York

Ichiro Akiguchi, M.D.
Division of Neurological and Cerebrovascular Disease Center, Takeda Hospital, Kyoto, Japan

Konstantinos Arfanakis, Ph.D.
Department of Biomedical Engineering, Illinois Institute of Technology, Chicago, Illinois

Chawki Benkelfat, M.D., D.E.R.B.H.
Department of Psychiatry, McGill University, Montreal, Quebec, Canada

Erin D. Bigler, Ph.D.
Department of Psychology, Brigham Young University, Provo, Utah

Deborah N. Black, M.D.
Department of Neurology, University of Vermont, Burlington, Vermont; Department of Psychiatry, University of Montreal, Quebec, Canada

Kevin J. Black, M.D.
Departments of Psychiatry, Neurology, and Radiology, Washington University School of Medicine, St. Louis, Missouri

Mathew M. Blurton-Jones, M.S.
Department of Neurobiology and Behavior, University of California at Irvine

William G. Bradley Jr., M.D., Ph.D.
Department of Radiology, University of California at San Diego

Jonathan B. Chalk, M.B.B.S., F.R.A.C.P., Ph.D.
School of Medicine and Centre for Magnetic Resonance, The University of Queensland, Brisbane, Australia

Pietro Cortelli, M.D., Ph.D.
Dipartimento di Scienze Neurologiche, Universita'di Bologna, Bologna, Italy

Luis Del Valle, M.D.
Center for Neurovirology and Cancer Biology, Temple University, Philadelphia, Pennsylvania

Thomas Ernst, Ph.D.
Department of Medicine, John A. Burns School of Medicine, University of Hawaii at Manoa, Honolulu, Hawaii

Ronald E. Fisher, M.D., Ph.D.
Department of Radiology, Baylor College of Medicine, Houston, Texas

Jaqueline N.W. Friedman, Ph.D.
Veterans Affairs Mid Atlantic Mental Illness Research, Education, and Clinical Center, Mental Health Service Line, Salisbury Veterans Affairs Medical Center, Salisbury, North Carolina

Glen O. Gabbard, M.D.
Department of Psychiatry and Behavioral Sciences, Baylor College of Medicine, Houston, Texas

Robert E. Hales, M.D., M.B.A.
Department of Psychiatry and Behavioral Sciences, University of California–Davis School of Medicine, and Sacramento County Mental Health Services, Sacramento, California; American Psychiatric Publishing, Inc., Arlington, Virginia

William Hart, B.S.R.S., R.T.
Plaza Medical Center of Fort Worth, Fort Worth, Texas

L. Anne Hayman, M.D.
Medical Clinic of Houston, Houston, Texas

Sabine C. Herpertz, M.D.
Department of Psychiatry and Psychotherapy, Rostock University, Rostock, Germany

Rudolf Hoehn-Saric, M.D.
Department of Psychiatry, Johns Hopkins School of Medicine, Baltimore, Maryland

Ramona O. Hopkins, Ph.D.
Department of Psychology, Brigham Young University, Provo, Utah

Robin A. Hurley, M.D., F.A.N.P.A.
Veterans Affairs Mid Atlantic Mental Illness Research, Education, and Clinical Center, Mental Health Service Line, Salisbury Veterans Affairs Medical Center, Salisbury, North Carolina; Departments of Psychiatry and Radiology, Wake Forest University School of Medicine, Winston-Salem, North Carolina; Departments of Radiology and of Psychiatry and Behavioral Sciences and the Herbert J. Frensley Center for Imaging Research, Baylor College of Medicine, Houston, Texas; Psychiatry Service, Houston Veterans Affairs Medical Center, Houston, Texas

Edward F. Jackson, Ph.D.
Department of Imaging Physics, The University of Texas M.D. Anderson Cancer Center, Houston, Texas

Peter A. Johnson, M.D. (B.A. at original publication)
Menninger Department of Psychiatry and Behavioral Sciences, Baylor College of Medicine, Houston, Texas

Derek K. Jones, Ph.D.
Institute of Psychiatry, King's College London, United Kingdom

Gregory M. Jones, Ph.D.
State Science Advisor, Salt Lake City, Utah

Kamel Khalili, Ph.D.
Center for Neurovirology and Cancer Biology, Temple University, Philadelphia, Pennsylvania

Asra Khan, M.D.
Department of Radiology, University of Michigan, Ann Arbor, Michigan

Ruth A. Lanius, M.D., Ph.D., F.R.C.P.C.
Department of Psychiatry, London Health Sciences Centre, University of Western Ontario, London, Ontario, Canada

Maryse Lassonde, Ph.D.
Centre de Recherche en Neuropsychologie et Cognition, University of Montreal, Quebec, Canada

Haleema T. Latifi, M.D.
Private practice, Houston, Texas

Jeffrey David Lewine, Ph.D.
Department of Radiology, University of Utah School of Medicine, Salt Lake City, Utah

David A. Lewis, M.D.
Department of Psychiatry, University of Pittsburgh, Pittsburgh, Pennsylvania

Joseph C. McGowan, Ph.D.
Managing Engineer, Exponent, Philadelphia, Pennsylvania

Cecilia V. Mendez, M.D.
Department of Psychiatry, Wake Forest University School of Medicine, Winston-Salem, North Carolina

Mario F. Mendez, M.D., Ph.D.
Departments of Neurology and Psychiatry and Biobehavioral Sciences, David Geffen School of Medicine, University of California at Los Angeles

Lisa A. Miller, M.D.
Menninger Department of Psychiatry and Behavioral Sciences, Baylor College of Medicine and Houston-Galveston Psychoanalytic Institute, Houston, Texas

Diane D. Murphy, Ph.D.
National Institute of Neurological Disorders and Stroke, National Institutes of Health, Bethesda, Maryland

William W. Orrison Jr., M.D.
Department of Radiology, University of Utah, Salt Lake City, Utah and Department of Psychology, Brigham Young University, Provo, Utah

Carlo Pierpaoli, M.D., Ph.D.
Section on Tissue Biophysics & Biomimetics, National Institute of Child Health & Human Development, National Institutes of Health, Bethesda, Maryland

Bernice Porjesz, M.D.
Department of Psychiatry, SUNY Downstate Medical Center, Brooklyn, New York

Anis Rashid, M.D.
Department of Psychiatry, The University of Texas M.D. Anderson Cancer Center, Houston, Texas

Scott L. Rauch, M.D.
Departments of Psychiatry and Radiology, Massachusetts General Hospital, Charlestown, Massachusetts

Liesbeth Reneman, M.D.
School of Neurosciences, Academic Medical Center, Amsterdam, The Netherlands

Stephen E. Rose, Ph.D.
Centre for Magnetic Resonance, The University of Queensland, Brisbane, Australia

Fergus J. Rugg-Gunn, M.D.
Department of Clinical and Experimental Epilepsy, Institute of Neurology, University College London, Queen Square, United Kingdom

Sanjaya Saxena, M.D.
Department of Psychiatry, University of California at San Diego

Andreea L. Seritan, M.D.
Department of Psychiatry and Behavioral Sciences, University of California–Davis, Sacramento, California

Daniel H.S. Silverman, M.D., Ph.D.
Department of Molecular and Medical Pharmacology, David Geffen School of Medicine, University of California at Los Angeles

Isabella Laura Simone, M.D.
Department of Neurological and Psychiatric Sciences, University of Bari, Bari, Italy

Wolfgang Staffen, M.D.
Department of Neurology, Christian Doppler Clinic and Center for Neurocognitive Research, Paracelsus Private Medical University, Salzburg, Austria

Emmanuel Stip, M.D.
Departments of Psychiatry and Pharmacology, Centre de Recherche Fernand-Seguin, Hôpital Louis-Hippolyte Lafontaine, University of Montreal, Quebec, Canada

Peter L. Strick, Ph.D.
Research Service Line, Pittsburgh Veterans Affairs Medical Center and Departments of Neurobiology, Neurological Surgery, and Psychiatry, University of Pittsburgh, Pennsylvania

Katherine H. Taber, Ph.D., F.A.N.P.A.
Veterans Affairs Mid Atlantic Mental Illness Research, Education, and Clinical Center, Mental Health Service Line, Salisbury Veterans Affairs Medical Center, Salisbury, North Carolina; Departments of Radiology, Physical Medicine and Rehabilitation, and of Psychiatry and Behavioral Sciences and the Herbert J. Frensley Center for Imaging Research, Baylor College of Medicine, Houston, Texas; School of Health Information Sciences, University of Texas Health Science Center, Houston, Texas

Hidekazu Tomimoto, M.D.
Department of Neurology, Graduate School of Medicine, Kyoto University, Kyoto, Japan

Deborah L. Warden, M.D.
Defense and Veterans Brain Injury Center, Walter Reed Army Medical Center, Washington, DC; Departments of Psychiatry and Neurology, Uniformed Services University of the Health Sciences, Bethesda, Maryland

Christopher Wen, M.D.
Private practice, Orange, California

Howard Yonas, M.D.
Department of Neurosurgery, University of New Mexico School of Medicine, Albuquerque, New Mexico

Stuart C. Yudofsky, M.D.
Menninger Department of Psychiatry and Behavioral Sciences, Baylor College of Medicine, Houston, Texas

Jingwu Zhang, M.D., Ph.D.
Department of Neurology, Baylor College of Medicine, Houston, Texas

Liying Zhang, Ph.D.
Bioengineering Center, Wayne State University, Detroit, Michigan

Jana G. Zimmerman, Ph.D.
Plaza Medical Center of Fort Worth, Fort Worth, Texas

Foreword

One avenue of understanding the history of medicine and of assaying the future of medicine is to identify and elucidate the applications of technological advances of a particular era to the diagnosis and treatment of human illnesses. Consider, for example, the glass magnifying lens. When Leeuwenhoek created the microscope by joining two convex lenses at the disparate ends of a hollow tube, he was paving the way for the advent of microbiology, antibiotic treatments, and even, arguably, evidence-based medicine. For the first time in history, physicians and scientists could visualize, and thereby study, classify, and link microorganisms to human disease states. Manifestly, the countless lives that have been saved based on these and related discoveries are monumental. However, the conceptual changes brought about the advances in medicine that can be traced to the applications of lens-based technology may be even more far-reaching. Prior to our ability to visualize microorganisms, the idea that invisible (evil?) particles from the air could enter the human body, infect and destroy human tissue, and take human life would be more closely related to metaphysics and superstition. Did these invisible particles come from gods? Were these flotsams dispatched to wreak havoc on particular individuals or mankind in general, because we had sinned against the gods? Were they the work of evil-doers amongst us who were spreading destructive spells, poisoning our drinking wells? How should we placate the gods to obviate these plagues—Excommunication? Sacrifice those among us who seem different? How should we punish those responsible aliens—wars, imprisonment, burning them on crosses? More constructively, and most important to our consideration in this book, what new technologies—beyond the glass lens—could be applied to the visualization of the human organism and the external agents that affect such towards the purpose of enhanced understanding of normative and disordered/diseased organic function?

In 1987, with the encouragement and generous support of the American Psychiatric Press, Inc., we (SCY and REH) founded and were appointed Editor and Deputy Editor, respectively, of *The Journal of Neuropsychiatry and Clinical Neurosciences* (*JNP*), a new peer-reviewed journal devoted to exploring and expanding the interface of psychiatry and neurology. Several years later, *JNP* was afforded the honor of being designated the official journal of the American Neuropsychiatric Association, the leading American association devoted to the advancement of neuropsychiatry and behavioral neurology.

The 1990s were designated the "Decade of the Brain," with the extravagant hope that scientific research would lead to a markedly enhanced understanding of human brain function and the pathogeneses of brain dysfunctions and the concomitant forging of major headways in the diagnosis and treatment of neuropsychiatric illnesses. Leading the charge in this ambitious enterprise were three extraordinary scientific enterprises: genetics, cellular and molecular biology, and neuroimaging.

During the first half of the 1990s, enormous excitement in the fields of neuropsychiatry and behavioral neurology was generated by the potential impact of technological advances in neuroimaging—particularly functional brain imaging—on the diagnosis and treatment of neuropsychiatric illnesses. *JNP* was receiving steadily increasing numbers of submissions related to neuroimaging, and many of these were innovative, interesting, and important contributions. Nonetheless, we believed that the role and promise of neuroimaging in neuropsychiatry was of sufficient importance that our readership could benefit from regular updates and overviews of advances in this realm. Of particular interest was how these neuroimaging advances were affecting—or might soon affect—the everyday practice of neuropsychiatry and behavioral neurology.

In 1996, we approached two brilliant young scientists who, as assistant professors at Baylor College of Medicine, were collaborating productively on a vast array of research and educational projects. Robin A. Hurley, M.D., is as gifted, energetic, and creative a neuropsychiatrist as we have seen in the combined half century that we have had leadership positions in academic institutions. Even as an assistant professor, Dr. Hurley was an accomplished scholar who had achieved an almost incomparable mastery of neuroanatomy, neurocircuitry, and neurophysiology, and was applying her vast knowledge to the ever-enlarging scope of neuroimaging. Katherine H. Taber, Ph.D., was a highly regarded neurobiologist with a keen interest in the emerging field of medical informatics—with the focus on understanding of the intersection between neuroradiology and neuropsychiatric disease. We asked Drs. Hurley and Taber to develop a regularly appearing column in each of the quarterly issues of *JNP* that would "bring to life" the clinical applications of the advances in neuroimaging for the practicing neuropsychiatrist, behavioral neurologist, and neuropsychologist. Prototypically modest and understated, this dynamic duo initially declined our offer, as they believed that they did not have the experience to take on such a challenge. We persisted, and they acceded to write several columns for *JNP* "on a trial basis." That was about 10 years—and 40 columns—ago.

Drs. Hurley and Taber decided to name their new column "Windows to the Brain" and to limit the lengths of the articles to 5–10 pages. Their stated goal was to craft unique pieces that were timely, original, interesting, entertaining, and, most importantly, clinically applicable. They would emphasize new neuroimaging technologies and their innovative applications to neuropsychiatry. To add dimension and diversity to their columns, Drs. Hurley and Taber, inveterate collaborators, selected authors and co-authors from international pioneers in brain imaging. The net result has been a product that has exceeded the both authors' and our own ambitious goals and our own high expectations for quality and relevance. The images presented in "Windows to the Brain" are clearly explained, clinically relevant, and often quite beautiful. Soon these images became the "cover art" for *JNP*, a practice broadly emulated by other fine scientific journals. The response of the *JNP* readership was uniformly and wildly enthusiastic, with many communicating to us that the column is their favorite component to the journal.

At the Annual Meeting of the American Neuropsychiatric Association (ANPA), one ANPA member surprised SCY by reporting the following:

> "Windows to the Brain" is the primary way I keep up with advances in clinical neuropsychiatry. It's not just the images, but the pithy case reports that describe both rare and common neuropsychiatric disorders and how to go about working patients up with these conditions. It is a very, very, efficient way to stay current.

SCY shared this comment with REH, and we both thought that, given all of the other resources by which to keep current, the member's enthusiasm was somewhat overstated. Although we had read—with enthusiasm—every word of every "Windows to the Brain" column, we were not prepared for the impact of the present volume, wherein all of the articles have been collected and organized into the coherent and integrating units of 1) imaging techniques, 2) specific diseases, 3) anatomy and circuitry, and 4) treatment. "The whole," in truth, is far greater than the sum of its parts. Let us consider several chapters as examples of this contention.

Chapter 1, "Blood Flow Imaging of the Brain: 50 Years' Experience," is a concise summary of the origins and step-by-step development of blood flow imaging techniques and applications. The authors dissect lucidly the limitations of the technologies and precisely how these were overcome. Differences among and relative advantages of differing imaging techniques such as cerebral blood flow (CBF), positron emission tomography (PET), single photon emission computed tomography (SPECT), computed tomography (CT), functional magnetic resonance imaging (fMRI), and others are illuminated. Chapter 2, "Functional Magnetic Resonance Imaging: Application to Posttraumatic Stress Disorder," immediately applies the basic information provided in Chapter 1 to a highly prevalent and disabling anxiety disorder. More details are provided about the underlying mechanistic principles of fMRI, and how this can be applied to study and understand changes in brain functioning in patients suffering from posttraumatic stress disorder (PTSD). The authors review and explicate the published literature, comparing changes in regional brain function in patients with PTSD with those in matched controls and concluding that "this finding is consistent with the finding that PTSD involves a failure of medial frontal regions to properly inhibit the amygdala...With fMRI techniques, the delicate balance between the structures of the emotion and memory tracts becomes more evident." Chapter 4 introduces the reader to another imaging modality, diffusion tensor imaging, and its applications to neuropsychiatry, while Chapter 6 discusses magnetoencephalography and how it can be applied to the study of people with autism, and Chapter 7 reviews applications of xenon computed tomography to general neuropsychiatric practice. We know of no other book that presents this information, vital to the practice of clinical neuropsychiatry or behavioral neurology, so concisely and clearly.

As revealed in Part 2 of *Windows to the Brain,* diagnostic neuroimaging has truly "come of age" in neuropsychiatry. From diagnosing the subtle and rare dementia, cortical basal degeneration, utilizing fluorodopa PET, to assaying the extent of brain damage secondary to carbon monoxide poisoning utilizing CT, MRI, and SPECT, understanding the role of new brain imaging technologies has become essential to the modern neuropsychiatrist and behavioral neurologist's diagnostic and prognostic armamentarium. In our opinion, no other book, to our knowledge, is as up-to-date, comprehensive, or as clear in this domain. The presentations and clinical descriptions of the neuropsychiatric conditions that are considered are tours de force in clarity and brevity. We invite you to peruse the descriptions of autism, Huntington's disease, mild (sports-related) traumatic brain injury, traumatic axonal injury, corticobasal degeneration, metachromic leukodystrophy, HIV-related progressive multifocal leukoencephalography, prion disease, Binswanger's disease, normal pressure hydrocephalus, multiple sclerosis, and a vast array of conditions conventionally considered to be psychiatric such as bipolar disorder, panic disorder, and obsessive compulsive disorder. The authors have succeeded in providing descriptive "snapshots" of these conditions that are useful for review, preparation for board examinations, and bedside applications. These chapters are veritable modern versions of clinical pathological conferences.

We indicated earlier our belief that one can gain a glimpse of the future of medicine by speculating about the applications of the cutting edge technologies of the present. Nowhere is this more manifest than in Part 4 of *Windows to the Brain,* which focuses on treatment. Chapter 30, "Predicting Treatment Response in Obsessive-Compulsive Disorder," provides a hint of the "personalized treatments" that neuroimaging and neurogenetics will help to bring about. Surgical treatments of neuropsychiatric diseases will revolutionize the treatments of neuropsychiatric conditions by providing more focal interventions than are possible by our current approach of "flooding the brain" with pharmacologic agents. Paving the way for and enabling these breakthroughs will be the full array of neuroimaging that will localize lesions, guide the placements of electrical devices, and measure brain responses to the neurosurgical interventions. We believe that procedures such as stereotactic neurosurgical ablation procedures and deep brain stimulation are barely the "tip of the iceberg" of future opportunities to treat a panoply of neuropsychiatric conditions that, heretofore, have been considered intractable.

We look forward with enormous enthusiasm to Drs. Hurley and Taber documenting and explicating this exciting new therapeutic world in succeeding "Windows to the Brain" *JNP* columns, while expressing our fathomless admiration and appreciation for their peerless prior contributions that are offered in this book.

Stuart C. Yudofsky, M.D.
Robert E. Hales, M.D., M.B.A.

PREFACE

The 1990s were designated the "Decade of the Brain." During this time, the scientific understanding of mental illness grew considerably. Psychiatry began to grasp the contributions of genetics, substance abuse, and stress to mental illness. Many new neurotransmitters were identified as having significant roles in these conditions as well. The study and classification of dementias flourished, as did a small but growing subspecialty, "neuropsychiatry." However, the contributions of neuroanatomy and the emotion/memory circuits remained more challenging. Parallel to the developments in psychiatry, radiology was also undergoing a technical revolution, with advances in computed tomography and the initial foray of clinical magnetic resonance imaging (MRI) into brain pathology. It only seemed natural that the two specialties would meet to advance our understanding of psychiatric disease. As the 21st century arrived, the pace of technological advances in radiological imaging accelerated with the development of MRI sequences to more clearly separate normal from pathological tissue, to view images in three dimensions, and to view the living brain as it functions. In fact, the technology advanced so quickly that it outstripped the clinicians' ability to use that information at the bedside. These new technologies made it possible to study the brain as a person thinks a thought, feels an emotion, or even has a hallucination. However, these incredible scientific tools and new discoveries were only "academic" if they could not be applied to patient care. Most practicing psychiatrists, at that point in time, had limited training in and understanding of how to use radiologic tools in mental health. Thus, the need to educate clinicians in order to apply this knowledge became imperative.

A single patient with new-onset psychosis after a recent motor vehicle accident created the environment that brought a neuroradiologist, a neurobiologist, and a psychiatry resident together. The three soon realized that they shared a common interest in advancing the understanding of neuroanatomy and neuroimaging as applied to psychiatric disease. One major challenge was how to present large amounts of scientific data in a clinician-friendly format. To meet this challenge, the neurobiologist (KHT) had been studying the new field of medical informatics, particularly the principles of information design. These concepts became readily useful to the group for both radiological publications and local teaching. Seeing the results of these efforts, Drs. Yudofsky and Hales encouraged the group to expand to a larger audience and thus, "Windows to the Brain" was created. Since that time, we have been fortunate to continue the series for seven years and expand into anatomical teaching charts, models, posters, lectures, and now, this textbook. It contains all of the "Windows to the Brain" papers (1999–2006), with the accompanying cover art and updates on the subject matter as available to date.

Within this book, we have separated the "Windows" papers into four sections to assist the reader in organizing the knowledge and to increase appreciation of the wide range of research and clinical applications for imaging in neuropsychiatry (imaging techniques, specific diseases, anatomy and circuitry, and treatment). The imaging chapters each largely focus on a particular imaging technique, its underlying principles, strengths and weaknesses, and applications to an example disease; the disease chapters each largely focus on a particular disease and the range of investigative techniques that are being utilized; the anatomy and circuitry chapters each largely focus on a particular brain structure or a functional neuropsychiatric circuit; the treatment-focused chapters each largely focus on a particular imaging-based approach to understanding or selecting best treatment options.

As neuropsychiatry continues to grow, and the understanding of anatomy and imaging continues to expand, it is our hope to continue to create this series. We want to bring that excitement and new knowledge to our clinicians and to our patients. This work could not have happened without the initial and continual mentorship of Drs. Yudofsky and Hales. It is under their leadership and guidance that we have succeeded. In addition, the series would not have been possible if it were not for our multitude of co-authors and helpful field experts. We have been fortunate over the years to be able to collaborate with many of the world's authorities in anatomy and imaging research.

We have always asked of them to assure that we have validity and accuracy when forging into a new area. We thank them immensely and wish each of them continual successes in their work. In addition, we are very appreciative of our supporting medical schools (Baylor College of Medicine and Wake Forest University) and the Veterans Health Administration, without which we could not have completed these papers. Finally, we wish to thank our patients, their families, and our own families, for they are our inspirations and motivations to pursue an understanding of our brains and how we can improve our lives.

Robin A. Hurley, M.D.
Katherine H. Taber, Ph.D.

Part 1

IMAGING TECHNIQUES

The human brain can be imaged both structurally and functionally. Structural imaging allows the clinician to view the normal anatomical landmarks, gray matter, white matter, and ventricles, as well as bony landmarks. Structural imaging is generally presented to the clinician in traditional x-ray format. Most importantly, this type of imaging allows for identification of pathology large enough for visualization. Traditional structural clinical imaging includes computed tomography (CT) and magnetic resonance imaging (MRI). CT is the preferred imaging modality when acute bleeding or skull fracture is suspected. MRI is preferred for visualization of more chronic pathological conditions. Functional imaging allows visualization of the living brain. The most common techniques are single-photon emission computed tomography (SPECT) and positron emission tomography (PET). Although some clinicians view these techniques as research tools, the last decade has proven many clinical uses. Functional imaging of the human brain has become a rapidly expanding field with such new techniques as functional MRI (fMRI), xenon CT, magnetoencephalography (MEG), neurotransmitter receptor imaging, diffusion tensor imaging (DTI), magnetization transfer imaging, and MR spectroscopy. Although the clinical utility of all these techniques is not fully understood, the applications are growing continuously. For a more general review of the basic principles of structural and functional imaging techniques and common clinical applications, the novice is referred to a general neuropsychiatry or imaging textbook.

In this section of the book, the reader will be exposed to many of these structural and functional methods from a more advanced neuropsychiatric point of view. Each of the papers largely focuses on one particular imaging technique at a time, its basic underlying principles, strengths and weaknesses, and applications to an example disease. As the reader reviews these techniques, he/she should be mindful that the disease/lesion process mentioned is only a single example of how to apply the technique. The papers were written to be read either in sequence as a group or as a single reference to a particular method of interest. Each paper contains references where the advanced scientist may go for more details and technical information, as well as a brief summary of pertinent literature that has been published since the original release of the *Windows* paper. By the conclusion of this section, the reader should have a basic understanding of the imaging methods available for neuropsychiatric practice or research.

Chapter 1

Blood Flow Imaging of the Brain

50 Years' Experience

Katherine H. Taber, Ph.D.
Kevin J. Black, M.D.
Robin A. Hurley, M.D.

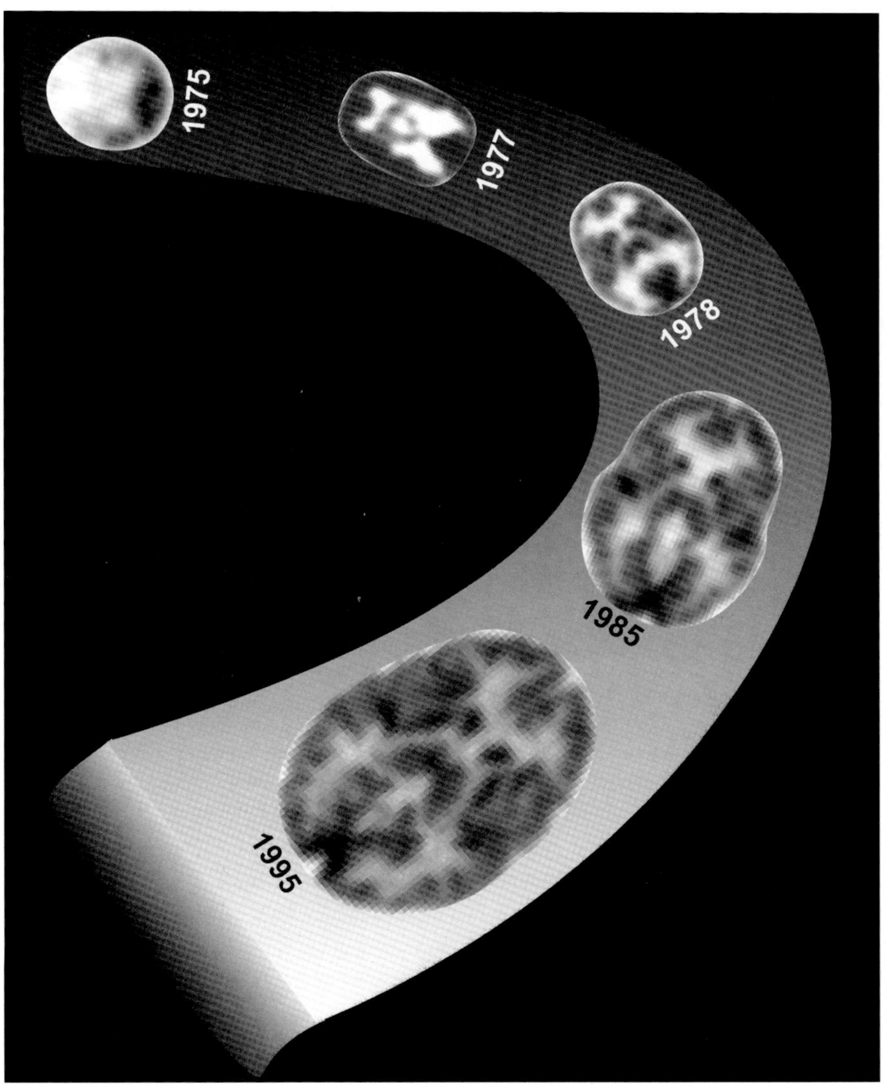

Representative axial cerebral blood flow images are labeled with the year they were made, illustrating the steady improvement in resolutions over the past two decades.

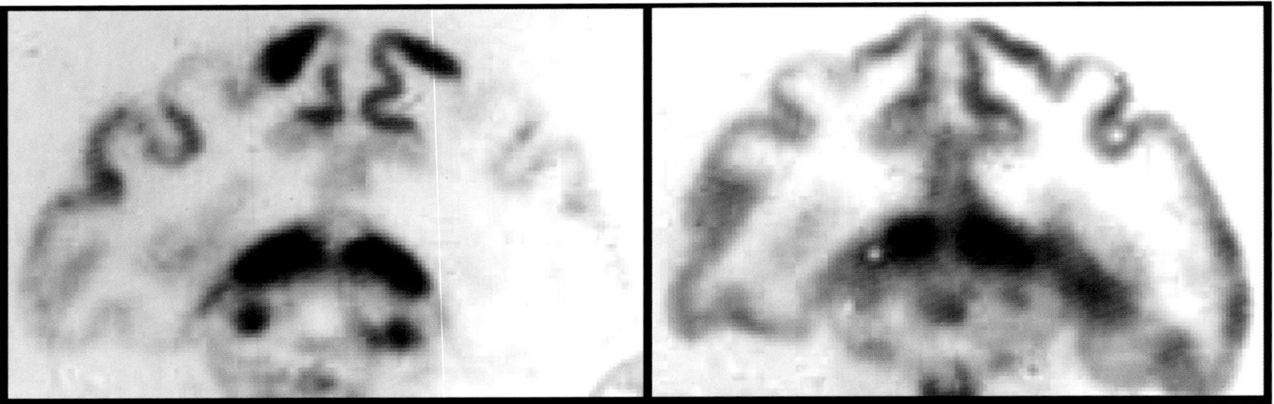

FIGURE 1–1. The first regional CBF images were acquired using the autoradiographic method (darker indicates higher flow).[1] The image on the right is a coronal CBF image from a cat sedated with thiopental anesthesia. The image on the left is from an awake cat. Note the much higher regional CBF in the awake animal. Images from the study kindly provided by Drs. Bill Landau and Marc Raichle.

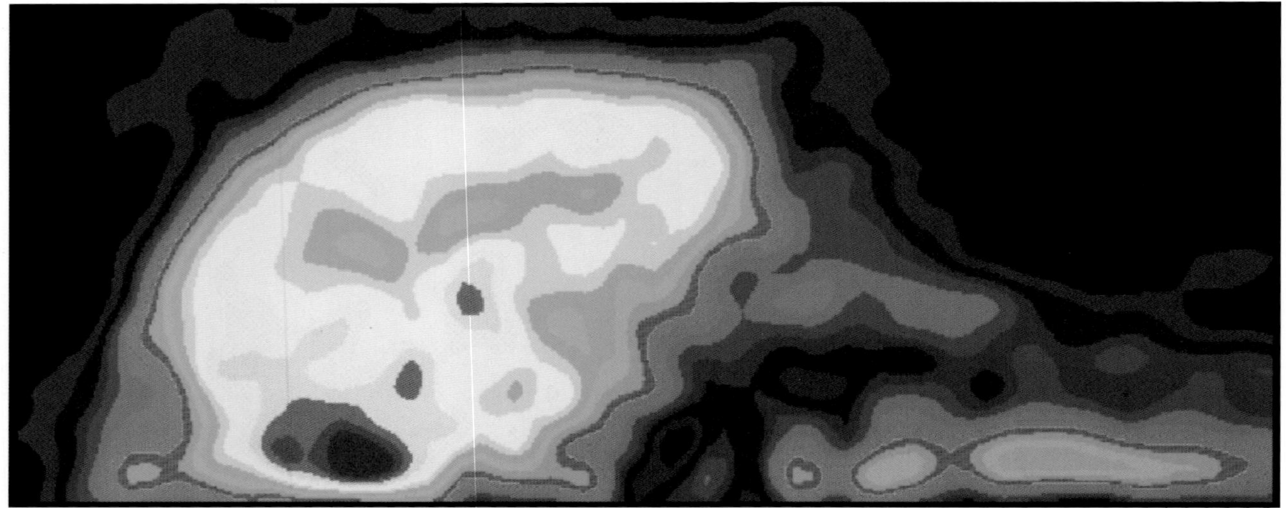

FIGURE 1–2. A midsagittal image of CBF using the [^{15}O] water PET technique in an awake macaque, acquired using a micro-PET scanner. Unpublished data courtesy of Dr. Kevin Black from work supported by NIH grant R01 NS044598.

The year 2005 marks the 50th anniversary of presentation of the first cerebral blood flow (CBF) image. An exciting new era opened in 1955 with the publication of "The local circulation of the living brain," an ex vivo study of the feline brain using a soluble gaseous radioactive tracer, trifluoroiodomethane.[1] This technique was called *autoradiography* because images were acquired by laying radioactive brain sections directly onto x-ray film.[4] The study included CBF images showing clear changes between a baseline (sedated) and stimulated (awake, restrained) state (Figure 1–1). This seminal study, which built upon earlier work from the same group demonstrating that CBF is locally regulated, set the stage for the development of the field of functional brain imaging.[5] The volatile nature of the gaseous tracer used initially created challenges.[4] Handling procedures were developed to prevent loss of the gas from tissue. The frozen brain had to be sectioned very rapidly, so sections were necessarily rather thick (~5 mm). These were stored in liquid nitrogen until placed between layers of x-ray film, surrounded by solid CO_2, and stored in darkness for the 10-hour exposure. Another challenge with this tracer was that its solubility in blood was influenced by both hematocrit and lipid content. The resultant individual differences in blood level of the tracer meant that a calibration curve had to be created for each subject. This group continued to refine the measurement of CBF. They introduced new radiotracers, first ^{131}I-antipyrine, followed by ^{14}C-antipyrine.[6,7] ^{14}C-antipyrine had many

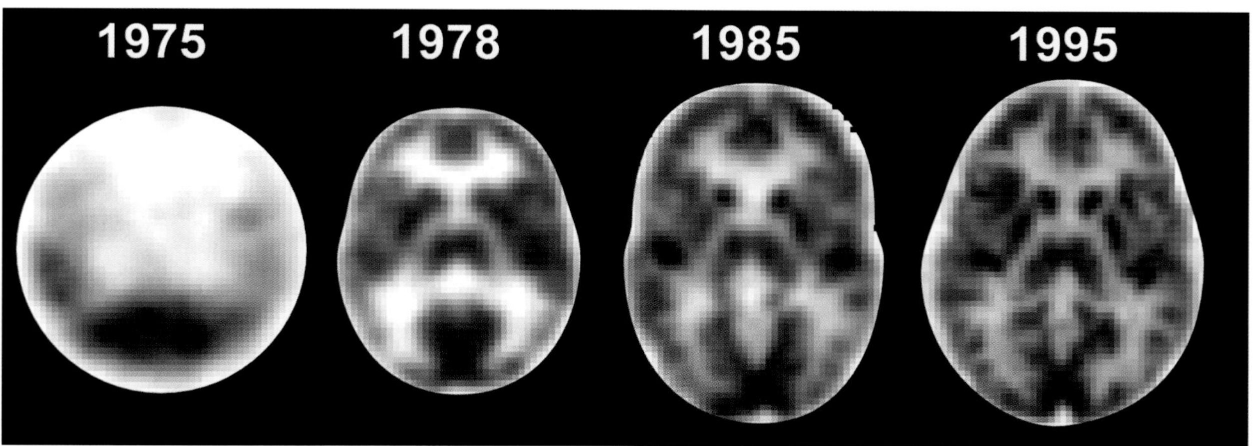

FIGURE 1–3. Axial PET images of brain acquired in 1975, 1978, 1985, and 1995. Note the significant improvement in resolution since the 1970s. To date, the number of detector elements has doubled ~ every 2 years.[2] Graphics courtesy of CTI Molecular Imaging, Inc.

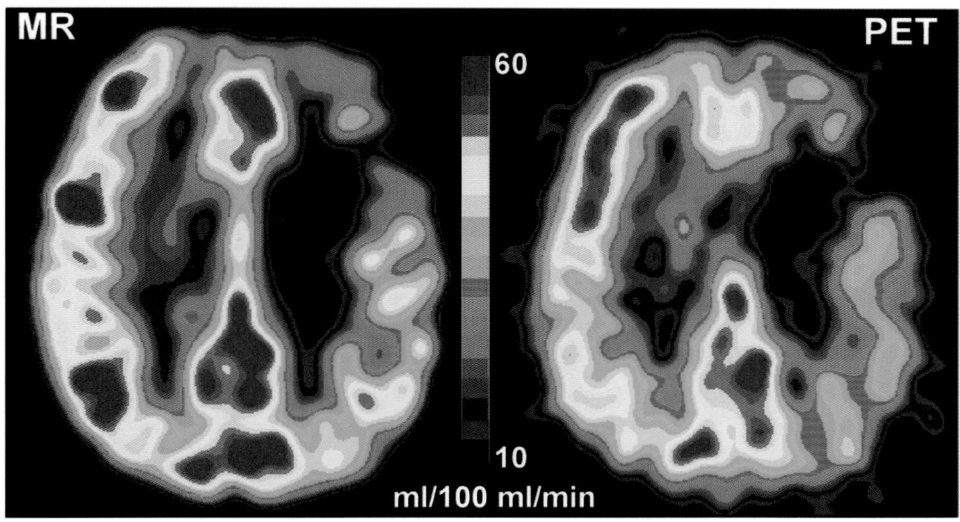

FIGURE 1–4. A comparison of axial CBF images acquired using dynamic susceptibility contrast-enhanced perfusion magnetic resonance imaging (left) and quantitative [^{15}O] water PET imaging (right) in a patient with chronic carotid occlusive disease. Both methods provide clear visualization of decreased CBF in the left hemisphere and an area of absent flow indicating chronic infarction in the frontal lobe. Close comparison of the two images shows areas of both over- and underestimation of CBF in the MR image. Used with permission from Mukherjee et al.[3]

advantages over previous tracers.[7] It was inert and freely diffusible. With a stable (nonvolatile) tracer it was possible to collect thin (~20 μm) sections and expose the x-ray film at room temperature. In addition, the much longer half-life made it possible to create permanent calibration standards. It also provided much higher resolution images, although exposure times were much longer (~2–4 weeks).[8] Interestingly, the authors themselves preserved a marked skepticism on the subject during presentation of the initial study. "Of course we recognize that this is a very secondhand way of determining physiological activity; it is rather like trying to measure what a factory does by measuring the intake of water and the output of sewage. This is only a problem of plumbing and only secondary inferences can be made about function. We would not suggest that this is a substitute for electrical recording in terms of easy evaluation of what is going on."[1] The past half-century of studies have clearly shown that CBF imaging can, in fact, produce valuable information about brain function.[9]

The critical next step was development of techniques during the early 1970s that allowed imaging of CBF in the living brain, making functional imaging in human subjects possible. This method was initially called *positron emission transaxial tomography* (PETT), later shortened to *positron emission tomography* (PET) (because it was possible to reconstruct images in planes other than transaxial).[2] Soon after the invention of PET, the new technique was applied to the measurement of regional CBF using radiolabeled water ($^{15}O-H_2O$).[10–12] Advances in physics and engineering have allowed production of PET images of very high resolution (microPET) for animal work (Figure 1–2). Animal imaging remains important for both prospective study of experimental models and development of new methods.

The prototype PET scanner suitable for human imaging was built in 1974, and commercial systems became available in 1978 (Figure 1–3).[2] Single-photon emission computed tomography (SPECT) was introduced soon after.[13] Both methods were quickly applied to studies of human cognition and of neurological and psychiatric disease, providing insights into processes previously unobtainable.[13–15] It was found, for example, that in nor-mal awake individuals the frontal lobes consistently had the highest CBF and that these regions were responsive to many conditions. In contrast, individuals with schizophrenia often had reduced frontal CBF (hypofrontality) and decreased responsiveness in these regions.[13]

A major challenge during these early years was development of standardized methods for comparisons within and across individuals and groups. Image resolution was too low for accurate visual identification of anatomical regions. One solution was development of mathematical methods that allowed translation of each individual's brain scans into the standard stereotactic system used by neurosurgeons.[16] With this conversion in place, it became possible to select regions for analysis based upon the stereotactic atlas of the brain and to identify regions by consultation with the atlas.[16,17] This refinement in technique allowed group studies that had more statistical power, better representation of the population, and examined the whole brain.[18] Imaging of CBF continues to be the major application of SPECT, although receptor studies are becoming more common.[19–21] PET quickly diversified with the development of new radiotracers for a wide variety of measurements, including cerebral metabolism and neurotransmitter receptor binding. Now, the majority of PET studies utilize these new tracers.[19–22]

The most commonly used tracer for PET CBF imaging is radiolabeled water ($^{15}O-H_2O$). This tracer has a very short half-life (~2 minutes), so a bolus injection provides a snapshot of CBF that can be repeated, if required, every 12–15 minutes.[22] This technique has been particularly useful clinically in the study of acute stroke.[23] Decreased perfusion (misery perfusion) is found in areas near the infarct during the first few hours after onset, followed by increases (luxury perfusion) over the first week. PET has been used to monitor the effectiveness of thrombolytic therapy and other interventions. Inhalation of ^{15}O provides several measures, including oxygen consumption, oxygen extraction ratio, and cerebral blood volume (CBV). This is not considered a clinical technique, as it is quite complex.

SPECT regional cerebral blood flow (rCBF) imaging is quite valuable in many neuropsychiatric conditions, including dementias, seizures, trauma, movement disorders, anxiety, obsessive-compulsive disorder, and schizophrenia.[24,25] It is widely available, as the same nuclear medicine cameras and software that are used for clinical scans of thyroids, prostates, or hearts are also used for brains. Three-dimensional images can be reconstructed, as well as the traditional axial, sagittal, and coronal planes of section. The most commonly used SPECT brain blood flow tracer remains ^{99m}Tc-hexamethylpropyleneamine oxime (HMPAO), followed by L,L-ethyl cysteinate dimer (ECD). Once injected under quiet, dimly lit standard conditions, HMPAO allows for immediate fixation in the brain and scanning up to several hours later.[20] A recent review article provides an excellent in-depth introduction to the science of brain perfusion in SPECT imaging.[26]

The most widely studied and most common neuropsychiatric use for SPECT imaging is in the differential diagnosis of Alzheimer's disease (AD) from vascular and other dementing diseases (e.g., Lewy body dementia, frontotemporal dementia, or Parkinson's disease).[27,28] A recent metaanalysis found SPECT to have a higher specificity than clinical criteria in discerning AD from other dementias (91% vs. 70%), although clinical criteria have a higher sensitivity.[27] Other applications under extensive study with dementia include the staging of the cognitive decline and mild cognitive impairments in patients likely to develop AD, and new looks at treatment response patterns with the cholinesterase inhibitors.[29–31]

Localization of seizure foci in epilepsy patients for evaluation of surgical candidacy remains an area of extensive use of brain SPECT. Medication-resistant seizures can cause extreme debilitation to patients, and surgical resection after lesion localization can be curative. If the tracer is administered while a seizure is occurring (ictal scan), the ictal focus will have hyperperfusion as compared to the resting or interictal hypoperfusion state.[24,32,33]

Cerebrovascular conditions such as hypoperfusion, cerebrovascular accidents, transient ischemic attacks, and post-vascular interventions are also imaged with highly successful lesion localization.[24] Other clinical uses for SPECT include identification of areas of abnormal blood flow in vasculitis and multiple sclerosis, and in documentation of poor brain function after trauma.[34–36] Evidence of altered brain function via grossly abnormal blood flow pictures can assist with symptom explanation, diagnostic clarification, and biopsychosocial treatment plan changes in patients with normal structural imaging.[34–36] Investigational uses of SPECT for blood flow in psychiatric diseases include extensive imaging of obsessive-compulsive disorder patients with hyperperfusion patterns and hypoperfusion in schizophrenia, Gilles de la Tourette's syndrome, and unipolar depression.[24]

The PET and SPECT methods for acquiring CBF images provided much of the data that is key to our modern understanding of brain and behavior. These methods continue to be valuable, but clinical applications are limited by their reliance on radioisotope production and administration of ionizing radiation. More recently, several different approaches to imaging CBF have been developed that do not require administration of radiotracers.

Within a decade of the introduction of computed tomography (CT) two methods for evaluating CBF were developed, both based on administration of a contrast agent. The simple addition of a rapid injection of an iodine-containing contrast agent to the CT protocol (first-pass or bolus perfusion CT) allows simultaneous assessment of several parameters, including CBF, CBV, mean transit time (MTT), and blood-brain barrier (BBB) permeability.[37–39] A major advantage of this technique is that it requires no special equipment. The software required to calculate these maps is available from all major CT companies. Its addition to the imaging examination requires only a few extra minutes. First-pass perfusion CT is valuable for examination of acute stroke, providing a rapid method for assessing the extent and severity of ischemia. The combination of CBF, CBV, and BBB permeability assessment has also shown potential for grading of cerebral tumors. At present, the major limitation of this technique is coverage. On most CT scanners only a few sections can be obtained. An alternative method of perfusion CT uses a slow administration of contrast agent in order to maintain a steady concentration over a sufficient time to allow imaging of the entire brain. This method, however, provides only CBV measurement.[38]

The other CT contrast agent that is used to measure CBF is stable xenon gas (Xe).[38,40] When inhaled, this radio-dense, lipid-soluble gas dissolves into the blood and passes into the brain, providing a quantitative measure of CBF. Like perfusion CT, XeCT adds very little time to the exam time. Unlike most methods of imaging CBF, XeCT is truly quantitative and has been found to be accurate even at very low and very high flow rates. An additional advantage is its rapid elimination, which makes repeated scanning under different conditions (e.g., drug challenge) possible. Xe is a narcotic gas, however, and even in the low doses presently used, some euphoric or dysphoric side effects are seen. XeCT is valuable in the management of acute stroke, allowing differentiation of the salvageable ischemic penumbra from the core. This is critical information, for if no area within the stroke is still viable, then thrombolytic therapy should not be commenced. Management of severe traumatic brain injury is also enhanced by use of XeCT CBF studies to identify development of conditions (e.g., cerebral swelling) that can lead to secondary brain injury. In February of 2001 the use of Xe as an x-ray contrast agent was temporarily halted by the FDA, pending completion of required studies that are currently under way at many academic medical centers.

Magnetic resonance (MR) imaging also provides two approaches to measuring CBF.[38,39] Like first-pass perfusion CT, one approach uses administration of a contrast agent (this technique is variously called *dynamic susceptibility contrast, first-pass,* or *bolus perfusion MR imaging*). Unlike XeCT, however, MR contrast agents remain intravascular. In addition, MR contrast agents alter image intensity indirectly by the effect of the contrast agent on surrounding tissues. These differences complicate quantification. A weakness of this technique is that at the present time only approximate measures of CBV, CBF, and MTT can be derived. Quantifying the tracer in a given volume of magnetic resonance imaging (MRI) space is not as straightforward as quantification of a radiolabeled tracer with PET. This is an active area of research.[41] Direct comparison studies indicate that there is good qualitative but not quantitative agreement between CBF measurement made with PET and dynamic susceptibility contrast perfusion MRI (Figure 1–4).[3,42] A major advantage of this technique is the absence of exposure to radiation of any sort. The most common clinical application is evaluation of acute stroke.[38,39] Recent work suggests that it may also be useful in monitoring of multiple sclerosis.[43]

The other MRI method for imaging CBF does not require administration of a contrast agent; rather, water molecules in the carotid arteries are "tagged" by radiofrequency pulses, which change the signal from the water in blood, making the blood itself into a contrast agent.[44] The altered signal is imaged shortly thereafter as the tagged blood flows upward through the brain. This approach is called *arterial spin labeling* (ASL). Multiple ASL MRI methods have been developed. While this way of CBF imaging is still considered an experimental technique, it has great potential for future clinical and research applications. Most importantly, it requires neither exposure to any form of radiation nor administration of a contrast agent, and measures can be repeated as often as required.

The development and application of methods to measure local brain blood flow in living humans revolutionized neuroscience and has captured substantial public interest. Functional imaging has significantly increased our understanding of the emotion and behavior circuits of the brain. As always, caution must be used in interpreting individual data. Many factors can influence functional studies including comorbidities, technical factors, medications, individual patient state, and tracer injection conditions. More extreme care is needed when medicolegal issues arise. One recent review notes the limitations of such imaging in forensic testimony.[45]

References

1. Landau WM, Freygang WH Jr, Roland LP, et al: The local circulation of the living brain: values in the unanesthetized and anesthetized cat. Trans Am Neurol Assoc 1955; 80:125–129
2. Nutt R: The history of positron emission tomography. Mol Imaging Biol 2002; 4:11–26
3. Mukherjee P, Kang HC, Videen TO, et al: Measurement of cerebral blood flow in chronic carotid occlusive disease: Comparison of dynamic susceptibility contrast perfusion MR imaging with positron emission tomography. Am J Neuroradiol 2003; 24:862–871
4. Kety SS: Measurement of local blood flow by the exchange of an inert, diffusible substance. Methods Med Res 1960; 8:228–236
5. Small SA: Quantifying cerebral blood flow: regional regulation with global implications. J Clin Invest 2004; 114:1046–1048
6. Kety SS: Measurement of local contribution within the brain by means of inert, diffusible tracers: examination of the theory, assumptions and possible sources of error. Acta Neurol Scand Suppl 1965; 14:20–23
7. Reivich M, Jehle J, Sokoloff L, et al: Measurement of regional cerebral blood flow with antipyrine-14C in awake cats. J Applied Physiol 1969; 27:296–300
8. Ullberg S, Larsson B, Tjälve H, et al: Autoradiography, in Biologic Applications of Radiotracers. Edited by Glenn HJ. Boca Raton, FL, CRC Press, 1982, pp 55–108
9. Raichle ME: Behind the scenes of functional brain imaging: A historical and physiological perspective. Proc Natl Acad Sci 1998; 95:765–772
10. Ginsberg MD, Lockwood AH, Busto R, et al: A simplified in vivo autoradiographic strategy for the determination of regional cerebral blood flow by positron emission tomography: Theoretical considerations and validation studies in the rat. J Cereb Blood Flow Metab 1982; 2:89–98
11. Herscovitch P, Markham J, Raichle ME: Brain blood flow measurement with intravenous $H_2{}^{15}O$. I: Theory and error analysis. J Nucl Med 1983; 24:782–789
12. Raichle ME, Martin W, Herscovitch P, et al: Brain blood flow measured with intravenous $H_2{}^{15}O$. II: Implementation and validation. J Nucl Med 1983; 24:790–798
13. Ingvar DH: History of brain imaging in psychiatry. Dement Geriatr Cogn Disord 1997; 8:66–72
14. Maurer AH: Nuclear medicine: SPECT comparisons to PET. Radiol Clin North Am 1988; 26:1059–1074
15. Jamieson DJ, Alavi A, Jolles P, et al: Positron emission tomography in the investigation of central nervous system disorders. Radiol Clin North Am 1988; 26:1075–1088
16. Fox PT, Perlmutter JS, Raichle ME: A stereotactic method of anatomical localization for positron emission tomography. J Comput Assist Tomogr 1985; 9:141–153
17. Perlmutter JS, Herscovitch P, Powers WJ, et al: Standardized mean regional method for calculating global positron emission tomographic measurements. J Cereb Blood Flow Metab 1985; 5:476–480
18. Ball MJ, Fisman M, Hachinski V, et al: A new definition of Alzheimer's disease: a hippocampal dementia. Lancet 1985; 1:14–16
19. Frankle WG, Laruelle M: Neuroreceptor imaging in psychiatric disorders. Ann Nucl Med 2002; 16:437–446
20. Warwick JM: Imaging of brain function using SPECT. Metab Brain Dis 2004; 19:113–123
21. Lingford-Hughes AR: Human brain imaging and substance abuse. Curr Opin Pharmacol 2005; 5:42–46
22. Parsey RV, Mann JJ: Applications of positron emission tomography in psychiatry. Semin Nucl Med 2003; 33:129–135
23. Newberg AB, Alavi A: The role of PET imaging in the management of patients with central nervous system disorders. Radiol Clin North Am 2005; 43:49–65
24. Camargo EE: Brain SPECT in neurology and psychiatry. J Nucl Med 2001; 42:611–623
25. Gupta A, Elheis M, Pansari K: Imaging in psychiatric illness. Int J Clin Pract 2004; 58:850–858
26. Catafau AM: Brain SPECT in clinical practice, Part I: Perfusion. J Nucl Med 2001; 42:259–271
27. Dougall NJ, Bruggink S, Ebmeier KP: Systematic review of the diagnostic accuracy of 99mTc-HMPAO-SPECT in dementia. Am J Geriatr Psychiatry 2004; 12:554–570
28. Trollor JN, Sachdev PS, Haindl W, et al: Regional cerebral blood flow deficits in mild Alzheimer's disease using high resolution single photon emission computerized tomography. Psychiatry Clin Neurosci 2005; 59:280–290
29. Cabranes JA, De Juan R, Encinas M, et al: Relevance of functional neuroimaging in the progression of mild cognitive impairment. Neurol Res 2004; 26:496–501
30. Ceravolo R, Volterrani D, Tognoni G, et al: Cerebral perfusional effects of cholinesterase inhibitors in Alzheimer disease. Clin Neuropharmacol 2004; 27:166–170
31. Tanaka M, Namiki C, Thuy DH, et al: Prediction of psychiatric response to donepezil in patients with mild to moderate Alzheimer's disease. J Neurol Sci 2004; 225:135–141
32. Henry TR, Van Heertum RL: Positron emission tomography and single photon emission computed tomography in epilepsy care. Semin Nucl Med 2003; 33:88–104
33. Van Paesschen W: Ictal SPECT. Epilepsia 2004; 45:35–40
34. Hurley RA, Taber KH, Zhang J, et al: Neuropsychiatric presentation of multiple sclerosis. J Neuropsychiatry Clin Neurosci 1999; 11:5–7
35. Abu-Judeh HH, Parker R, Singh M, et al: SPECT brain perfusion imaging in mild traumatic brain injury without loss of consciousness and normal computed tomography. Nucl Med Commun 1999; 20:505–510
36. Anderson KE, Taber KH, Hurley RA: Functional imaging, in Textbook of Traumatic Brain Injury. Edited by Silver JM, McAllister TW, Yudofsky SC. Washington, DC, American Psychiatric Press, 2005; 107–133
37. Miles KA: Brain perfusion: computed tomography applications. Neuroradiology 2004; 46:194–200
38. Latchaw RE: Cerebral perfusion imaging in acute stroke. J Vasc Interv Radiol 2004; 15:S29–S46

39. Sunshine JL: CT, MR imaging, and MR angiography in the evaluation of patients with acute stroke. J Vasc Interv Radiol 2004; 15:S47–S55
40. Levy EI, Yonas H: Xenon-enhanced computed tomography: technique and clinical applications, in Imaging of the Nervous System. Edited by Latchaw RE, Kucharczyk J, Moseley ME. Elsevier, Philadelphia, PA, 2005; 259–272
41. Jackson A: Analysis of dynamic contrast enhanced MRI. Br J Radiol 2004; 77:S154–S166
42. Grandin CB, Bol A, Smith AM, et al: Absolute CBF and CBV measurements by MRI bolus tracking before and after acetazolamide challenge: repeatability and comparison with PET in humans. Neuroimage 2005; 26:525–535
43. Ge Y, Law M, Johnson G, et al: Dynamic susceptibility contrast perfusion MR imaging of multiple sclerosis lesions: Characterizing hemodynamic impairment and inflammatory activity. Am J Neuroradiol 2005; 26:1539–1547
44. Detre JA, Alsop DC: Arterial spin labeled perfusion magnetic resonance imaging, in Imaging of the Nervous System. Edited by Latchaw RE, Kucharczyk J, Moseley ME. Elsevier, Philadelphia, PA, 2005; 323–331
45. Reeves D, Mills MJ, Billick SB, et al: Limitations of brain imaging in forensic psychiatry. J Am Acad Psychiatry Law 2003; 31:89–96

Recent Publication of Interest

Wintermark M, Sesay M, Barbie E, et al: Comparative overview of brain perfusion imaging techniques. J Neuroradiol 2005; 32:294–314

Presents a comparative overview of the main techniques used for imaging cerebral blood flow in the clinical setting. It is intended as a guide for clinicians, to help them choose the most appropriate technique for a given clinical situation.

Reprinted from Taber KH, Black KJ, Hurley RA: "Blood Flow Imaging of the Brain: 50 Years Experience." *Journal of Neuropsychiatry and Clinical Neurosciences* 17:441–446, 2005. Used with permission.

Chapter 2

FUNCTIONAL MAGNETIC RESONANCE IMAGING

Application to Posttraumatic Stress Disorder

KATHERINE H. TABER, PH.D.
SCOTT L. RAUCH, M.D.
RUTH A. LANIUS, M.D., PH.D., F.R.C.P.C.
ROBIN A. HURLEY, M.D.

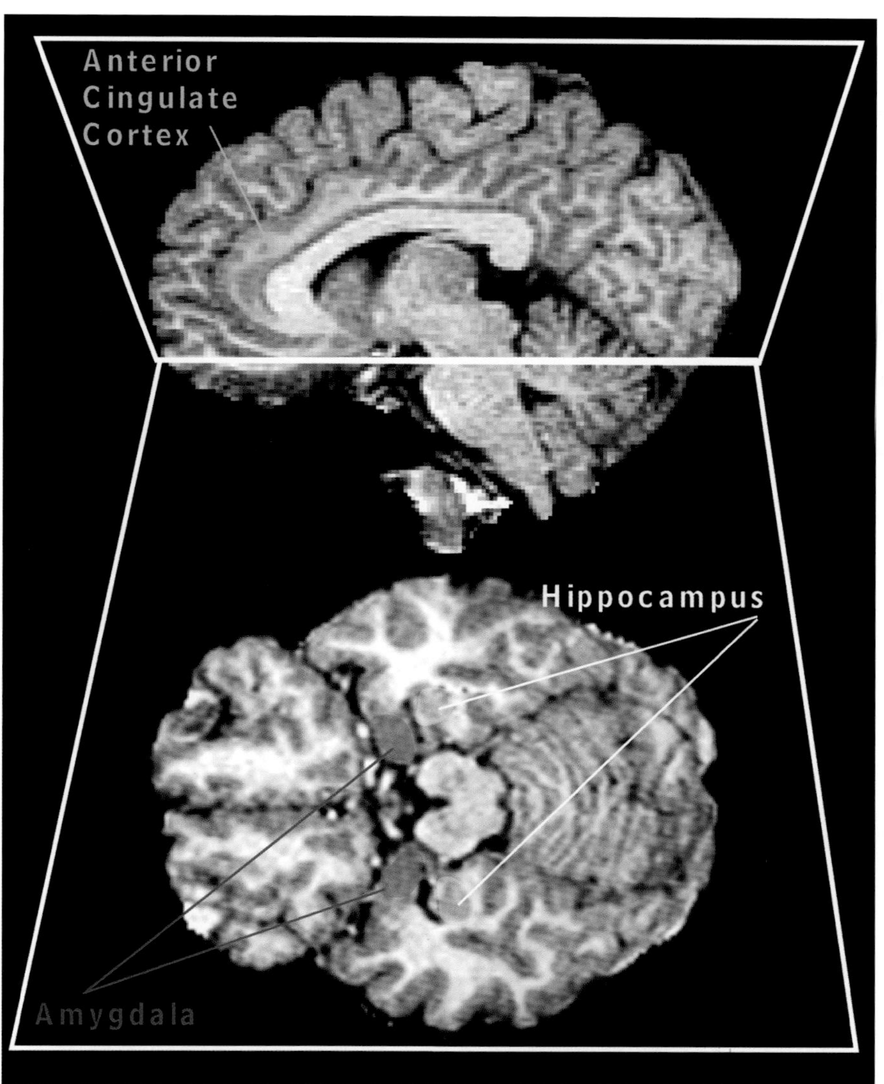

Several areas believed to be important in PTSD are indicated in color on sagittal (upper image) and axial (lower image) T_1-weighted MR images from a normal individual: rostral anterior cingulate cortex (*blue*), amygdala (*pink*), hippocampus (*yellow*). The approximate location of the axial section is indicated on the midline sagittal MR image. Broca's area (not illustrated) has also been implicated.

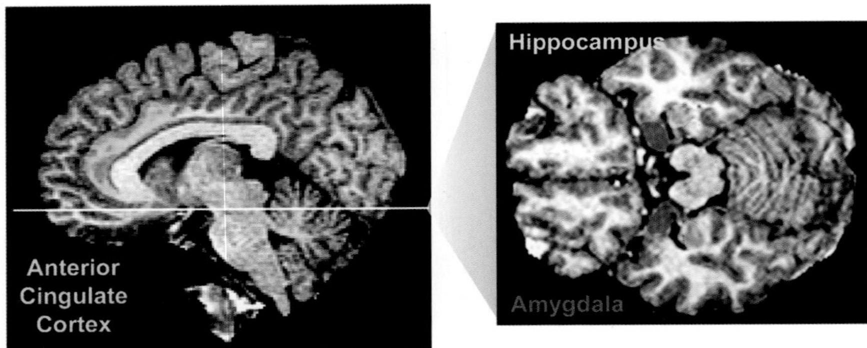

FIGURE 2–1. The locations of the rostral anterior cingulate (*blue*), amygdala (*pink*), and hippocampus (*yellow*) are indicated on midline sagittal (left image) and axial (right image) MR images from a normal individual. The approximate location of the axial section is indicated on the sagittal image.

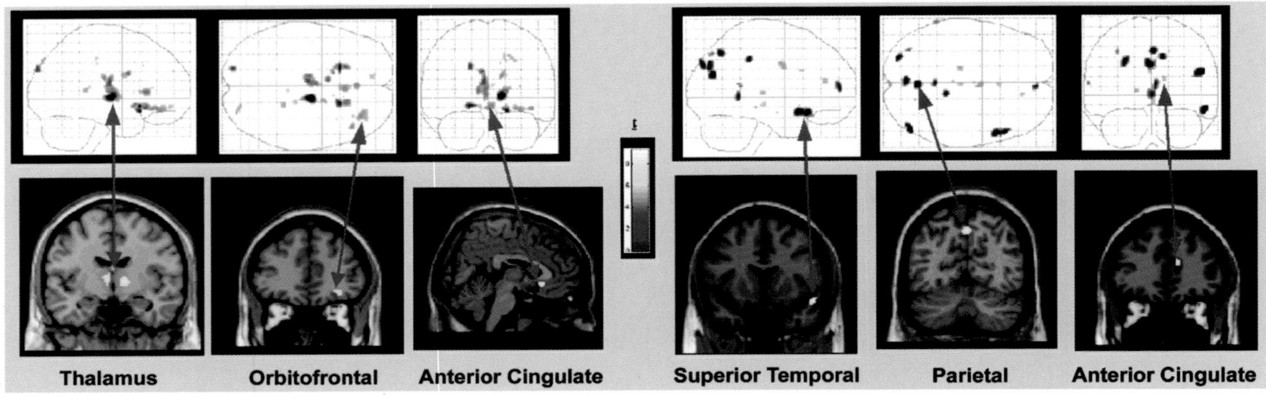

FIGURE 2–2. Areas of significantly increased blood-oxygen-level-dependent (BOLD) response (measured by fMRI) during traumatic script recall versus baseline between groups are superimposed on T_1-weighted MR images and schematics of the brain. Patients with PTSD (as a result of sexual abuse or assault or motor vehicle accidents) who had increased heart rate during remembering, an indication of autonomic arousal, had less activation than controls in the thalamus, orbitofrontal cortex, and subgenual anterior cingulate cortex (left panel). PTSD patients who did not have increased heart rate during remembering, an indication of dissociation, had more activation than controls in the superior temporal cortex, parietal cortex, and rostral anterior cingulate cortex (right panel). The control group had similar trauma exposure to both PTSD groups but did not have PTSD. The color bar illustrates the corresponding t values.

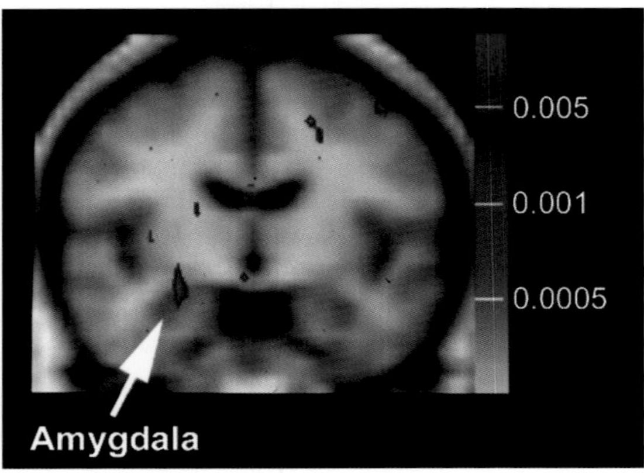

FIGURE 2–3. (left) Brain activation was measured by fMRI during exposure to masked-fearful versus masked-happy faces, a task designed to activate the amygdala in isolation (i.e., in the absence of frontal cortical activation). The areas of greater activation in combat-exposed men with PTSD ($n = 8$) compared with a similar group of combat-exposed men without PTSD are superimposed on averaged structural MRI data. The color bar illustrates the corresponding *P* values. Note the significantly greater activation evident in the right amygdala. Reprinted with permission from Rauch et al.[1]

Posttraumatic stress disorder (PTSD) is classified as an anxiety disorder that occurs in approximately 8% of the population.[2] It is frequently chronic and often co-occurs with other psychiatric disorders, such as major depression and substance abuse.[2,3] This disorder involves exposure to a life-threatening event along with intrusive reexperiencing of the event, persistent avoidance of stimuli associated with the event, increased arousal, duration of symptoms exceeding one month, and clinically significant impairment in general life functioning.

PTSD has been studied from many aspects, including searches for the neurochemical and neuroanatomical changes that occur. This work has produced many conflicting results because of variations in the population studied, study design, outcome measures, and comorbid variables such as preexisting conditions. Newport and Nemeroff provide a review of documented neurobiological abnormalities.[4] Neurochemical abnormalities have been most often reported in the hypothalamic-pituitary-adrenal axis, particularly increased levels of norepinephrine and epinephrine. Patients with PTSD have been found to produce elevated levels of corticotropin-releasing factor but low levels of cortisol. Other possible abnormalities include increased levels of triiodothyronine (T_3) and thyroxine (T_4), serotonin dysfunction, impaired γ-aminobutyric acid (GABA) function, increased cellular immune activation, sensory processing abnormalities, and dysregulation of the endogenous opioid system.[4]

The neuroanatomical correlates of PTSD using neuroimaging have been less well studied. A PubMed search produced only 65 references for neuroimaging and PTSD. Three recent reviews summarize results from these preliminary studies.[5–7] As with the neurochemical literature, study designs vary, study populations differ, and a variety of outcome measures have been used. Thus, given the early stage of imaging research in PTSD, it would be premature to draw any conclusions.

Study tools have included magnetic resonance imaging (MRI), magnetic resonance spectroscopy, single-photon emission computed tomography (SPECT), positron emission tomography (PET), ligand studies with radioisotopes that tag neurotransmitters or medications, and, more recently, functional magnetic resonance imaging (fMRI). Together these studies have examined both brain morphology and brain functioning in subjects with PTSD. Comparison groups have included individuals who have not experienced trauma and subjects with traumatic exposures who did not develop PTSD. Hull has summarized the central findings of these studies; they include decreased hippocampal volume, increased amygdala activity, decreased anterior cingulate cortex activation, decreased Broca's area activity, right hemispheric lateralization, decreased *N*-acetylaspartate in medial temporal regions, and activation of the visual cortex.[5] Theories to explain these findings include the pivotal role of the amygdala in fear conditioning coupled with roles of the anterior cingulate and the hippocampus to extinguish fear, as well as the role of Broca's area in attaching meaning or significance to experiences that can be translated into words.[5,7] Bremner, reviewing both published and unpublished data, noted in addition a significant role for the orbitofrontal cortex and the posterior cingulate.[6] Although these are exciting findings, as noted earlier, replication of results and a clear understanding of the relationships between brain structures are still lacking. Many unanswered questions await further study with both the older and the newer imaging tools. Among the newer tools is fMRI, which combines brain function and matching anatomical images.

Functional Magnetic Resonance Imaging

The principle underlying fMRI is that deoxygenated hemoglobin (deoxyhemoglobin) is paramagnetic and thus acts as a natural MR contrast agent.[8–12] The signal intensity of blood in a functional magnetic resonance (MR) image is therefore dependent on the local balance between oxygenated and deoxygenated hemoglobin—hence the term *blood-oxygen-level-dependent (BOLD) response* in describing the MR technique used to acquire the images. The presence of deoxyhemoglobin within the blood vessel creates a small magnetic field gradient, affecting an area of perhaps 1–2 radii beyond the vessel wall. Numerous different approaches are used to make the MRI sensitive to the presence of deoxyhemoglobin (susceptibility-weighted images).[8,10] One problem with the most commonly used methods of obtaining susceptibility weighting is the presence of susceptibility-related artifacts in areas of magnetic field inhomogeneity, such as the interfaces between brain, bone, and air. Thus regions of importance in neuropsychiatry that are adjacent to bone, such as the orbitofrontal cortex and the inferior temporal region, are difficult to assess.

When an area of brain suddenly becomes more active, such as when it is participating in the performance of a cognitive task, the increase in local blood flow is larger than that required to meet metabolic demand. The level of deoxyhemoglobin in the blood decreases, causing a slight (1%–5%) increase in signal intensity in that small area of brain. Although this is too small a change to see in the image by eye, it can be measured when the signal intensity under a baseline (resting) condition is compared with the signal intensity under an activated condition. Thus, unlike PET, in which actual blood flow or metabolic rate can be measured, all fMRI measurements are relative to a baseline condition. Defining and creating a baseline state for comparison is a considerable challenge.[13] For example, if the brain area of interest is abnormally active under baseline conditions, further activation may not be measurable, resulting in an apparent absence of activation when the image sets are analyzed.

Areas of higher signal intensity are presumed to indicate areas of higher neuronal activation. Previously it was assumed that the BOLD response was correlated with action potential generation and thus could be used as a measure of connectivity between activated brain regions. However, several lines of evidence, including acquisition of functional MR images at the same time as electrophysiological recording of both neuronal spiking and local field potentials, indicate that this may not be the case.[12,14,15] Rather, the BOLD response correlates best with the local field potential (which reflects incoming activity and local processing) rather than with action potential generation (output). Changes in local cerebral blood flow are also correlated with local field potentials, not with spike rate.[14] Thus an fMRI activation could be present without an increase in the firing rate of the projection neurons. In addition, an increase in local cerebral blood flow and therefore a BOLD response would be expected for both excitatory and inhibitory processing, because energy demand is increased in both.

There are many ways of analyzing fMRI data.[8,9] The simplest is to subtract the average of the baseline images from the average of the activated images. A more sophisticated approach is to correlate the signal intensity of each voxel with the stimulus condition, identifying voxels in which the signal intensity is highly correlated with the stimulus presentation. Other approaches are also used, including use of a voxelwise *t* test or calculation of the hemodynamic response to the stimulus for each voxel. All of these approaches can be spatially filtered to eliminate voxels that appear activated as a result of random noise (not part of a larger group of activated voxels). Neuroanatomical localization is provided by overlaying areas that either are greater than the chosen signal intensity threshold or meet particular statistical criteria onto companion structural MR images obtained during the same session.

There are several methodological issues of importance in fMRI. A major challenge is differentiating areas of increased signal intensity that are within the microvasculature of the parenchyma of the brain and due to brain activity from those that are within slightly larger draining veins that are at some distance from the area of brain activation.[12,16] One approach to this problem is to collect an MR angiogram along with the structural and functional data sets. The locations of angiographically identified vessels are compared with the locations of areas of increased signal intensity in the fMRI data set. Those that coincide can be excluded from further analyses. Another approach is to alter the fMRI acquisition so that it is much more sensitive to the signal from the microvasculature and less sensitive to the signal from larger vessels. Motion artifacts are also a problem in fMRI. Any movement, including minor head movements and movements related to respiration and speech, can create spurious areas of activation or mask areas of true activation.[9] Head restraints and postprocessing are both important in this regard.[8,16]

The environment of the MR scanner has aspects that are particularly troublesome in neuropsychiatric research. The scanner bore is a long, narrow tube. During imaging, loud noise is created by gradient switching. Thus, the subject is in a very loud, uncomfortable, confined space that is liable to induce a claustrophobic response. Even some control subjects have difficulty tolerating these conditions. This is a substantial problem in neuropsychiatric research, because many of the populations of interest have difficulty remaining perfectly still for long periods. In addition, the physical limitations of the MR environment coupled with the need to prevent motion make the presentation/response conditions challenging, particularly for the more complex cognitive tasks (as opposed to simple sensory or motor tasks).

fMRI has several advantages over other techniques for functional imaging of the brain. Most important, it is totally noninvasive and requires no ionizing radiation or radiopharmaceuticals. Minimal risk makes it appropriate for use in children as well as adults. Multiple imaging sessions can be conducted with individuals for longitudinal studies. The anatomic resolution of fMRI is higher than in other techniques as well. In addition, the required equipment is widely available. However, fMRI is not easy to implement and analyze, and this may limit its clinical usefulness. At present, it should be considered a research technique.

As noted earlier, a typical fMRI study requires comparison of a baseline with an activated state. In some cases the baseline condition is simply the absence of a specific cognitive task or stimulation condition. In other cases it is a variation on the cognitive task or stimulus condition, such as changing a single variable. The activation can be anything from a simple sensory stimulation to a complex cognitive task. The baseline and activated conditions are usually presented several times in alternating sequence. These repetitions allow averaging of data, thus increasing statistical power and making it possible to analyze data from individuals (as opposed to averaging across a group).[16] However, an underlying assumption is that the brain activations in each repetition occur in the same regions. In some cases this may not be true.

In PTSD research, reminders of the traumatic event are often used as stimuli either to induce PTSD symptoms or to probe the network of brain regions responsible for processing trauma-related information. Although exposure to generic stimuli can be used, use of a script that is individualized for each subject increases the likelihood of a strong reexperiencing. This approach has been criticized because the stimuli do not necessarily affect all subjects to the same degree. The psychological impact may differ across subjects or between groups. If so, differences in brain activation may be due to differing degrees of fear experienced rather than differences in brain processing of fear.[17]

One group has used script-driven imagery to evoke traumatic memories in conjunction with fMRI measurement of brain activation (Figure 2–2).[18,19] In this series of experiments, subjects listened to 30 seconds of their script, then spent 30 seconds remembering the traumatic event as clearly as possible, and then spent 120 seconds relaxing and recovering. This cycle was repeated three times. Baseline images were collected 60 seconds before each period of recollection. Activation images were collected during the final 30 seconds of each period of recollection. The final fMRI data sets were an average of all three cycles. Heart rate was recorded as an indicator of autonomic state.

In their first study the authors reported that patients with PTSD (six whose PTSD was a result of sexual abuse or assault, three because of motor vehicle accidents) showed less activation in the thalamus, medial frontal cortex (Brodmann's area 10/11), and anterior cingulate cortex (Brodmann's area 32) during trauma remembering than control subjects with similar trauma exposure but without PTSD.[18] The PTSD group also had increases in heart rate during remembering, an indication of autonomic reactivity. The authors suggested that higher levels of arousal in the patients with PTSD (as indicated by increased heart rate) may alter thalamic processing, disrupting information flow to the cortex.

In their second study the authors selected patients with PTSD (all seven as a result of sexual or physical abuse) who did not have an increase in heart rate during remembering of traumatic events. The authors noted that approximately 30% of their patients show this type of dissociative response. The PTSD and control groups had similar levels of thalamic activation. The PTSD group had higher activations (predominantly on the right) in the superior and middle temporal gyri (Brodmann's area 38), occipital lobe (Brodmann's area 19), parietal lobe (Brodmann's area 7), inferior frontal gyrus (Brodmann's area 47), medial frontal and prefrontal cortex (Brodmann's areas 9 and 10), and anterior cingulate cortex (Brodmann's areas 24 and 32). The authors noted that activation of the superior and middle temporal gyri is consistent with the temporal lobe theory of dissociation, and activation of frontal areas is somewhat consistent with the corticolimbic model of depersonalization. They also emphasized the importance of categorizing patients with PTSD according to their response to traumatic memories (e.g., hyperarousal versus dissociation), since it is likely that the areas of the brain involved differ.

Another group has used fMRI in conjunction with cognitive tasks designed specifically to activate areas of the brain implicated in PTSD to assess responsivity.[1,20] Both the amygdala and the medial frontal cortex are activated during passive viewing of fearful faces. The group's first study employed a cognitive task designed to probe the responses of the amygdala to fearful faces in the absence of cortical modulation.[1] To accomplish this they presented emotionally expressive faces by the technique of backward masking (masked-faces paradigm). Alternating blocks of 56 masked-fearful, 56 masked-happy, and a fixation condition are shown, with each type of stimulus presented twice per second (for a total of 28 seconds per block). Each of the 56 presentations consisted of a short exposure (33 msec) to a fearful or a happy face (target) followed by a longer exposure (167 msec) to a neutral face (mask). Previous studies have shown that this approach activates the amygdala but not the medial frontal cortex. Eight men with combat-related PTSD were compared with eight men with similar exposure who did not have PTSD. Vascular contamination was minimized by using MR angiography to identify larger vessels and collecting the fMRI with an asymmetric spin-echo sequence to minimize contributions from smaller vessels. Only the areas of the amygdala, medial frontal cortex, and fusiform gyrus were analyzed. As expected, the two groups showed a similar level of fusiform gyrus activation in response to faces, indicating that overall hemodynamic responses were similar. Neither group had medial frontal activation in response to fearful faces. Both groups had amygdala activation in response to fearful faces, but the level of activation was significantly higher in the PTSD group (Figure 2–3). In addition, the level of activation in the amygdala was correlated with PTSD symptom severity but not with severity of trauma exposure. The authors noted that this protocol distinguished the two groups with 100% specificity and 75% sensitivity.

In a second study, the same group measured the responsivity of the rostral anterior cingulate cortex.[20] This brain region is thought to have a role in the processing of emotional stimuli, and it has been shown to be activated in normal individuals during performance of an emotional variant of the Stroop task, in which emotionally negative words are viewed and counted (as compared with neutral words). Previous studies have shown that individuals with PTSD have slower response times to trauma-related negative words in this task (as compared with general negative words). Eight men with combat-related PTSD were compared with eight men with similar exposure who did not have PTSD. Blocks of neutral words alternated with blocks of general negative words and blocks of trauma-related words, with all blocks being 30 seconds in duration. For each trial, subjects viewed (for 1.45 seconds) a set of one to four identical words and were required to press a button to indicate how many words were displayed. Comparisons were made of response times, error rates, and areas of activation to neutral, generally negative, and trauma-related words.

The PTSD group had slower response times and made more errors in response to all three types of words. Activation of the insular cortex was found in both groups. Unlike the control group, the PTSD group did not have significant activation of the rostral anterior cingulate region. The authors noted that this finding is consistent with the hypothesis that PTSD involves a failure of medial frontal regions to properly inhibit the amygdala.

Conclusion

Although functional magnetic resonance imaging is in its early stages of application in psychiatry, there is certainly promise for its use in investigating many disorders, including PTSD. With fMRI techniques, the delicate balance between the structures of the emotion and memory tracts becomes more evident. As our understanding of this balance evolves, it is hoped that treatment interventions may be developed to alleviate symptoms such as intrusive memories, avoidance, and heightened arousal.

References

1. Rauch SL, Whalen PJ, Shin LM, et al: Exaggerated amygdala response to masked facial stimuli in posttraumatic stress disorder: a functional MRI study. Biol Psychiatry 2000; 47:769–776
2. First MB, Frances A, Pincus HA: DMS-IV-TR: Handbook of Differential Diagnosis. Washington, DC, American Psychiatric Publishing, Inc, 2002, pp 463–468
3. Kessler RC, Sonnega A, Bromet E, et al: Posttraumatic stress disorder in the National Comorbidity Survey. Arch Gen Psychiatry 1995; 52:1048–1060
4. Newport DJ, Nemeroff CB: Neurobiology of posttraumatic stress disorder. Curr Opin Neurobiol 2000; 10:211–218
5. Hull A: Neuroimaging findings in post-traumatic stress disorder: systematic review. Br J Psychiatry 2002; 181:102–110
6. Bremner J: Neuroimaging studies in post-traumatic stress disorder. Curr Psychiatry Rep 2002; 4:254–263
7. Pitman R, Shin L, Rauch S: Investigating the pathogenesis of posttraumatic stress disorder with neuroimaging. J Clin Psychiatry 2001; 62:47–54
8. Menon RS, Gati JS, Goodyear BG, et al: Spatial and temporal resolution of functional magnetic resonance imaging. Biochem Cell Biol 1998; 76:560–571
9. Forster BB, Mackay AL, Whittall KP, et al: Functional magnetic resonance imaging: the basics of blood-oxygen-level-dependent (BOLD) imaging. Can Assoc Radiol J 1998; 49:320–329
10. Howseman AM, Bowtell RW: Functional magnetic resonance imaging: imaging techniques and contrast mechanisms. Phil Trans R Soc Lond B 1999; 354:1179–1194
11. Cacace AT, Tasciyan T, Cousins JP: Principles of functional magnetic resonance imaging: application to auditory neuroscience. J Am Acad Audiol 2000; 11:239–272
12. Logothetis NK: The neural basis of the blood-oxygen-level-dependent functional magnetic resonance imaging signal. Phil Trans R Soc Lond B 2002; 357:1003–1037
13. Gusnard DA, Raichle ME: Searching for a baseline: functional imaging and the resting human brain. Nat Rev Neurosci 2001; 2:685–694
14. Lauritzen M: Relationship of spikes, synaptic activity, and local changes of cerebral blood flow. J Cereb Blood Flow Metab 2001; 21:1367–1383
15. Logothetis NK, Pauls J, Augath M, et al: Neurophysiological investigation of the basis of the fMRI signal. Nature 2001; 412:150–157
16. Turner R, Howseman A, Rees GE, et al: Functional magnetic resonance imaging of the human brain: data acquisition and analysis. Exp Brain Res 1998; 123:5–12
17. Grossman R, Buchsbaum MS, Yehuda R: Neuroimaging studies in post-traumatic stress disorder. Psychiatr Clin North Am 2002; 25:317–340
18. Lanius RA,Williamson PC, Densmore M, et al: Neural correlates of traumatic memories in posttraumatic stress disorder: a functional MRI investigation. Am J Psychiatry 2001; 158:1920–1922
19. Lanius RA, Williamson PC, Boksman K, et al: Brain activation during script-driven imagery induced dissociative responses in PTSD: a functional magnetic resonance imaging investigation. Biol Psychiatry 2002; 52:305–311
20. Shin LM, Whalen PJ, Pitman RK, et al: An fMRI study of anterior cingulate function in posttraumatic stress disorder. Biol Psychiatry 2001; 50:932–942

Recent Publications of Interest

Vieweg WV, Julius DA, Fernandez A, et al: Posttraumatic stress disorder: clinical features, pathophysiology, and treatment. Am J Med 2006; 119:383–390
Provides an overview of posttraumatic stress disorder that includes prevalence, symptomatology and diagnosis, common comorbid disorders, and principles of treatment.

Savoy RL: Experimental design in brain activation MRI: cautionary tales. Brain Res Bull 2005; 67:361–367
Reviews the fundamentals of designing an fMRI experiment, with an emphasis on the difficulties involved, using illustrative examples from the literature.

Kim DS: The cutting edge of fMRI and high-field fMRI. Int Rev Neurobiol 2005; 66:147–166
Includes an in-depth discussion of the relationship between the BOLD response (the present basis for fMRI) and neuronal activity.

Ballenger JC, Davidson JRT, Lecrubier Y, et al: Consensus statement update on posttraumatic stress disorder from the International Consensus Group on Depression and Anxiety. J Clin Psychiatry 2004; 65 Suppl 1:55–66
Updates the previous (2000) consensus statement on posttraumatic stress disorder by the International Consensus Group on Depression and Anxiety. Fruitful areas for new research are detailed.

Nutt DJ, Malizia AL: Structural and functional brain changes in posttraumatic stress disorder. J Clin Psychiatry 2004; 65 Suppl 1:11–17
An excellent synthesis of the neuroimaging literature related to posttraumatic stress disorder.

Reprinted from Taber KH, Rauch SL, Lanius RA, et al: "Functional Magnetic Resonance Imaging: Application to Posttraumatic Stress Disorder." *Journal of Neuropsychiatry and Clinical Neurosciences* 15:125–129, 2003. Used with permission.

Chapter 3

Ecstasy in the Brain
A Model for Neuroimaging

Robin A. Hurley, M.D.
Liesbeth Reneman, M.D.
Katherine H. Taber, Ph.D.

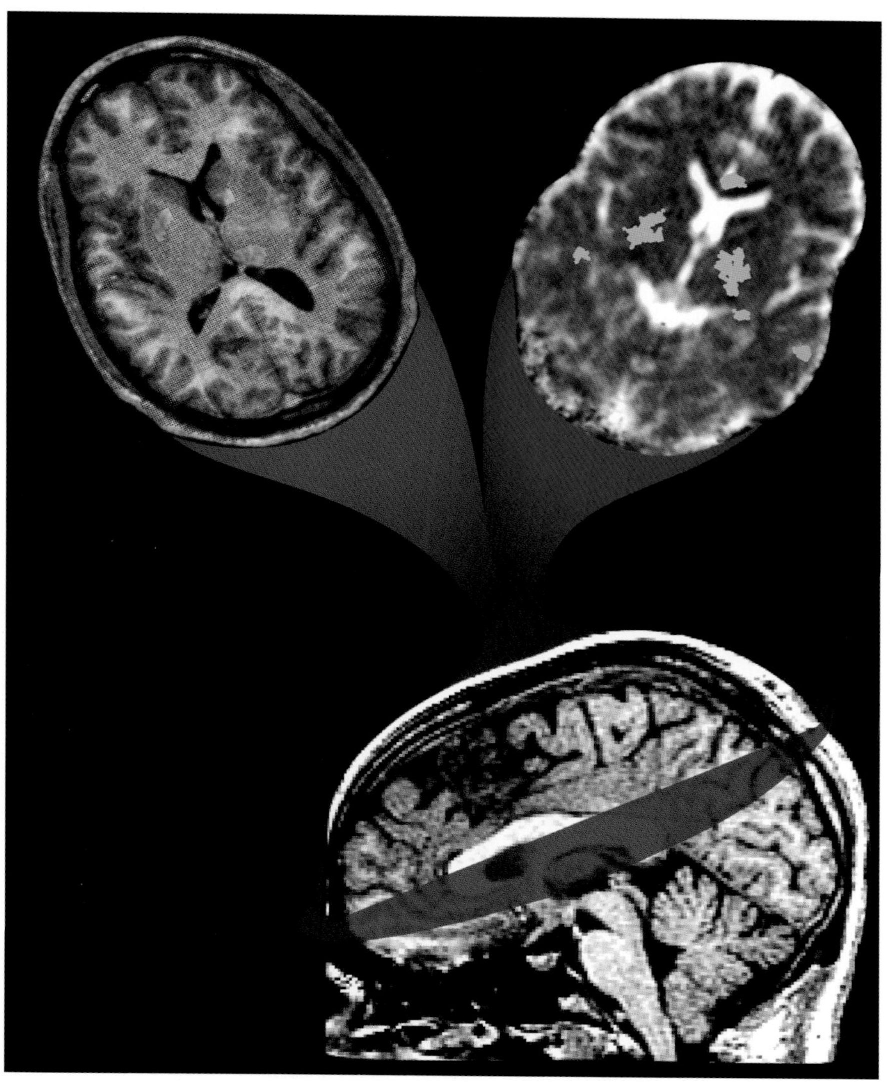

Images show serotonin receptor binding overlaid on a magnetic resonance image in a control subject (upper left) and apparent diffusion coefficient changes in an abstinent ecstasy user (upper right). The approximate location of the axial sections is marked on the sagittal magnetic resonance image.

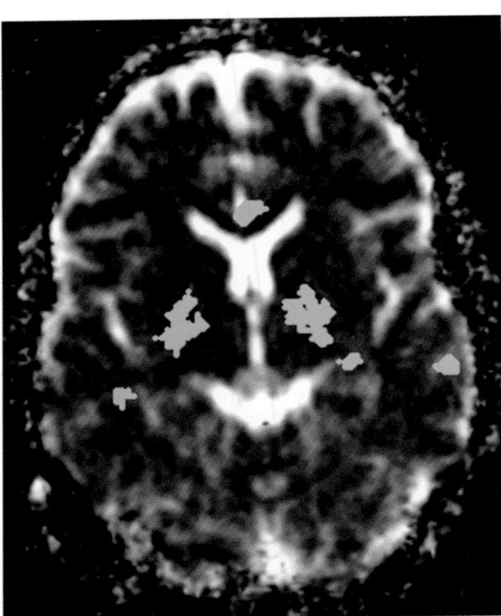

FIGURE 3–1. Diffusion-weighted imaging. In a recent study the ADC was significantly higher in 8 ecstasy users (abstinent for at least 3 weeks), as compared with control subjects, in many regions (*green*), including the globus pallidus and cingulate cortex. Reprinted with permission from Reneman et al.[1]

Ecstasy is the most common street name for 3,4-methylenedioxymethamphetamine (MDMA) or its analogues. It is also known as "xtc," "adam," "eve," or "x." It is a ring-substituted amphetamine that was first produced by a German pharmaceutical company, Merck, in 1912 as an appetite suppressant for German soldiers in World War I. However, it was quickly discarded because the empathic side effects observed on the battlefield were not considered desirable.[2] MDMA is classified as both a stimulant and a mild hallucinogen. Morgan[3] extensively reviewed the cognitive and emotional aspects of ecstasy exposure. Acutely, MDMA produces positive feelings, including euphoria, increased self-confidence, increased sensory perceptions, empathy, intimacy, and openness. Negative acute effects include bruxism, tachycardia, hyperthermia, trismus (severe enough that users commonly resort to pacifiers or lollipops), and, more rarely, psychosis or death. The "crash" occurs 24–48 hours later, with muscle aches, depression, fatigue, and decreased concentration. The long-term effects are more controversial and probably relate to extent of use. Symptoms more consistently found in heavier users include depression, insomnia, anxiety, impulsivity, aggression, decreased learning and memory performance (recall and working memory), and, less frequently, decreased attention. Some or all of these symptoms may improve with prolonged abstinence.[3]

Doyon[4] recently reviewed the basic pharmacology and acute management of MDMA toxicity. Onset is in 30 minutes, with maximum effects in 1–3 hours and a half-life of 16–31 hours. Most commonly, ecstasy is ingested in the form of tablets or capsules, but it can also be smoked, injected, or absorbed as a suppository. The street drug is made in basements or garages, often with many additives to intensify the effect, including dextromethorphan (most frequently), caffeine, ephedrine, pseudoephedrine, and salicylates.[5] One interesting analysis of "ecstasy pills" revealed that 29% of tested samples contained no MDMA and 8% contained no psychoactive drugs.[5]

During the 1960s and 1970s, there were a few reports advocating use of MDMA in psychotherapy, but its major popularity was in the party circles of Europe. MDMA was declared illegal by the U.S. Drug Enforcement Agency in 1985. Use increased during the 1990s and early 2000s at teen and young adult "raves" or all-night dance parties. In different studies, 0.5%–39% of young adults reported at least one ecstasy use.[6–8]

Many users consider ecstasy to be harmless. Medical literature on MDMA suggests otherwise. Mortality as a result of ecstasy is unusual, but it occurs.[9,10] Deaths have been attributed to hyperthermia, disseminated intravascular coagulation, fatal arrhythmias, acute myocardial infarctions, ischemic myocardial necrosis, and cerebral edema with cerebellar herniation and hepatic necrosis. MDMA may have a strongly nonlinear pharmokinetic profile. If so, a small increase in dose could lead to a substantial increase in plasma level and toxicity.[11]

Lasting effects in recreational users are under active investigation. MDMA causes significant serotonin toxicity in a variety of animal species.[12] Release of serotonin (and to a lesser extent dopamine) and decreased reuptake of the neurotransmitters are followed by an acute depletion. At certain doses, MDMA causes destruction of serotonin terminals. The extent to which these findings are applicable to humans is controversial. This is an important debate because these monoaminergic neurotransmitters are of vital importance to cognitive and emotional functioning.

A major challenge is the difficulty in designing studies that can clearly answer the question, "Is there anatomical injury from ecstasy use?" Inherent difficulties include unknown premorbid serotonin functioning; the effect of concomitant drug use (most users are polydrug users); reliability of self-reported usage; wide ranges in reported lifetime dose; variability in time from last dose; small group size; and difficulty recruiting a comparable control group. With these significant limitations in mind, a brief review and synthesis of existing imaging studies may aid the neuropsychiatrist in understanding the postulated effects of MDMA on the serotonin system, the potential secondary and tertiary effects mediated by vascular and other mechanisms, and possible implications for future health care demands. These reports on the effects of ecstasy

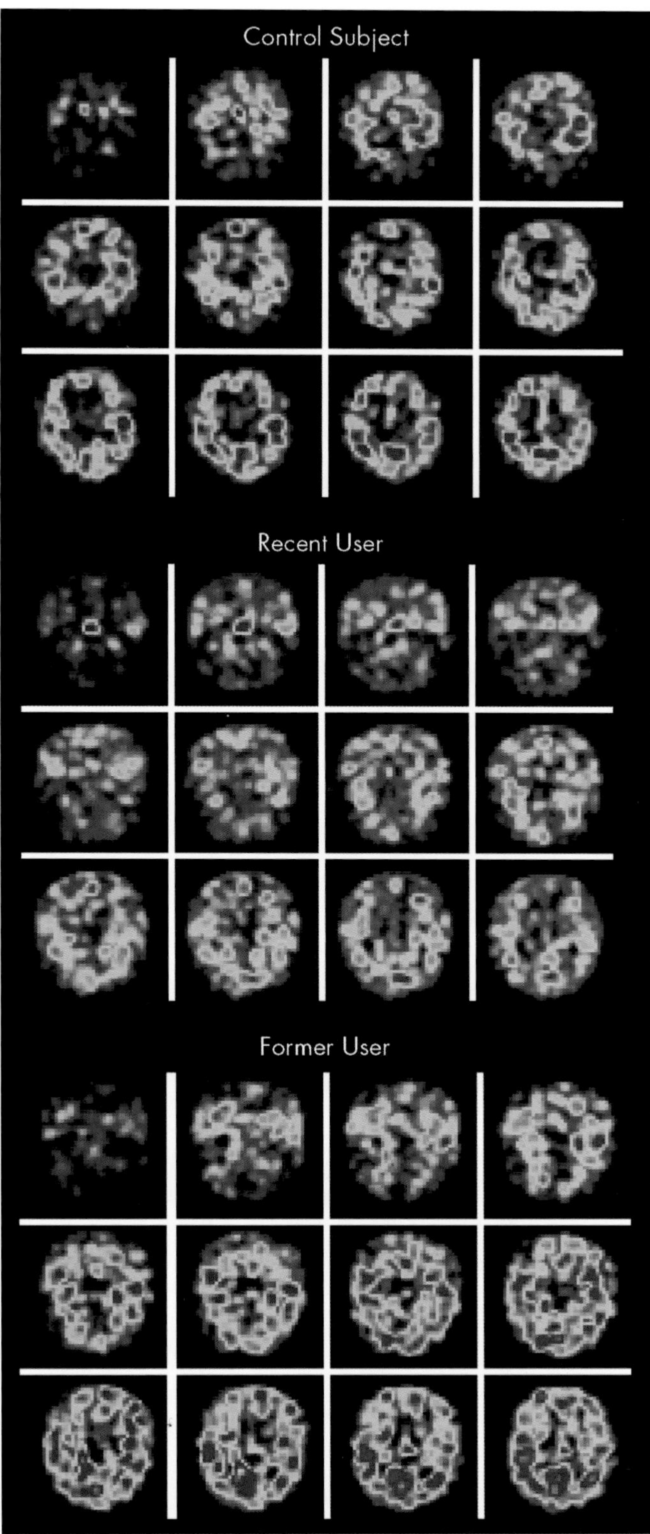

FIGURE 3–2. Serotonin receptor imaging using SPECT. The postsynaptic serotonin receptor 5-HT_{2A} was imaged with SPECT (using [^{123}I]-5-I-R91150) in recent and former ecstasy users. The level of binding (*black* is low, *blue* is moderate, *orange* is high) was significantly decreased in frontal, parietal, and occipital cortex in recent ecstasy users as compared with former ecstasy users and control subjects. The former users had slightly higher binding ratios than control subjects; this correlated with impaired performance on a delayed memory task.

demonstrate the progress being made in the study of brain functioning from an anatomical and neurochemical perspective.

Magnetic Resonance (MR) Imaging and MR Spectroscopy

Most functional imaging studies include standard MR imaging, yet do not report any brain abnormalities in their ecstasy users. One study has reported a negative correlation between duration of ecstasy use and individual global brain volume (gBV), although there was no difference in mean gBV between the ecstasy and control groups.[13] Abnormal imaging findings (in globus pallidus and subcortical white matter) have been reported in ecstasy users who have survived initial toxic reactions.[14–16]

It may be that lesions result from serotonin-induced vasoconstriction within the microcirculation, with the area affected often too small to be seen on standard imaging. Diffusion MR imaging measures the microscopic movement of water within tissue and is quite sensitive to microstructural changes. In a recent study, the apparent diffusion coefficient (ADC) was higher in some regions in 8 ecstasy users (abstinent for 3 or more weeks) compared with control subjects (Figure 3–1).[1] In the same study, regional cerebral blood volume (rCBV) measured by contrast-enhanced MR imaging was also higher in these ecstasy users. The authors suggest that initially, ecstasy causes a release of serotonin and a decrease in blood volume due to serotonin-induced vasoconstriction. Serotonin is then depleted and a rebound vasodilation occurs.

Proton MR spectroscopy (^{1}H MRS) provides a way of measuring certain brain metabolites, presented as the spectrum of the amount of signal produced by the metabolites contained within a volume of brain. An MRS study of 21 ecstasy users (abstinent 0.5–26 months) found a significant increase in *myo*-inositol (MI) content in parietal white matter of users compared with control subjects.[17] In addition, MI concentrations in both parietal white matter and occipital cortex were significantly higher in those users with the highest cumulative lifetime exposures. MI is thought to be a glial marker. Increases may reflect glial hypertrophy, perhaps an indication of brain insult or ongoing repair processes. Levels of *N*-acetylaspartate (NAA, a neuronal marker), glutamate, and lactate were normal, suggesting that axonal degeneration had not occurred, at least not at a level measurable by this technique. In another study, the ratios of NAA to creatine and choline were lower in the frontal gray matter of users compared with nonusers, and reductions correlated with the extent of previous ecstasy use.[18] NAA levels in occipital gray matter and parietal white matter did not differ from the levels in control subjects. The discrepancy between these studies may, in part, be explained by higher ecstasy exposure in the second study.

Functional Brain Imaging

Both single-photon emission computed tomography (SPECT) and positron emission tomography (PET) are nuclear medicine techniques that use radioactive tracers to image some aspect of brain function. SPECT has the advantage of wider availability; PET provides better image resolution but is performed only in research settings. Relatively few functional imaging studies of ecstasy users have been published, and the available literature encompasses several very different measures. There is little in the way of replication of findings.

An important premise in functional imaging is that blood flow and metabolism rise and fall with brain activity. Thus, regional cerebral glucose uptake reflects regional cerebral metabolism and therefore neuronal activity. Several PET studies (using 2-[^{18}F]-fluoro-2-deoxy-D-glucose; FDG) have looked for changes in regional brain metabolism related to MDMA exposure. A double-blind, placebo-controlled study examined the acute effects of MDMA in 14 drug-naive physicians and psychologists.[19] Subjects were evaluated with psychometric testing prior to and 90 minutes after drug or placebo intake, followed by FDG administration. During PET scanning, an auditory task was used to provide a more constant and reproducible mental state. Global glucose uptake was similar in the two groups. Regionally, the drug group had decreased glucose uptake bifrontally, and increased uptake bilaterally in the cerebellum and in the right putamen. Changes in cognition were correlated with decreased uptake in the frontal cortex, cingulate, and amygdala. The cortical results parallel known effects of other psychotropic substances and psychiatric illnesses. The authors note that these changes in the fronto-striatal (thalamic) cerebellar network argue for a cerebellar role in cognitive and emotional processes.

Another group has used FDG PET to examine the relationship between total lifetime consumption of ecstasy, time since last dose, and regional cerebral glucose uptake in prefrontal cortex (Brodmann's areas 10 and 11), striatum (caudate and putamen), and limbic areas (cingulate cortex, amygdala, hippocampus).[20,21] Their preliminary study found decreased uptake in the limbic areas and increased uptake in both frontal cortex and striatum. Their later, larger study found decreased uptake in all areas except area 10, where uptake was increased. They found no relationship between total lifetime dose and regional glucose uptake. A correlation between time from last dose and regional glucose uptake was found only for the cingulate cortex. Interestingly, uptake was more severely depressed in those who started ecstasy use prior to age 18.

Regional cerebral blood flow (rCBF) is also considered to be indicative of neuronal activity. A double-blind, placebo-controlled study examined the acute effects of MDMA on rCBF measured with $H_2{}^{15}O$ PET in 16 drug-naive students and hospital staff in two sessions separated by at least 2 weeks.[22] During imaging, all subjects performed a visual task to provide a more constant and reproducible mental state. The MDMA group had decreased rCBF in the precentral and paracentral lobule, dorsal anterior and posterior cingulate, superior temporal gyrus, insula, and thalamus. Increased rCBF was found in the ventromedial prefrontal, ventral anterior cingulate, inferior temporal, and cerebellar cortices. These blood flow changes were concomitant with elevated mood and changes in sensory/somatic perceptions. A later study from the same group found no differences in rCBF in 16 regular users versus control subjects while performing a simple cognitive activation task.[23] However, the study did not control for time since last drug intake.

Another group has used SPECT to evaluate rCBF, using xenon-133 (^{133}Xe) and technetium-99m hexamethylpropyleneamine oxime ([^{99m}Tc]HMPAO) in 21 abstinent (0.5–26 months) users and matched control subjects.[13] They found no significant differences in rCBF and 2.3% lower global CBF in the abstinent users. Neither global CBF nor rCBF correlated with duration, frequency, or recency of ecstasy use. Ten of these users were then given MDMA and rescanned (8 subjects at 2 weeks post-use and 2 subjects at 2 months post-use). The subjects rescanned at 2 weeks had decreased rCBF in most brain regions, with the largest decreases bilaterally in caudate and superior parietal cortex and the right dorsolateral frontal cortex (areas rich in serotonergic neurons). The decreases were more noticeable in the subjects given higher doses of MDMA. The 2 subjects scanned at 2 months showed increased global CBF. The authors suggested that these results may be related to the acute/ subacute vasoconstrictive effects of MDMA-induced serotonin release. With time, an adaptive or neuronal recovery process may occur.

Another type of functional imaging directly evaluates neurotransmitter systems by measuring receptor binding. One group has imaged the postsynaptic serotonin receptor 5-HT_{2A} with SPECT (using [^{123}I]-5-I-R91150) in recent and former ecstasy users.[24,25] Binding was significantly decreased in frontal, parietal, and occipital cortex in 10 recent ecstasy users (abstinent 1–8 weeks, mean 7 weeks) as compared with 5 former ecstasy users (abstinent 8 or more weeks, mean 18 weeks) and 10 control subjects. The former users had slightly higher binding ratios than the control subjects; this correlated with impaired performance on a delayed memory task (Figure 3–2). In a companion rCBV study (using contrast-enhanced MRI) of a subset of each group, decreased rCBV and serotonin receptor binding were positively correlated in the globus pallidus and occipital cortex in 3 recent ecstasy users. Increased rCBV was found in 2 former ecstasy users. The authors suggest that ecstasy induces acute vasoconstriction via a large serotonin release that floods the postsynaptic receptors and triggers down-regulation; the resulting serotonin depletion causes a subacute up-regulation of receptors and vasodilation.[24] Both conditions could leave the user vulnerable to cerebral vascular accidents, especially in areas with a "watershed" blood supply (e.g., basal ganglia, subcortical white matter).

Both SPECT (using [^{123}I]-2β-carbomethoxy-3β-(4-iodophenyl)tropane, [^{123}I]β-CIT) and PET (using [^{11}C] McN-5652) have been used to image the serotonin presynaptic transporter (SERT).[26–29] In one study, 10 long-term ecstasy users were compared with control subjects matched for other recreational drug use. Ecstasy users had decreased binding in posterior cortical regions and a positive correlation between time from last dose and binding in the cingulate.[26,28] These investigators also found a decrease in cortical binding in current users (abstinent 3 weeks), but not in former users (abstinent 1 year or longer), compared with control subjects. Both the recent and former users had significant deficits in verbal memory, although these were not correlated with the SPECT findings.

The authors proposed several theories to account for these results, including the possibility of reversible injury; deficits not measurable by the current SPECT [^{123}I]β-CIT binding studies; abnormal reinnervation; or the deficits being postsynaptic in nature. Critics argue that SPECT [^{123}I]β-CIT binding is not reliable enough to make any firm conclusions and that concomitant marijuana use may have affected the results.[30]

In a related study, the same group found significant differences in the SPECT [^{123}I]β-CIT binding in female, but not male, ecstasy users as compared with female control subjects.[27] Decreased binding in females was dose-related and was evident even in the former users, but was not statistically different from levels seen in control subjects. The authors proposed that females are more susceptible to the effects of ecstasy and that these effects might be reversible. However, no sex-related difference was found in a PET study using [^{11}C]McN-5652.[29] SERT binding was decreased both globally and regionally (cingulate, frontal, occipital, and parietal cortices; striatum, cerebellum) in 14 ecstasy users (abstinent 3 weeks to >1 year) compared with control subjects. Binding correlated with extent of MDMA exposure, but not with time since last dose.

Conclusion

Although most users believe it to be harmless, most researchers agree that MDMA is to some extent toxic to human serotonergic (and perhaps dopaminergic) neurons. They also agree that some of the toxicity may be long-lasting. Imaging studies have examined structure, metabolites, blood flow, blood volume, glucose uptake, and serotonin receptor binding. Although results do not always agree, the most consistently implicated structures belong to the frontostriatal (thalamic) cerebellar network.

These studies are timely and crucial because some researchers are now advocating use of MDMA as an adjunct to treatment of posttraumatic stress disorder.[31] The findings may also have other public health implications. In particular, if permanent loss of serotonergic terminals occurs in some ecstasy users, this may pose clinically significant problems in later life as a result of decreased "serotonergic reserve."[26] Finally, these neuroimaging techniques may give a way to further understand the complex interrelationships of the emotion and memory circuits and the role of serotonin in the human brain.

References

1. Reneman L, Majoie CB, Habraken JB, et al: Effects of ecstasy (MDMA) on the brain in abstinent users: initial observations with diffusion and perfusion MR imaging. Radiology 2001; 220:611–617
2. Goss J: Designer drugs: assess and manage patients intoxicated with ecstasy, GHB or rohypnol—the three most commonly abused designer drugs. J Emerg Med Serv 2001; 26:84–93
3. Morgan MJ: Ecstasy (MDMA): a review of its possible persistent psychological effects. Psychopharmacol (Berl) 2000; 152:230–248
4. Doyon S: The many faces of ecstasy. Curr Opin Pediatr 2001; 13:170–176
5. Baggott M, Heifets B, Jones RT, et al: Chemical analysis of ecstasy pills (letter). JAMA 2000; 284:2190
6. Christophersen AS: Amphetamine designer drugs: an overview and epidemiology. Toxicol Lett 2000; 112–113:127–131
7. Murray JB: Ecstasy is a dangerous drug. Psychol Rep 2001; 88:895–902
8. Pope HG Jr, Ionescu-Pioggia M, Pope KW: Drug use and life style among college undergraduates: a 30-year longitudinal study. Am J Psychiatry 2001; 158:1519–1521
9. Fineschi V, Centini F, Mazzeo E, et al: Adam (MDMA) and Eve (MDEA) misuse: an immunohistochemical study on three fatal cases. Forensic Sci Int 1999; 104:65–74
10. O'Connor A, Cluroe A, Couch R, et al: Death from hyponatraemia-induced cerebral oedema associated with MDMA ("Ecstasy") use. N Z Med J 1999; 112:255–256
11. de la Torre R, Ortuno J, Mas M, et al: Fatal MDMA intoxication (letter). Lancet 1999; 353:593
12. Ricaurte GA, Yuan J, McCann UD: (+/-)3,4-Methylenedioxymethamphetamine ("Ecstasy")-induced serotonin neurotoxicity: studies in animals. Neuropsychobiology 2000; 42:5–10
13. Chang L, Grob CS, Ernst T, et al: Effect of ecstasy [3,4-methylenedioxymethamphetamine (MDMA)] on cerebral blood flow: a co-registered SPECT and MRI study. Psychiatry Res 2000; 98:15–28
14. Bitsch A, Thiel A, Rieckmann P, et al: Acute inflammatory CNS disease after MDMA ("ecstasy"). Eur Neurol 1996; 36:328–329
15. Bertram M, Egelhoff T, Schwarz S, et al: Toxic leukencephalopathy following "ecstasy" ingestion. J Neurol 1999; 246:617–618
16. Spatt J, Glawar B, Mamoli B: A pure amnestic syndrome after MDMA ("ecstasy") ingestion. J Neurol Neurosurg Psychiatry 1997; 62:418–419
17. Chang L, Ernst T, Grob CS, et al: Cerebral (1)H MRS alterations in recreational 3,4-methylenedioxymethamphetamine (MDMA, "ecstasy") users. J Magn Reson Imaging 1999;10:521–526
18. Reneman L, Majoie CBLM, Flick H, et al: Reduced *N*-acetylaspartate levels in the frontal cortex of 3,4-methylenedioxymethamphetamine (ecstasy) users: preliminary results. AJNR Am J Neuroradiol 2002; 23:231–237
19. Schreckenberger M, Gouzoulis-Mayfrank E, Sabri O, et al: "Ecstasy"-induced changes of cerebral glucose metabolism and their correlation to acute psychopathology: an 18-FDG PET study. Eur J Nucl Med 1999; 26:1572–1579
20. Obrocki J, Buchert R, Vaterlein O, et al: Ecstasy: long-term effects on the human central nervous system revealed by positron emission tomography. Br J Psychiatry 1999; 175:186–188
21. Buchert R, Obrocki J, Thomasius R, et al: Long-term effects of "ecstasy" abuse on the human brain studied by FDG PET. Nucl Med Commun 2001; 22:889–897
22. Gamma A, Buck A, Berthold T, et al: 3,4-Methylenedioxymethamphetamine (MDMA) modulates cortical and limbic brain activity as measured by [H(2)(15)O]-PET in healthy humans. Neuropsychopharmacology 2000; 23:388–395
23. Gamma A, Buck A, Berthold T, et al: No difference in brain activation during cognitive performance between ecstasy (3,4-methylenedioxymethamphetamine) users and control subjects: a [H2(15)O]-positron emission tomography study. J Clin Psychopharmacol 2001; 21:66–71
24. Reneman L, Habraken JB, Majoie CB, et al: MDMA ("Ecstasy") and its association with cerebrovascular accidents: preliminary findings. AJNR Am J Neuroradiol 2000; 21:1001–1007
25. Reneman L, Booij J, Schmand B, et al: Memory disturbances in "Ecstasy" users are correlated with an altered brain serotonin neurotransmission. Psychopharmacol (Berl) 2000; 148:322–324
26. Semple DM, Ebmeier KP, Glabus MF, et al: Reduced in vivo binding to the serotonin transporter in the cerebral cortex of MDMA ("ecstasy") users. Br J Psychiatry 1999; 175:63–69
27. Reneman L, Booij J, de Bruin K, et al: Effects of dose, sex, and long-term abstention from use on toxic effects of MDMA (ecstasy) on brain serotonin neurons. Lancet 2001; 358:1864–1869

28. Reneman L, Lavalaye J, Schmand B, et al: Cortical serotonin transporter density and verbal memory in individuals who stopped using 3,4-methylenedioxymethamphetamine (MDMA or "ecstasy"): preliminary findings. Arch Gen Psychiatry 2001; 58:901–906
29. McCann UD, Szabo Z, Scheffel U, et al: Positron emission tomographic evidence of toxic effect of MDMA ("Ecstasy") on brain serotonin neurons in human beings. Lancet 1998; 352:1433–1437
30. McCann UD, Ricaurte GA, Molliver ME: "Ecstasy" and serotonin neurotoxicity: new findings raise more questions. Arch Gen Psychiatry 2001; 58:907–908
31. Imperio WA: Ecstasy research okayed. Clinical Psychiatry News 2001; 29:44

Recent Publications of Interest

Parrott AC, Marsden CA: MDMA (3,4-methylenedioxymethamphetamine) or ecstasy: the contemporary human and animal research perspective. J Psychopharmacol 2006; 20:143–146
Summarizes the review papers published in the March 2006 and May 2006 issues of this journal, providing an excellent overview of clinical and animal research on 3,4-methylenedioxymethamphetamine (MDMA), also known as ecstasy. Individual articles can be consulted for more detailed presentations.

Dumont GJ, Verkes RJ: A review of acute effects of 3,4-methylenedioxymethamphetamine in healthy volunteers. J Psychopharmacol 2006; 20:176–187
Reviews the literature on the acute effects of MDMA in healthy volunteers.

Easton N, Marsden CA: Ecstasy: are animal data consistent between species and can they translate to humans? J Psychopharmacol 2006; 20:194–210
Compares the results of animal and human studies of the acute and chronic effects of MDMA exposure.

Parrott AC: MDMA in humans: factors which affect the neuropsychobiological profiles of recreational ecstasy users, the integrative role of bioenergetic stress. J Psychopharmacol 2006; 20:147–163
Explores a wide range of both drug-related and other factors that are likely to modulate the neuropsychobiological effects of ecstasy use.

Reneman L, de Win MM, van den Brink W, et al: Neuroimaging findings with MDMA/ecstasy: technical aspects, conceptual issues and future prospects. J Psychopharmacol 2006; 20:164–175
Reviews functional neuroimaging studies that have evaluated the effects of MDMA on the human brain.

Reprinted from Hurley RA, Reneman L, Taber KH: "Ecstasy in the Brain: A Model for Neuroimaging." *Journal of Neuropsychiatry and Clinical Neurosciences* 14:125–129, 2002. Used with permission.

Chapter 4

The Future for Diffusion Tensor Imaging in Neuropsychiatry

Katherine H. Taber, Ph.D.
Carlo Pierpaoli, M.D., Ph.D.
Stephen E. Rose, Ph.D.
Fergus J. Rugg-Gunn, M.D.
Jonathan B. Chalk, M.B.B.S., F.R.A.C.P., Ph.D.
Derek K. Jones, Ph.D.
Robin A. Hurley, M.D.

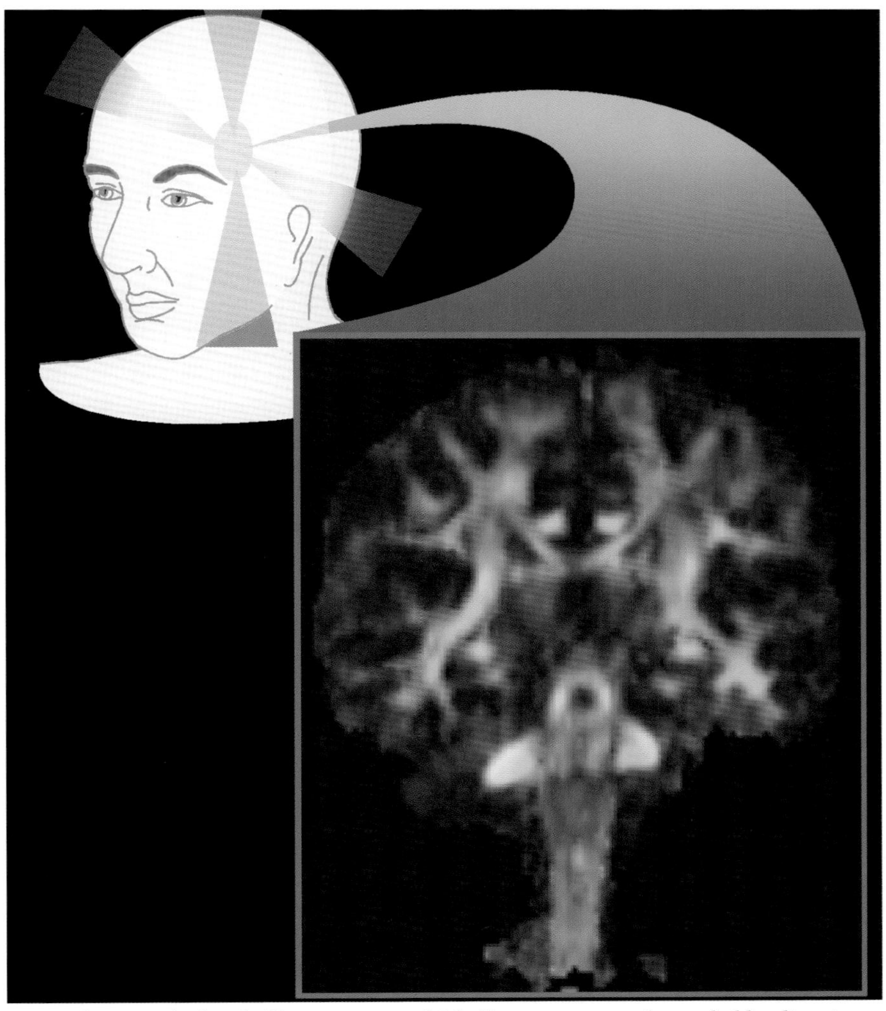

Coronal DTI at the level of brainstem in which fiber tracts are color-coded by direction as indicated by the colored triangles (superior–inferior, *blue*; left–right, *red*) and the colored oval (anterior–posterior, *green*) within the human head.[1] These also mark the approximate location of the coronal section.

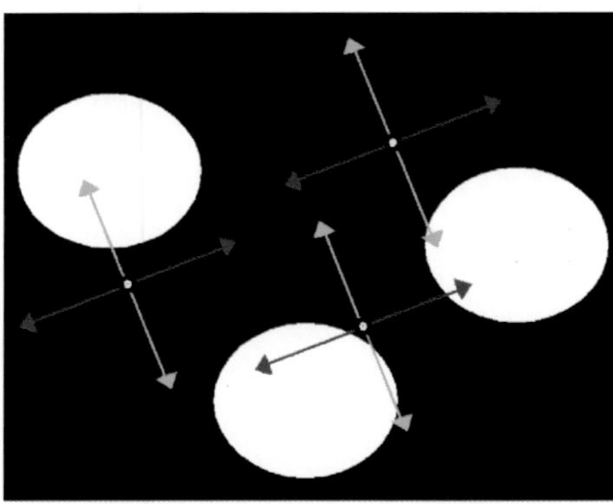

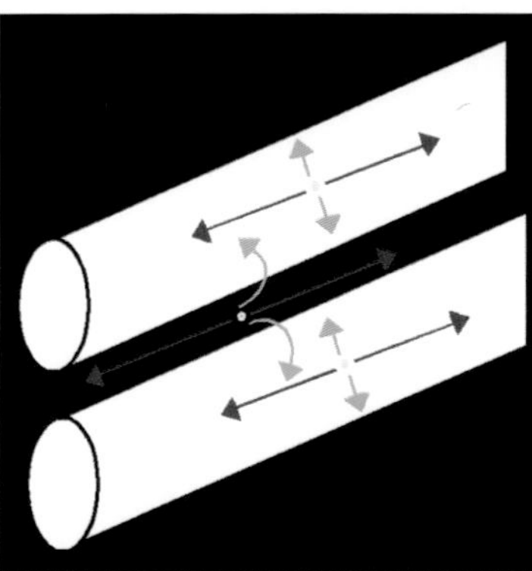

FIGURE 4–1. Isotropic diffusion (left): water diffusion is the same in all directions in gray matter (cell bodies and processes), as indicated by the similar length of the colored arrows. Anisotropic diffusion (right): in white matter (fiber tracts), water diffusion is faster parallel to axons (*red arrows*) than across (*green arrows*).

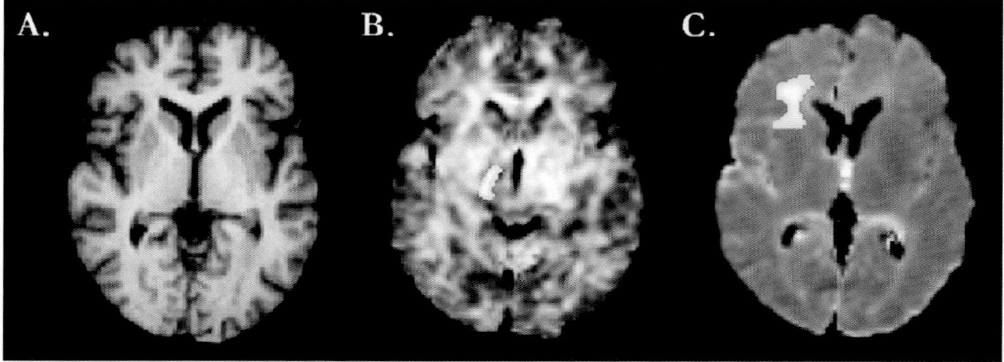

FIGURE 4–2. Standard T_1 (A) and T_2 (not shown)–weighted MRI were normal following a motor vehicle accident. Clinical symptoms included left-sided motor signs, severe frontal lobe dysfunction, and personality change. Abnormal areas were present on DTI (B, C). B: An area of significantly reduced anisotropy was identified in the posterior limb of the right internal capsule (*yellow*), concordant with the patient's motor signs. C: An area of increased mean diffusivity in the right frontal white matter (*yellow*) was concordant with the patient's neuropsychological findings. Adapted with permission from Rugg-Gunn et al.[2]

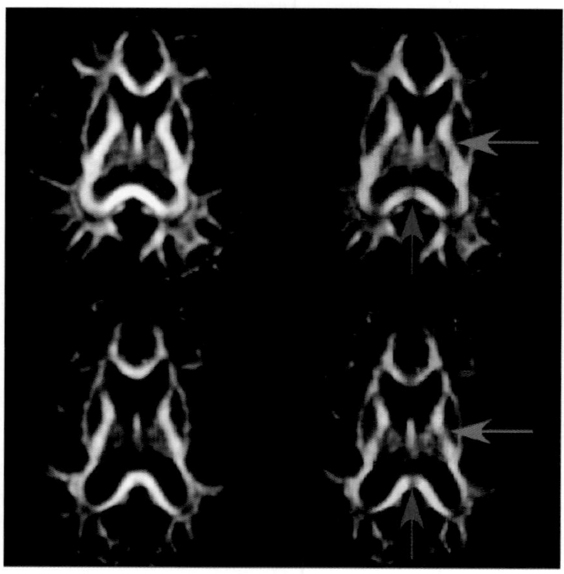

FIGURE 4–3. (left) Representative images from an age-matched control subject (top row) and a patient with probable Alzheimer's disease (bottom row; MMSE = 18) at the level of the internal capsule. On the left are maps of anisotropy; on the right, fiber direction has been color-coded (see image at opening to this chapter). The anisotropy of the pyramidal tract is similar in both (*purple arrows*). Decreased anisotropy in the splenium of the corpus callosum (*red arrows*) in the patient indicates decreased organization in this portion of the corpus callosum, perhaps due to loss of axons.

The phenomenon of nuclear magnetic resonance was discovered in the 1940s, leading to the development of magnetic resonance (MR) imaging of human patients in the 1970s. The 1980s and 1990s were years of learning to adapt this tool to clinical use. Advances made its use easier and broadened the range of clinically useful information that could be obtained. The most commonly encountered types of MR imaging in clinical practice are the T_2-weighted images that provide visualization of many pathologies and the T_1-weighted images that show anatomy best. As researchers discover ways to visualize different aspects of tissue structure, new methods of MR imaging are developed. One such advance was the development of diffusion tensor imaging (DTI), a more sophisticated version of diffusion-weighted (DW) MR imaging.[3–5] Although this technique has been under study since the mid-1980s, it is now just beginning to find clinical usefulness.

DTI provides a way to examine the microstructure of the brain, particularly of the white matter.[6,7] It is based on the finding that water diffuses differently along (parallel to) than across (perpendicular to) axons (Figure 4–1). Thus the direction and integrity of fibers can be assessed. A basic understanding of the principles of DTI will help the clinician follow the development of this technique as a useful clinical tool.

Fundamentals of Diffusion Tensor Imaging

In clinical DW imaging, two scans are collected for each brain section. One scan is simply a standard T_2-weighted image. The second image is modified during collection to make it sensitive to water movement (diffusion) in the chosen direction. An analysis is then done of the signal intensity change from the first to the second image for every location (volume element; voxel) within the brain section. The differences between the two images are used to calculate an index of the average speed of water diffusion (apparent diffusion constant or coefficient) for each voxel in the image. DW MR imaging is quite sensitive to processes that alter the size of the extracellular space, such as the development of cytotoxic edema in an area of ischemia.[7,8] It has proven very valuable, particularly in the imaging of acute stroke.[9] However, DW MR images provide limited information about the direction of water diffusion.

In DTI a minimum of seven images is acquired for each brain section. As in DW MR imaging, one image is simply a standard T_2-weighted image as is used in clinical imaging. The rest of the images are modified during collection to make them sensitive to water movement in different directions. From the complete set of seven images, a matrix that describes diffusional speed in each direction is calculated for every voxel in the image. This matrix is the *diffusion tensor* and gives the technique its name. It can take 20–30 minutes to collect all the images, depending on the number of diffusion-sensitive images acquired. In gray matter, the speed of diffusion is usually similar in all directions. This is termed *isotropic diffusion* (Figure 4–1, left). In white matter, the diffusion of water is significantly faster parallel to axons than across axons; it is directional. This is termed *anisotropic diffusion* (Figure 4–1, right). It is not yet clear what factors about white matter contribute to the constrained (and therefore directional) diffusion of water, but it is present prior to myelination, although it does increase as myelin is formed.[10–12]

Many quantities related to diffusion can be calculated from the tensor (matrix). The trace of the tensor provides a measure of average diffusion that is better than what can be obtained from simple DW imaging because it is not influenced by patient positioning or fiber orientation. Average diffusion is altered in areas of ischemia and may also be sensitive to gliosis. The degree of anisotropy within each voxel provides information on structural integrity of white matter. It can be used to identify areas of pathology or damage, as occur in multiple sclerosis or following traumatic brain injury. The principal direction of diffusion (eigenvector of the tensor associated with the largest eigenvalue) provides information about fiber direction. It can be used for mapping fiber tracts, which may be altered in areas of pathology or damage and by developmental changes. This technique also allows visualization of fiber tracts too small to be seen on conventional MR images.[1,13,14] One way of displaying this information is by using directionally encoded color (see Figure 4–3 and image at opening to this chapter). The principal direction of diffusion in each voxel is represented by a color scheme in which a set color is assigned to each major direction (anterior–posterior, left–right, superior–inferior).[1]

While promising, DTI is relatively early in its development and still suffers from some significant weaknesses. Most commonly the very fast echo-planar MR method is used to collect the images. This method results in artifacts in areas of magnetic field inhomogeneity, such as interfaces between brain, bone, and air. DTI requires combining information from many images and therefore is quite sensitive to patient movement. Most commonly the imaging matrix acquired is rather coarse (96×96, 128×128). As a result, voxels are large relative to some of the white matter structures that are being examined, and so images suffer from partial volume artifacts (inclusion of a mixture of tissues or fiber tracts within a voxel). Refinements are under development that will allow higher resolution while maintaining adequate signal in each voxel.[15] In addition, the measures average what is occurring within each voxel. In areas in which fibers are crossing or diverging, the resultant average can be quite misleading.[7,14,16,17] Techniques are being developed that extract measures of dispersion from each voxel, which should help with this problem.[14]

Clinical Applications

Although still in its infancy, DTI has the potential to expand our knowledge of the brain manyfold. Currently, reports exist in the literature that demonstrate its potential use in both the acute and the chronic patient. Below is a short summary of selected disease processes and cases in which DTI proved helpful clinically in either diagnosis, prognosis, or treatment planning.

Acquired Brain Injury (Acute and Chronic)

Jones et al. found changes in average diffusion similar to those found in acute stroke in the area surrounding sites of acute brain injury in all four cases they examined.[18] These areas appeared normal on standard T_2-weighted MR images, just as acute stroke does. The results suggest that these areas are ischemic and therefore might be responsive to treatment. The authors proposed that identification of such areas may lead to changes in acute treatment that render those brain areas "potentially salvageable." Rugg-Gunn et al. presented two cases of chronic traumatic brain injury in which diffuse axonal injuries distant from the major injury site were present on DTI that were not visible on conventional MR imaging.[2] Of great importance, the sites of diffuse axonal injury were consistent with the motor and neuropsychiatric deficits evident on examination. In another case report, the patient's excellent motor recovery by 18 months after traumatic brain injury correlated well with the preservation of normal anisotropy in a portion of the posterior limb of the internal capsule, an indication that the pathways were intact.[19] The authors suggested that this imaging method may well be able to differentiate between injuries that cause a transitory loss of function (as a result of temporary inflammation, edema, and/or shock) and permanent damage. If they are correct, this would allow patients to be separated into those who will recover function relatively quickly and those who will require extensive rehabilitation. Similarly, in another case, decreased anisotropy and increased diffusion were measured within the corticospinal tract for its entire length 18 months after cortical stroke.[20] In contrast, 3 weeks after hemorrhage into the putamen, anisotropy was decreased in the internal capsule but average diffusion was within normal limits.[20] These authors suggested that decreased anisotropy indicates axonal disruption, whereas increased diffusion indicates gliosis. Toxins can also alter the microstructure of the brain. A preliminary report of 15 patients with alcohol dependence indicates that DTI may provide insight into the anatomic basis of cognitive changes in alcoholism.[21]

Developmental Abnormalities

Mapping of alterations in fiber tracts that are related to particular functions is of primary interest in the application of DTI to the study of developmental disorders. Several groups have used DTI to test the theory that schizophrenia occurs as a result of frontal disconnection.[22–24] All three studies found decreases in the normal anisotropy of white matter, an indication of axonal disruption or disorganization. One found lower anisotropy in the prefrontal white matter of 5 patients with schizophrenia compared with normal subjects, as well as lower metabolic rates (as measured by positron emission tomography) in both frontal cortex and striatum.[22] In another study of 10 patients with schizophrenia, an overall decrease in anisotropy of white matter was found that was similar across all regions (prefrontal, temporal–parietal, parietal–occipital).[23] A third group looked only at the corpus callosum in a group of 20 patients with schizophrenia.[24] They found a reduction in anisotropy and an increased mean diffusivity in the splenium but not the genu of the corpus callosum in the patient group. DTI has also been used to show widespread abnormalities in tissue organization as a result of cortical maldevelopment with accompanying seizures.[25,26] Some of these areas of abnormal organization appeared normal on traditional imaging. Both authors note the significance of this in planning surgical correction of the accompanying epilepsy. DTI may also be sensitive to much more subtle white matter abnormalities. Adults with poor reading ability (previous diagnosis of developmental dyslexia) demonstrated decreased anisotropy in the left temporoparietal region that correlated well with reading skills.[27] No abnormalities were visible on high-resolution T_1-weighted MR images.

Degenerative Conditions

Rose et al. proposed DTI as a means to identify Alzheimer's disease (AD).[28] They imaged 11 patients who needed investigation for "dementia" and had been given a diagnosis of probable AD after meeting appropriate diagnostic criteria. When compared with nine age-matched control subjects, the patients with probable AD demonstrated reduced anisotropy in the splenium of the corpus callosum, superior longitudinal fasciculus, and left cingulum (Figure 4–3). Anisotropy of the splenium correlated well with the Mini Mental State Examination (MMSE) scores. The authors note that this region contains fibers that originated from the temporoparietal region—an area known to be affected in AD.

Ulug et al. included two patients with degenerative disease in their case series.[20] In the patient with amyotrophic lateral sclerosis, there was decreased anisotropy with no change in diffusion in the posterior limb of the internal capsule, although the area appeared normal on clinical imaging. In the patient with progressive bulbar paralysis, there was little change in anisotropy but an increase in diffusion. The authors suggest that this latter pattern may be associated with gliosis. Two studies suggest that DTI may help with the staging of lesions in multiple sclerosis and may provide insight into underlying disease mechanisms.[29,30] Wieshmann et al. report the examination of a patient with seizures and a tumor of the right frontal lobe.[31] DTI brought to light distant mass effect and displacement of white matter fibers adjacent to the tumor rather than destruction, a finding consistent with the patient's mild motor impairment. Again, the authors note the importance of this information in planning surgical interventions.

Summary

DTI is a powerful new imaging technique that provides a means to assess the integrity of white matter at the microstructural level. As the scattered case reports mentioned above indicate, it has broad applications in the study of both normal and abnormal brain development as well as acquired pathology. Some of these studies suggest an important role for DTI in guiding the planning of neurosurgical interventions based on the displacement or reorganization of fiber tracts around areas of pathology. If DTI can identify the extent of brain injuries and/or predict recovery potential, then traumatic brain injury treatment might be improved during both the acute and chronic stages. If lesions can be documented in patients with disease not generally respected by third-party payers or disability examiners, then patients may be able to receive benefits once denied them. And last but not least, patients and families may be comforted by seeing a lesion or abnormality on a clinical film that explains their symptoms.

References

1. Pajevic S, Pierpaoli C: Color schemes to represent the orientation of anisotropic tissues from diffusion tensor data: application to white matter fiber tract mapping in the human brain. Magn Reson Med 1999; 42:526–540
2. Rugg-Gunn FJ, Symms MR, Barker GJ, et al: Diffusion imaging shows abnormalities after blunt head trauma when conventional magnetic resonance imaging is normal. J Neurol Neurosurg Psychiatry 2001; 70:530–533
3. Taylor DG, Bushell MC: The spatial mapping of translational diffusion coefficients by the NMR imaging technique. Phys Med Biol 1985; 30:345–349
4. Le Bihan D, Breton E, Lallemand D, et al: MR imaging of intravoxel incoherent motions: application to diffusion and perfusion in neurologic disorders. Radiology 1986; 161:401–407
5. Basser PJ, Mattiello J, LeBihan D: Estimation of the effective self-diffusion tensor from the NMR spin echo. J Magn Reson B 1994; 103:247–254
6. Pierpaoli C, Jezzard P, Basser PJ, et al: Diffusion tensor MR imaging of the human brain. Radiology 1996; 201:637–648
7. Le Bihan D, Mangin JF, Poupon C, et al: Diffusion tensor imaging: concepts and applications. J Magn Reson Imaging 2001; 13:534–546
8. Sevick RJ, Kanda F, Mintorovitch J, et al: Cytotoxic brain edema: assessment with diffusion-weighted MR imaging. Radiology 1992; 185:687–690
9. Warach S, Dashe JF, Edelman RR: Clinical outcome in ischemic stroke predicted by early diffusion-weighted and perfusion magnetic resonance imaging: a preliminary analysis. J Cereb Blood Flow Metab 1996; 16:53–59
10. Beaulieu C, Allen PS: Determinants of anisotropic water diffusion in nerves. Magn Reson Med 1994; 31:394–400
11. Huppi PS, Maier SE, Peled S, et al: Microstructural development of human newborn cerebral white matter assessed in vivo by diffusion tensor magnetic resonance imaging. Pediatr Res 1998; 44:584–590
12. Prayer D, Barkovich AJ, Kirschner DA, et al: Visualization of nonstructural changes in early white matter development on diffusion-weighted MR images: evidence supporting premyelination anisotropy. AJNR Am J Neuroradiol 2001; 22:1572–1576
13. Nakada T, Nakayama N, Fujii Y, et al: Clinical application of three-dimensional anisotropy contrast magnetic resonance axonography: technical note. J Neurosurg 1999; 90:791–795
14. Wiegell MR, Larsson HB, Wedeen VJ: Fiber crossing in human brain depicted with diffusion tensor MR imaging. Radiology 2000; 217:897–903
15. Jones DK, Horsfield MA, Simmons A: Optimal strategies for measuring diffusion in anisotropic systems by magnetic resonance imaging. Magn Reson Med 1999; 42:515–525
16. Jones DK, Simmons A, Williams SC, et al: Non-invasive assessment of axonal fiber connectivity in the human brain via diffusion tensor MRI. Magn Reson Med 1999; 42:37–41
17. Virta A, Barnett A, Pierpaoli C: Visualizing and characterizing white matter fiber structure and architecture in the human pyramidal tract using diffusion tensor MRI. Magn Reson Imaging 1999; 17:1121–1133
18. Jones DK, Dardis R, Ervine M, et al: Cluster analysis of diffusion tensor magnetic resonance images in human head injury. Neurosurgery 2000; 47:306–313; discussion, 313–314
19. Werring DJ, Clark CA, Barker GJ, et al: The structural and functional mechanisms of motor recovery: complementary use of diffusion tensor and functional magnetic resonance imaging in a traumatic injury of the internal capsule. J Neurol Neurosurg Psychiatry 1998; 65:863–869
20. Ulug AM, Moore DF, Bojko AS, et al: Clinical use of diffusion-tensor imaging for diseases causing neuronal and axonal damage. AJNR Am J Neuroradiol 1999; 20:1044–1048

21. Pfefferbaum A, Sullivan EV, Hedehus M, et al: In vivo detection and functional correlates of white matter microstructural disruption in chronic alcoholism. Alcohol Clin Exp Res 2000; 24:1214–1221
22. Buchsbaum MS, Tang CY, Peled S, et al: MRI white matter diffusion anisotropy and PET metabolic rate in schizophrenia. Neuroreport 1998; 9:425–430
23. Lim KO, Hedehus M, Moseley M, et al: Compromised white matter tract integrity in schizophrenia inferred from diffusion tensor imaging. Arch Gen Psychiatry 1999; 56:367–374
24. Foong J, Maier M, Clark CA, et al: Neuropathological abnormalities of the corpus callosum in schizophrenia: a diffusion tensor imaging study. J Neurol Neurosurg Psychiatry 2000; 68:242–244
25. Eriksson SH, Rugg–Gunn FJ, Symms MR, et al: Diffusion tensor imaging in patients with epilepsy and malformations of cortical development. Brain 2001; 124:617–626
26. Wieshmann UC, Krakow K, Symms MR, et al: Combined functional magnetic resonance imaging and diffusion tensor imaging demonstrate widespread modified organisation in malformation of cortical development. J Neurol Neurosurg Psychiatry 2001; 70:521–523
27. Klingberg T, Hedehus M, Temple E, et al: Microstructure of temporo-parietal white matter as a basis for reading ability: evidence from diffusion tensor magnetic resonance imaging. Neuron 2000; 25:493–500
28. Rose SE, Chen F, Chalk JB, et al: Loss of connectivity in Alzheimer's disease: an evaluation of white matter tract integrity with colour coded MR diffusion tensor imaging. J Neurol Neurosurg Psychiatry 2000; 69:528–530
29. Werring DJ, Clark CA, Barker GJ, et al: Diffusion tensor imaging of lesions and normal-appearing white matter in multiple sclerosis. Neurology 1999; 52:1626–1632
30. Iannucci G, Rovaris M, Giacomotti L, et al: Correlation of multiple sclerosis measures derived from T_2-weighted, T_1-weighted, magnetization transfer, and diffusion tensor MR imaging. AJNR Am J Neuroradiol 2001; 22:1462–1467
31. Wieshmann UC, Symms MR, Parker GJ, et al: Diffusion tensor imaging demonstrates deviation of fibres in normal appearing white matter adjacent to a brain tumour. J Neurol Neurosurg Psychiatry 2000; 68:501–503

Recent Publications of Interest

Lee SK, Kim DI, Kim J, et al: Diffusion-tensor MR imaging and fiber tractography: a new method of describing aberrant fiber connections in developmental CNS anomalies. Radiographics 2005; 25:53–65
Uses clinical cases of developmental abnormalities to explore the usefulness of diffusion tensor imaging in visualizing aberrant connections. Specific topics discussed are the imaging protocol, abnormalities of the corpus callosum, malformations of cortical development, cerebral palsy, and posterior fossa malformations.

Kanaan RA, Kim JS, Kaufmann WE, et al: Diffusion tensor imaging in schizophrenia. Biol Psychiatry 2005; 58:921–929
Performed a systematic review of the diffusion tensor imaging literature in schizophrenia, and concluded that the results are not yet sufficiently consistent across studies to support specific white matter abnormalities.

Rovaris M, Gass A, Bammer R, et al: Diffusion MRI in multiple sclerosis. Neurology 2005; 65:1526–1532
Reviews and critically evaluates the literature on diffusion tensor imaging in patients with multiple sclerosis.

Sundgren PC, Dong Q, Gomez-Hassan D, et al: Diffusion tensor imaging of the brain: review of clinical applications. Neuroradiology 2004; 46:339–350
Provides an overview of diffusion tensor imaging techniques, and reviews common clinical applications (cerebral ischemia, brain maturation, traumatic brain injury) as well as its potential for use in other conditions (epilepsy, multiple sclerosis, Alzheimer's disease, brain tumors, metabolic disorders).

DaSilva AF, Tuch DS, Wiegell MR, et al: A primer on diffusion tensor imaging of anatomical substructures. Neurosurg Focus 2003; 15:E4
Gives a brief overview of this imaging technique and reviews its application to visualizing anatomy at high resolution, using brainstem and thalamus as illustrative examples.

Reprinted from Taber KH, Pierpaoli C, Rose SE, et al: "The Future for Diffusion Tensor Imaging in Neuropsychiatry." *Journal of Neuropsychiatry and Clinical Neurosciences* 14:1–5, 2002. Used with permission.

Chapter 5

Cortical Inhibition in Alcohol Dependence

Katherine H. Taber, Ph.D.
Robin A. Hurley, M.D.
Anissa Abi-Dargham, M.D.
Bernice Porjesz, M.D.

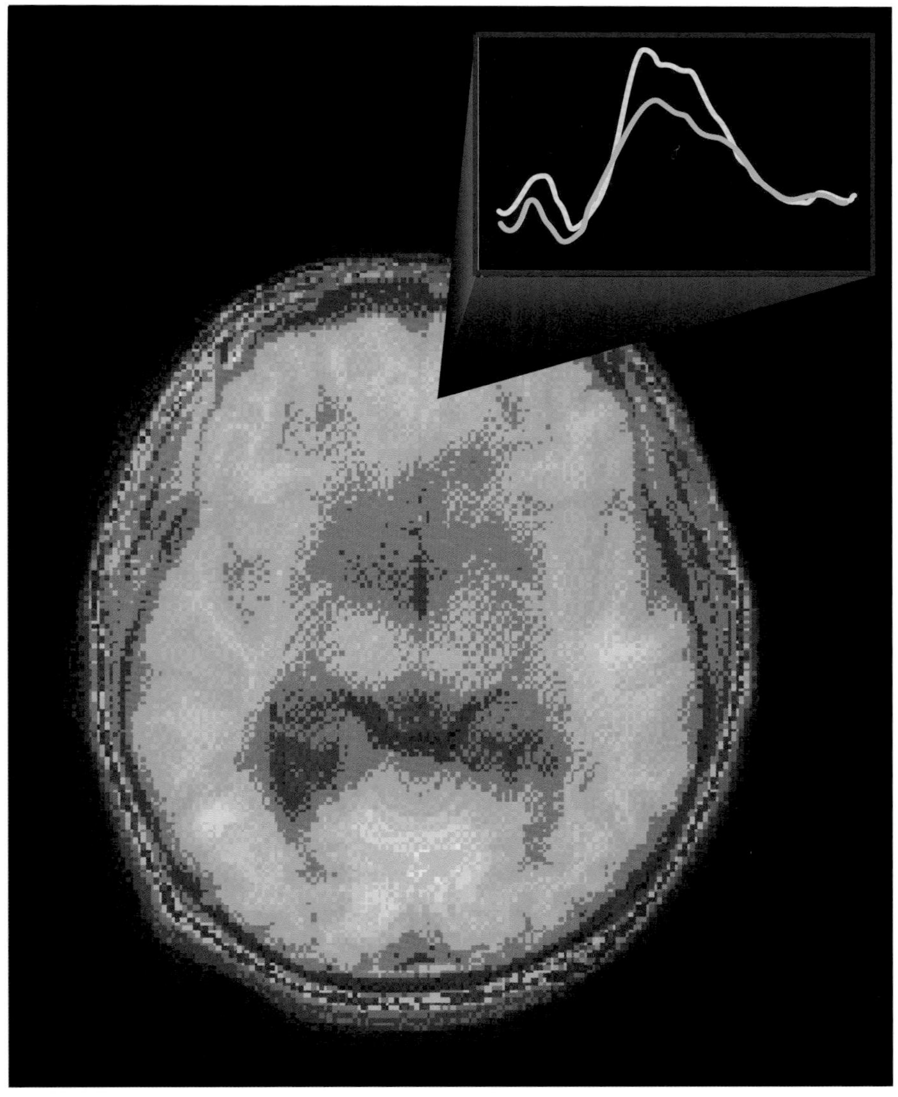

An axial image (bottom) of benzodiazepine receptor binding in an alcohol-dependent patient is overlaid with a comparison of event-related potentials (top) obtained during a Go/No-Go task from normal individuals (*gray*) and alcohol-dependent subjects (*green*).

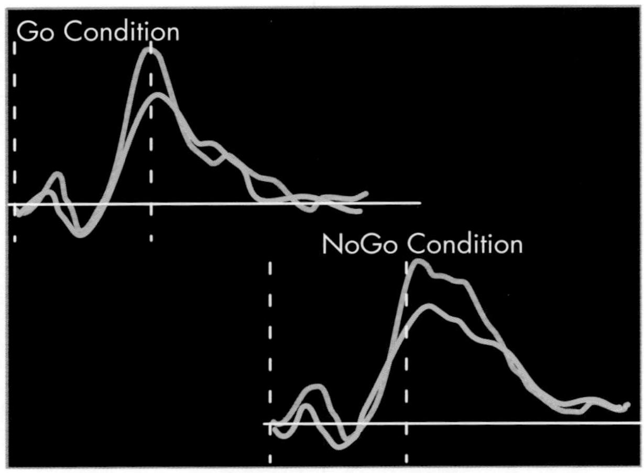

FIGURE 5–1. ERPs obtained by using a cued continuous performance test (Go/No-Go task). Note the decrease in the responses of the alcohol-dependent subjects (indicated in *green*) compared with control subjects (indicated in *gray*). The dashed lines indicate the time of target presentation and the time of peak response (300 ms, P300). The alcohol-dependent subjects had diminished frontal activation during both conditions, indicating diminished inhibition (disinhibition).

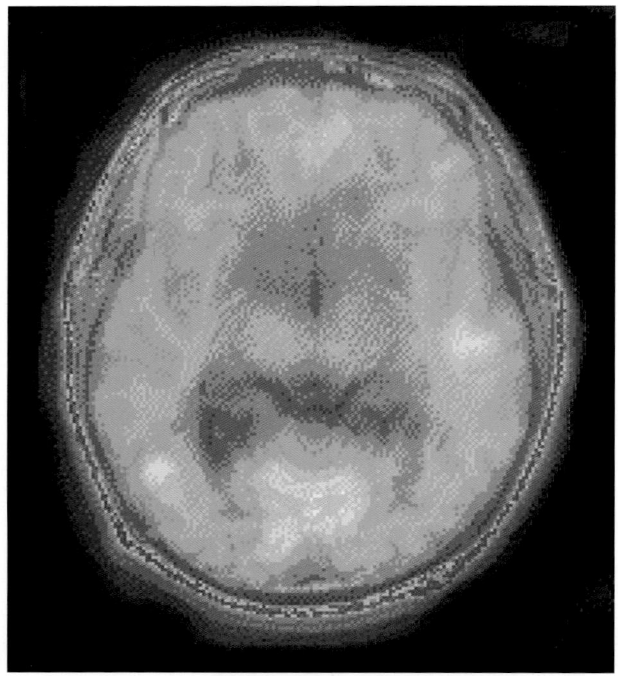

FIGURE 5–2. Transaxial slice of a SPECT study of BZD receptor binding (iomazenil [^{123}I]) superimposed on the corresponding MRI slice from a 56-year-old alcohol-dependent male who had been sober for 95 days. BZD binding in alcohol-dependent subjects is decreased in a number of brain regions compared with control subjects (see text for details).

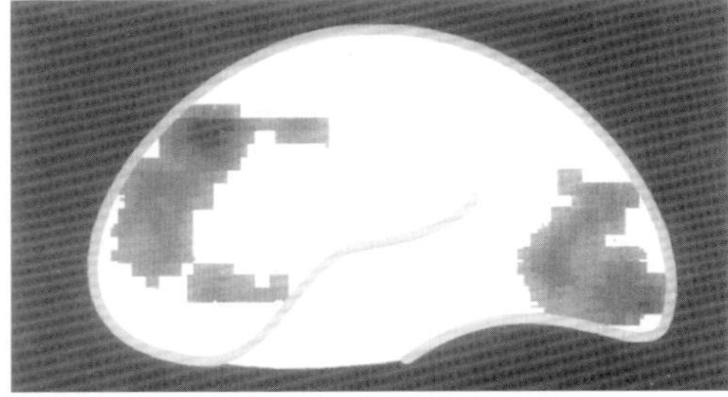

FIGURE 5–3. Sagittal projection view (frontal cortex to the left, occipital cortex to the right) summarizes regions where BZD receptor distribution was lower in alcohol-dependent subjects compared with control subjects. Although BZD receptor binding was lower in all regions, it was significantly lower in prefrontal cortex, anterior cingulate cortex, and cerebellum.

Alcohol dependence as defined by DSM-IV criteria is a psychiatric disorder that affects approximately 13% of the population at some point in life. This prevalence increases to 20% if individuals who have never consumed 12 or more drinks in any 1 year of life are excluded.[1] Approximately half of all homicides and motor vehicle–related deaths involve alcohol, as do one-fourth of all suicides. Comorbid psychiatric conditions are common. The estimated social impact of alcohol dependence is $100 billion in health care costs, lost wages, and family disruption.[2] To understand this enormous public health concern, researchers are studying alcoholism from the sociological to the molecular level. (A PubMed search on "alcohol" captures more than 68,000 references in the past 5 years alone.) A few research areas include the neurobiology of craving and tolerance, changes in cortical neurochemistry with dependence and withdrawal, and the development of medications to reverse intoxication and to prevent craving.

A genetic predisposition or vulnerability to development of alcohol dependence has been clearly demonstrated. There is a three- to ninefold increased risk in first-degree relatives of alcohol-dependent patients compared with the general population.[3] The genetic vulnerability to alcohol dependence is 0.50–0.60. Two chromosomal linkage studies have found strong evidence for possible candidate genes for alcohol dependence on chromosome 4 and lesser evidence for chromosomes 11, 1, 7, and 2.[4]

It has been recognized since the case of Phineas Gage was understood that the orbitofrontal cortex is a critical part of a circuit responsible for inhibition and for regulation of social behavior. It has been suggested that there is a relationship between alcohol dependence and the orbitofrontal cortex. This theory proposes a shift in the general excitability of the brain, perhaps as a result of decreased inhibition (disinhibition). Alcohol-dependent persons score high on several measures likely to reflect disinhibition, including exploratory excitability, impulsiveness, extravagance, and disorderliness.[5] In addition, there is evidence of abnormal brain processing in both persons who are alcohol dependent and individuals at high risk for alcoholism.

Evidence for abnormal processing has been obtained by using event-related potentials (ERPs). ERPs are the summed electrical activity recorded from scalp electrodes after a stimulus presentation. A variety of situations or tasks are used in this type of study, and the ERP has a characteristic shape for each. A very simple task commonly used requires monitoring a series of frequent visual shapes (e.g., squares) and responding by pushing a button whenever a designated different shape (e.g., a triangle) is presented ("oddball" task). The different, rarely occurring shape is the target. In normal individuals the positive waveform that occurs approximately 300 ms after the stimulus onset (P300 waveform) is much larger following presentation of a target compared with a nontarget in this task. In alcohol-dependent subjects, the P300 waveform to presentation of targets is much smaller than in normal individuals.[6] Importantly, it is reduced more in those with alcohol dependence who are from high-risk families than in those with no family history of alcohol abuse. It is also abnormal in individuals from high-risk families who are alcohol naive.[7] This waveform is thought to reflect inhibitory processes in cortex. Thus, the decreased size in patients with alcohol dependence and persons at risk may indicate a global or regional lack of cortical inhibition. The diminished increase when a target is presented may indicate deficits in processing of information.[8]

Electrophysiological studies of more complex tasks also support this view. Central nervous system inhibitory state can be assessed experimentally by use of a cued continuous performance test in which a motor response is required to one situation (Go condition) but must be suppressed to others (No-Go condition) (Figure 5–1). The ERP to each condition in this task is influenced by the complexity of the Go/No-Go decision.[9] In a simple version of this task a series of uppercase and lowercase letters is presented (usually all the same letter). One is designated the Go and the other the No-Go condition. In normal individuals the P300 waveform to the Go condition is larger than to the No-Go condition for this task, similar to results of the "oddball" task described previously. In contrast, subjects who are alcohol dependent do not show any increase in the P300 waveform to the Go condition, and they have lower P300 amplitudes overall.[9]

In a more difficult Go/No-Go task, a series of letters is presented in which one letter is designated as the primer. When the target letter follows the primer, the subject responds by pushing a button (Go condition). When any other letter follows the primer, the subject must inhibit responding (No-Go condition).[10] The P300 component of the ERP recorded following a stimulus in this task is localized to both frontal and parietal regions.[11] The frontal activation is larger in the No-Go condition than in the Go condition. A reasonable interpretation of this finding is that the frontal activation reflects the inhibition that is required for response suppression during the No-Go condition.[11] Persons who are alcohol dependent have less frontal activation during this task than normal individuals, an indication that frontal lobe control of response inhibition is reduced.[10]

Although alcohol interacts with many neurotransmitters in both excitatory and inhibitory pathways, its potentiation of benzodiazepines (BZDs) and interactions with γ-aminobutyric acid (GABA) provide key support for this theory. GABA is the major inhibitory neurotransmitter in the brain. Postmortem studies have found regional changes in BZD receptor density in alcohol-dependent persons.[12] The BZD receptor is a site on the $GABA_A$ receptor. Recent in vivo single-photon emission computed tomography (SPECT) and positron emission tomography (PET) studies have found decreased BZD receptor density in frontal, anterior cingulate, parietal, temporal, and cerebellar cortices in alcohol-dependent subjects compared with control subjects[13,14] (Figures 5–2 and 5–3). These differences were present even in alcohol-dependent subjects who had been abstinent for prolonged periods prior to the evaluation. A similar pattern of differences was found when abstinent alcohol-dependent subjects were compared with nondependent alcohol users—suggesting that the differences in BZD receptor density are intrinsic rather than a result of alcohol toxicity.[13] A pilot study using magnetic resonance spectroscopy found that cortical GABA levels were lower in alcohol-dependent subjects than in control subjects. In contrast, cortical glutamate levels were similar.[15] Because GABA is an inhibitory neurotransmitter, this decrease in GABAergic transmission (both receptors and absolute levels) might underlie the diminished inhibition or hyperexcitability that has been found in alcohol-dependent individuals and persons at high risk for substance abuse.

Parallel results have been found with PET: alcohol-dependent patients usually have decreased metabolism in frontal, temporal (left), and parietal cortices.[16,17] As alcohol-dependent patients undergo detoxification, cortical metabolism improves.[17] The greatest changes were obtained between 4 and 8 weeks after alcohol withdrawal. Orbitofrontal and dorsolateral prefrontal cortices showed the most recovery, basal ganglia the least.

Alcohol-dependent patients also have an altered cerebral metabolic response to BZD administration.[18] In normal subjects, BZD administration decreases both global and regional brain metabolism. Measures taken during the first month of detoxification found less than normal metabolic depression in response to lorazepam administration in the thalamus, basal ganglia, and orbitofrontal cortex in alcohol-dependent subjects.[18] Diminished responses may still be present at 11 weeks.[19] Interestingly, the early changes correlated with both cerebellar metabolism at baseline and BZD (and therefore $GABA_A$) receptor density. The cerebellum has direct GABAergic projections to thalamus, basal ganglia, and orbitofrontal cortex. Thus, it is possible that abnormalities in cerebellar input to the orbitofrontal circuit (which includes all three regions) lead to disinhibition and/or compulsive behaviors in alcohol-dependent patients. It is of interest that the depression in cerebellar function (as measured by both metabolic rate and motor coordination) normally induced by lorazepam administration is also diminished in alcohol-naive subjects with positive family histories for alcohol abuse.[20]

Although these studies are limited to small groups of subjects and many were performed early in detoxification, they may cast light on a portion of what underlies this devastating illness. The involvement with GABA is, of course, only one aspect of the effect of alcohol on the brain. Alcohol has major interactions with many aspects of brain function, including most or all of the major neurotransmitters. As the biological causes and effects of alcohol dependence come to be understood more fully, sophisticated and successful treatments can be developed—just as the discovery of cross-tolerance of alcohol and BZDs has led to decreased mortality from alcohol withdrawal.

References

1. Grant BF: Prevalence and correlates of alcohol use and DSM-IV alcohol dependence in the United States: results of the National Longitudinal Alcohol Epidemiologic Survey. J Stud Alcohol 1997; 58:464–473
2. Litten RZ, Allen JP: Advances in development of medications for alcoholism treatment. Psychopharmacol (Berl) 1998; 139:20–33
3. McCaul ME: Substance abuse vulnerability in offspring of alcohol and drug abusers. NIDA Res Monogr 1998; 169:188–208
4. Enoch MA, Goldman D: Genetics of alcoholism and substance abuse. Psychiatr Clin North Am 1999; 22:289–299
5. Wills TA, Vaccaro D, McNamara G: Novelty seeking, risk taking, and related constructs as predictors of adolescent substance use: an application of Cloninger's theory. J Subst Abuse 1994; 6:1–20
6. Porjesz B, Begleiter H: Genetic basis of event-related potentials and their relationship to alcoholism and alcohol use. J Clin Neurophysiol 1998; 15:44–57
7. Begleiter H, Porjesz B, Bihari B, et al: Event-related brain potentials in boys at risk for alcoholism. Science 1984; 225:1493–1496
8. Begleiter H, Porjesz B: What is inherited in the predisposition toward alcoholism? A proposed model. Alcohol Clin Exp Res 1999; 23:1125–1135
9. Cohen HL, Porjesz B, Begleiter H, et al: Neurophysiological correlates of response production and inhibition in alcoholics. Alcohol Clin Exp Res 1997; 21:1398–1406
10. Fallgatter AJ,Wiesbeck GA,Weijers HG, et al: Event-related correlates of response suppression as indicators of novelty seeking in alcoholics. Alcohol Alcohol 1998; 33:475–481
11. Strik WK, Fallgatter AJ, Brandeis D, et al: Three-dimensional tomography of event-related potentials during response inhibition: evidence for phasic frontal lobe activation. Electroencephalogr Clin Neurophysiol 1998; 108:406–413
12. Freund G, Ballinger WE: Loss of synaptic receptors can precede morphologic changes induced by alcoholism. Alcohol Alcohol Suppl 1991; 1:385–391
13. Lingford-Hughes AR, Acton PD, Gacinovic S, et al: Reduced levels of GABA-benzodiazepine receptor in alcohol dependency in the absence of grey matter atrophy. Br J Psychiatry 1998; 173:116–122
14. Gilman S, Koeppe RA, Adams K, et al: Positron emission tomographic studies of cerebral benzodiazepine-receptor binding in chronic alcoholics. Ann Neurol 1996; 40:163–171
15. Behar KL, Rothman DL, Petersen KF, et al: Preliminary evidence of low cortical GABA levels in localized ^{1}H-MR spectra of alcohol-dependent and hepatic encephalopathy patients. Am J Psychiatry 1999; 156:952–954
16. Volkow ND, Hitzemann R, Wang GJ, et al: Decreased brain metabolism in neurologically intact healthy alcoholics. Am J Psychiatry 1992; 149:1016–1022
17. Volkow ND, Wang GJ, Hitzemann R, et al: Recovery of brain glucose metabolism in detoxified alcoholics. Am J Psychiatry 1994; 151:178–183
18. Volkow ND, Wang GJ, Hitzemann R, et al: Decreased cerebral response to inhibitory neurotransmission in alcoholics. Am J Psychiatry 1993; 150:417–422
19. Volkow ND, Wang GJ, Overall JE, et al: Regional brain metabolic response to lorazepam in alcoholics during early and late alcohol detoxification. Alcohol Clin Exp Res 1997; 21:1278–1284
20. Volkow ND, Wang GJ, Begleiter H, et al: Regional brain metabolic response to lorazepam in subjects at risk for alcoholism. Alcohol Clin Exp Res 1995; 19:510–516

Recent Publications of Interest

Krystal JH, Staley J, Mason G, et al: Gamma-aminobutyric acid type A receptors and alcoholism: intoxication, dependence, vulnerability, and treatment. Arch Gen Psychiatry 2006; 63:957–968

Reviews the literature on the role of brain GABA systems in alcohol response, dependence, vulnerability, and pharmacotherapy.

Crews FT, Buckley T, Dodd PR, et al: Alcoholic neurobiology: changes in dependence and recovery. Alcohol Clin Exp Res 2005; 29:1504–1513

Reports the findings of a recent symposium that reviewed the brain changes that occur during active alcoholism as well as those that may occur during abstinence. Topics covered include findings from human neuroimaging, neuro-

physiology, and neuropsychological assessments; changes in human brain gene expression; and preclinical studies investigating mechanisms of alcohol-induced neurotoxicity and neuroprogenitor cells during dependence and recovery from alcohol dependence.

Sullivan EV, Pfefferbaum A: Neurocircuitry in alcoholism: a substrate of disruption and repair. Psychopharmacology (Berl) 2005; 180:583–594

Presents the evidence for both transitory and permanent alcoholism-related brain structural and functional modifications. The phenomena of restoration of function and volume loss with abstinence are discussed.

Criswell HE, Breese GR: A conceptualization of integrated actions of ethanol contributing to its GABAmimetic profile: a commentary. Neuropsychopharmacology 2005; 30:1407–1425

Provides a historical perspective of attempts to define ethanol's ability to influence the GABA system in brain, followed by an overview of findings from recent initiatives to clarify the means by which ethanol displays its GABAmimetic profile.

Hines LM, Ray L, Hutchison K, et al: Alcoholism: the dissection for endophenotypes. Dialogues Clin Neurosci 2005; 7:153–163

Discusses the evidence for a wide range of alcohol-related characteristics as potential endophenotypes of alcohol dependence. Alcohol metabolism, physiological and endocrine measures, neuroimaging, electrophysiology, personality, drinking behavior, and responses to alcohol and alcohol-derived cues are included.

Cohen HL, Ji J, Chorlian DB, et al: Alcohol-related ERP changes recorded from different modalities: a topographic analysis. Alcohol Clin Exp Res 2002; 26:303–317

Evaluates event-related potential (ERP) abnormalities in abstinent alcoholic patients to both visual and auditory versions of the "oddball" task. The results suggest that, in abstinent alcoholic patients, abnormalities in auditory ERPs may be localized to more anterior sources, while abnormalities in visual ERPs may be localized to more posterior sources.

Reprinted from Taber KH, Hurley RA, Abi-Dargham A, et al: "Cortical Inhibition in Alcohol Dependence." *Journal of Neuropsychiatry and Clinical Neurosciences* 12:173–176, 2000. Used with permission.

Chapter 6

APPLICATION OF MAGNETOENCEPHALOGRAPHY TO THE STUDY OF AUTISM

ROBIN A. HURLEY, M.D.
JEFFREY DAVID LEWINE, PH.D.
GREGORY M. JONES, PH.D.
WILLIAM W. ORRISON JR., M.D.
KATHERINE H. TABER, PH.D.

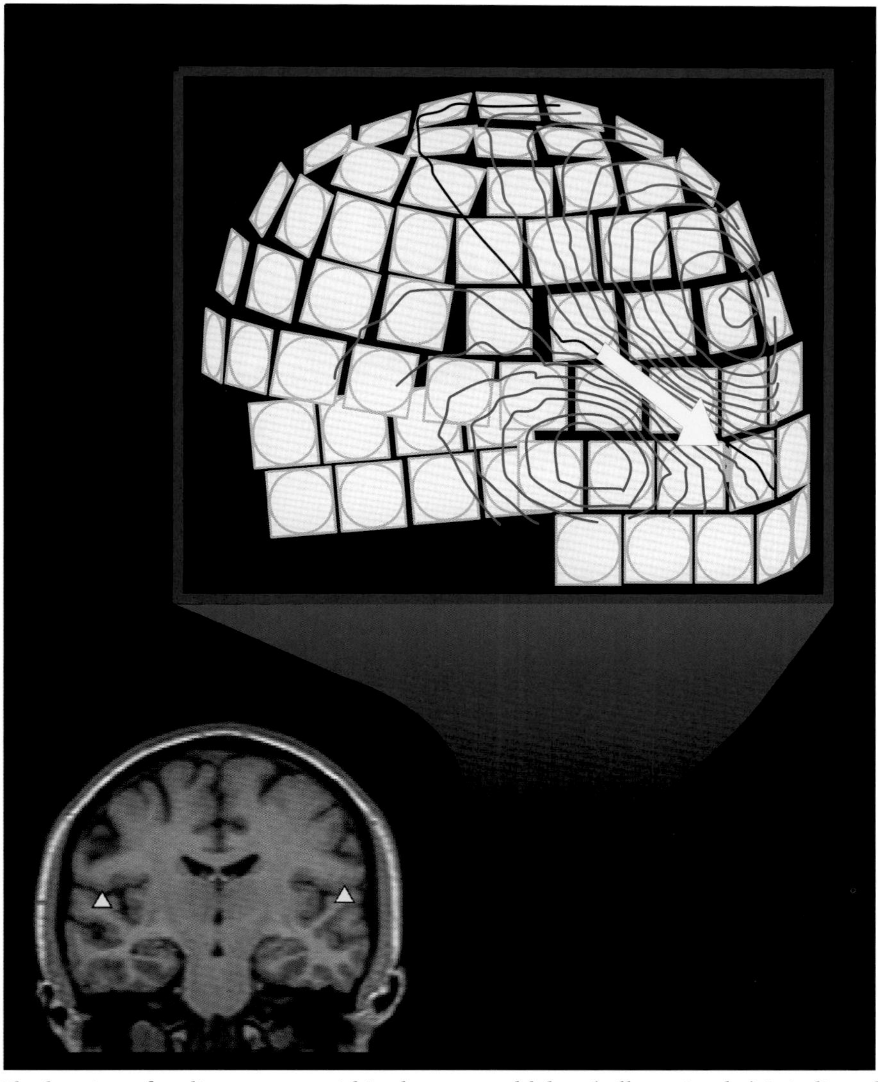

The location of auditory cortex within the temporal lobes (*yellow triangles*) is indicated on a coronal magnetic resonance image. The magnetic field lines recorded for one hemisphere of the brain by whole-head magnetoencephalography are shown above.

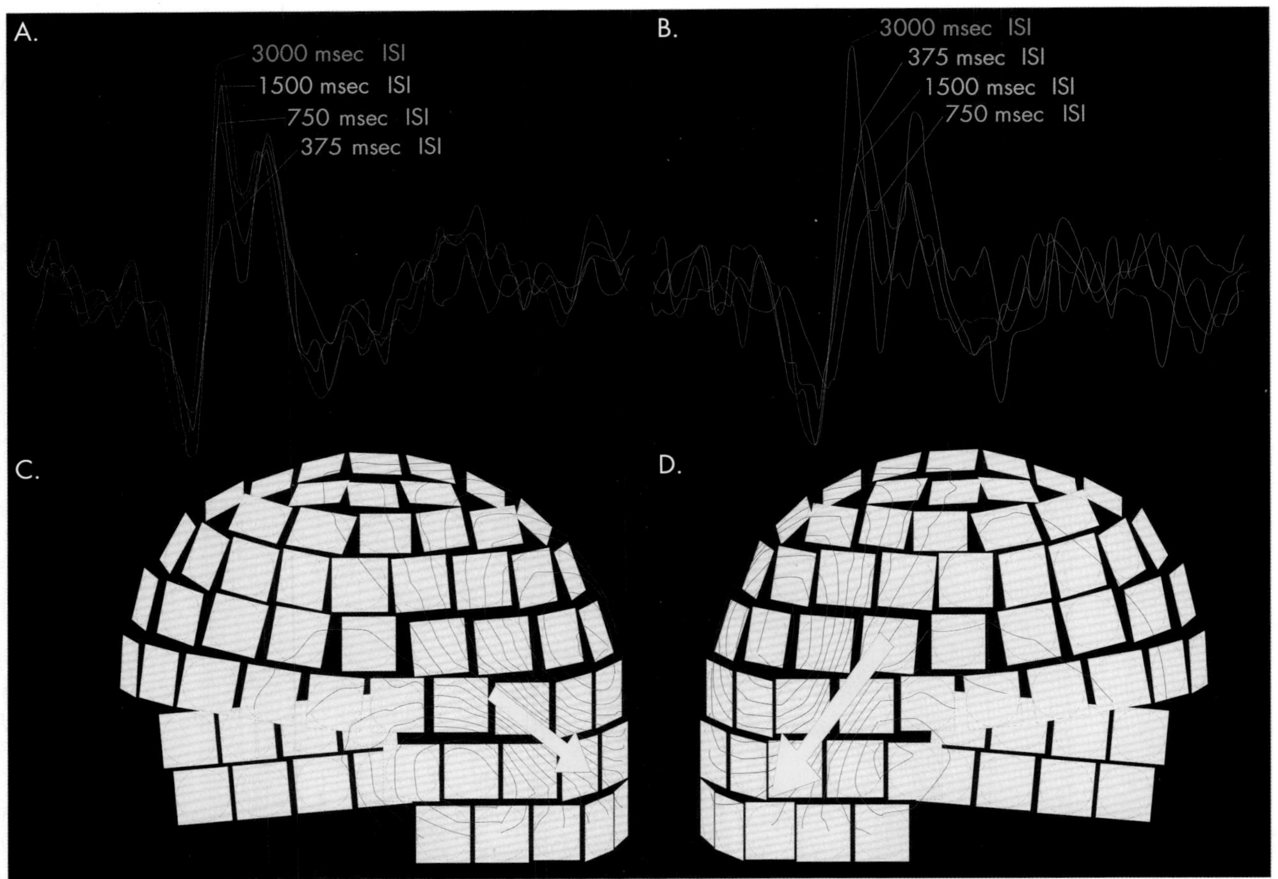

FIGURE 6–1. Whole-head MEG data were collected from a 33-year-old male who was diagnosed at 6 years of age with autism. Childhood symptoms included acquired aphasia, self-stimulatory behavior, poor eye contact, and social withdrawal. By parental report, the subject was highly agitated by a variety of sounds during his childhood years, although his level of sound sensitivity has decreased in adulthood. MEG involves noninvasive measurement of the magnetic signal generated by the brain's neuroelectric activity. The upper set of graphs (A, B) show the tracings from single representative sensors over the right (A) and left (B) temporal lobes. These data were collected during an auditory task where tones were presented with varying interstimulus intervals (ISIs). The lower set of drawings (C, D) represent magnetic field flux lines (*dark blue* represents magnetic flux flowing into the head; *red* represents magnetic flux flowing out of the head) and the mathematically derived magnetic field generators (*yellow arrows*) that are calculated from the sensor data (representative sensors from the full array of 306 sensors are shown in *gray*). The activity localizes to auditory cortex (indicated by triangles in the magnetic resonance image at opening to this chapter). Note that over the right hemisphere (A) there is the normal progressive decrease in the response at 100 ms as a function of decreasing ISI. In contrast, over the left hemisphere (B), the response at 100 ms in the shortest ISI condition (375 ms; *light blue*) is actually larger than that seen for longer ISI conditions (750 and 1,500 ms; *medium* and *dark blue*). There is also evidence of abnormal waveform morphology over the left hemisphere, especially for the 750-ms ISI condition. This demonstrates that patients with autism may have altered patterns in the decay of auditory memory traces and dysfunction of auditory sensory gating mechanisms.

Autistic disorder or infantile autism is a pervasive developmental disorder that occurs in 1–2 children per 1,000 live births, more commonly in males than females (2–4:1).[1–3] Its reported incidence has increased dramatically with the recent recognition of higher functioning individuals. Autism was first described by Kanner in 1943.[4] Since that time, it has been a disorder of extensive scientific interest and controversy.[5]

Current diagnostic standards require symptom presentation before 3 years of age. These children (and adults) display problems in three major areas: 1) social interaction, 2) communication, and 3) range of interests and activities.[2,3,5] Impairments in social interaction may include lack of person-to-person bonding (expressed as a lack of attachment to the primary caregiver or failure to develop appropriate peer relationships), and inability to interact socially and to share with others. Impairments in communication may include delay in, lack of, or loss of development of receptive or expressive language; difficulty with initiating and sustaining conversation; stereotyped or repetitive use of language; and lack of spontaneous make-believe play. Restrictions in the range of interests and activities may include preoccupation with repetitive or stereotyped patterns of interest (often with abnormally intense focus), inflexible adherence to exact schedules or routines, and stereotyped or repetitive movements (head banging, rocking, hand or finger flapping, or twisting). Executive dysfunction, decreased central coherence (the ability to integrate information into a whole versus individual pieces), and abnormal sensory sensitivity are also commonly seen.[6–8]

Prognosis in autism is generally poor. Longitudinal studies indicate that 90% of individuals with autism have clinical deficits that persist throughout adulthood.[9] Approximately 60%–70% of autistic individuals have an IQ below 70, and symptom severity is inversely related to IQ.[1,5,9] In one longitudinal study, 27% of autistic adults were employed, primarily in sheltered workshops or menial jobs. Almost all required assisted living, either with family members (47%) or in residential placements (53%).[9,10]

Whereas autism was once considered to be the result of poor parenting, it is now generally accepted that it is a biologically based neurodevelopmental disorder. Several lines of evidence suggest serotonergic abnormalities in autism. Autism is likely to have a polygenetic component, although concordance rates in twin studies indicate that other factors must also be important. A difficult challenge in both genetic and neurobiological research in autism is the possibility that there are many different core etiologies, each ultimately generating a similar cognitive and behavioral profile through a common final pathway. For example, there are several very different disease conditions (e.g., fragile X syndrome, congenital rubella, herpes simplex encephalitis, tuberous sclerosis, and fetal exposure to toxins) that are often associated with autism.[5,11]

Recent reviews of imaging studies in autism indicate that no focal brain injury has yet been consistently demonstrated, although a number of potentially important differences have been reported.[3,12] In brief, autopsy studies have found cerebellar pathology, including a decreased number of Purkinje and granular cells in posterior–inferior cerebellar cortex. Limbic structures were also abnormal, including increased neuronal density with small cell bodies and stunted dendrites. Some magnetic resonance imaging (MRI) studies have reported significantly smaller lobules VI and VII of the cerebellar vermis in autism, but this finding has not been replicated consistently. Generalized increases in brain volume have been reported from studies of head circumference and MRI-based measurements, but not from an autopsy study that measured brain weight.[3,12,13]

More promising are the results from various methods of functional brain imaging, which may provide insight into abnormalities in processing and functional organization. These include initial reports of globally elevated glucose utilization as well as focal metabolic or blood flow abnormalities in the anterior cingulate gyrus, temporal and parietal lobes, basal ganglia, thalamus, and cerebellum. There are also indications of atypical language dominance and decreased hemispheric functional specialization.[3,12,14,15]

Neuronal functioning can be recorded more directly by electroencephalography (EEG) and magnetoencephalography (MEG). Abnormalities in the spontaneous EEG are common in autism, and several studies have demonstrated that epilepsy develops in 20%–30% of autistic individuals.[10,16] A general limitation of EEG studies is a difficulty in relating EEG abnormalities to specific brain regions. This is because electrical conductivity barriers between the brain, cerebrospinal fluid, skull, and scalp distort the neuroelectric pattern recorded at the scalp. MEG uses superconducting sensors to noninvasively measure the neuromagnetic fields generated by the brain's electrical activity. It offers an attractive alternative to EEG because the above-described conductivity barriers cause only minimal neuromagnetic distortions. Thus, relatively simple mathematical models can be used to infer the spatiotemporal pattern of brain activities that generated specific neuromagnetic signals of interest, allowing good localization of the active brain regions.[17] In autism, MEG has recently shown a high incidence of sleep epileptiform activity in perisylvian brain regions, even in patients who have never experienced a clinical seizure.[10,16] MEG is also used to measure changes in brain activity in response to functional activation. In the case presented here, an auditory task was used to demonstrate abnormal auditory information processing (Figure 6–1).

As is the case with other neurodevelopmental disorders, there is no cure for autism. However, there have been recent advances and recommendations for the reduction of specifically targeted symptoms through behavioral and pharmacological strategies. The most successful advances have been achieved with behavior modification programs that incorporate therapist-trainers and parents in home-based programs such as TEACCH (Treatment and Education of Autistic and Related Communication-Handicapped Children) and educational day centers focused on activities of daily living, social skills, and communication (both auditory and visual).[18] Pharmacological interventions have also proved useful for reducing specific symptoms. Neuroleptics and mood stabilizers may decrease aggression and hyperactivity. Selective serotonin reuptake inhibitors such as fluoxetine and paroxetine have been reported to lessen ritualistic obsessive activities.[19,20] Use of other agents, such as vitamin B_6, immunoglobulin injections, clomipramine, naltrexone, and clonidine, has been more controversial, with some inconsistencies in the reproducibility of effects.[5,21,22] Medications such as sodium valproate can help to reduce autistic features, consistent with EEG and MEG observations of increased incidence of epileptiform activity in autism.[23] Through definition of specific cortical processing abnormalities in autism, functional brain imaging strategies may soon lead to the development of new therapeutic approaches to the pervasive developmental disorders.

References

1. Honda H, Shimizu Y, Misumi K, et al: Cumulative incidence and prevalence of childhood autism in children in Japan. Br J Psychiatry 1996; 169:228–235
2. Rapin I: Autism. N Engl J Med 1997; 337:97–104
3. Rapin I, Katzman R: Neurobiology of autism. Ann Neurol 1998; 43:7–14
4. Kanner L: Autistic disturbances of affective contact. Nervous Child 1943; 2:217–250
5. Rutter M: The Emanuel Miller Memorial Lecture 1998. Autism: two-way interplay between research and clinical work. J Child Psychol Psychiatry 1999; 40:169–188
6. Bailey A, Phillip W, Rutter M: Autism: towards an integration of clinical, genetic, neuropsychological, and neurobiological perspectives. J Child Psychol Psychiatry 1996; 37:89–126
7. Pring L, Hermelin B, Heavey L: Savants, segments, art and autism. J Child Psychol Psychiatry 1995; 36:1065–1076
8. Frith U, Happe F: Language and communication in autistic disorders. Philos Trans R Soc Lond B Biol Sci 1994; 346:97–104
9. Ballaban-Gil K, Rapin I, Tuchman R, et al: Longitudinal examination of the behavioral, language, and social changes in a population of adolescents and young adults with autistic disorder. Pediatr Neurol 1996; 15:217–223
10. Nordin V, Gillberg C: The long-term course of autistic disorders: update on follow-up studies. Acta Psychiatr Scand 1998; 97:99–108
11. DeLong GR: Autism: new data suggest a new hypothesis. Neurology 1999; 52:911–916
12. Deb S, Thompson B: Neuroimaging in autism. Br J Psychiatry 1998; 173:299–302
13. Courchesne E, Muller RA, Saitoh O: Brain weight in autism: normal in the majority of cases, megalencephalic in rare cases. Neurology 1999; 52:1057–1059
14. Ryu YH, Lee JD, Yoon PH, et al: Perfusion impairments in infantile autism on technetium-99m ethyl cysteinate dimer brain single-photon emission tomography: comparison with findings on magnetic resonance imaging. Eur J Nucl Med 1999; 26:253–259
15. Muller RA, Behen ME, Rothermel RD, et al: Brain mapping of language and auditory perception in high-functioning autistic adults: a PET study. J Autism Dev Disord 1999; 29:19–31
16. Lewine JD, Andrews R, Chez M, et al: Magnetoencephalographic patterns of epileptiform activity in children with regressive autism spectrum disorders. Pediatrics 1999; 104:405–418
17. Lewine JD, Orrison WW: Clinical electroencephalography and event-related potentials, in Functional Brain Imaging. Edited by Orrison WW, Lewine JD, Sanders JA, et al. St. Louis, MO, Mosby–Year Book, 1995, pp 327–368
18. Campbell M, Schopler E, Cueva JE, et al: Treatment of autistic disorder. J Am Acad Child Adolesc Psychiatry 1996; 35:134–143
19. Posey DI, Litwiller M, Koburn A, et al: Paroxetine in autism (letter). J Am Acad Child Adolesc Psychiatry 1999; 38:111–112
20. DeLong GR, Teague LA, McSwain KM: Effects of fluoxetine treatment in young children with idiopathic autism. Dev Med Child Neurol 1998; 40:551–562
21. Gupta S: Treatment of children with autism with intravenous immunoglobulin (letter). J Child Neurol 1999; 14:203–205
22. Sanchez LE, Campbell M, Small AM, et al: A pilot study of clomipramine in young autistic children. J Am Acad Child Adolesc Psychiatry 1996; 35:537–544
23. Childs JA, Blair JL: Valproic acid treatment of epilepsy in autistic twins. J Neurosci Nurs 1997; 29:244–248

Recent Publications of Interest

Kahkonen S: Magnetoencephalography (MEG): a noninvasive tool for studying cortical effects in psychopharmacology. Int J Neuropsychopharmacol 2006; 9:367–372
Reviews the basics of magnetoencephalography and its application to the study of pharmacological agents.

Lainhart JE: Advances in autism neuroimaging research for the clinician and geneticist. Am J Med Genet C Semin Med Genet 2006; 142:33–39
Provides an excellent synthesis of recent structural and functional imaging studies in autism.

Penn HE: Neurobiological correlates of autism: a review of recent research. Child Neuropsychol 2006; 12:57–79
Focuses on integrating research findings from histopathological, imaging, neurochemical, and animal lesion research with proposed neuropsychological frameworks for understanding autism.

Matson JL, Nebel-Schwalm M: Assessing challenging behaviors in children with autism spectrum disorders: a review. Res Dev Disabil 2006; epub ahead of print
Provides a useful synopsis of the available screening instruments for the autistic spectrum disorders, with an emphasis on early diagnosis. The origin, validation studies, and targeted age range for each are discussed.

Filipek PA, Steinberg-Epstein R, Book TM: Intervention for autistic spectrum disorders. NeuroRx 2006; 3:207–216
Reviews the epidemiology and diagnosis of autistic spectrum disorders and provides a quick guide to present laws related to education as a prelude to presentation of a psychopharmacologic treatment algorithm. Several case examples are included to illustrate the importance of careful identification and targeting of symptoms for medication.

Kagan-Kushnir T, Roberts SW, Snead OC III: Screening electroencephalograms in autism spectrum disorders: evidence-based guideline. J Child Neurol 2005; 20:197–206

Reviewed the literature from 1966–2003, and concluded that there is good evidence that seizure disorders are common in patients with autistic spectrum disorder, fair evidence that subclinical epileptiform activity is present in many patients without a history of seizures, and very little solid information on the clinical implications.

Chez MG, Chang M, Krasne V, et al: Frequency of epileptiform EEG abnormalities in a sequential screening of autistic patients with no known clinical epilepsy from 1996 to 2005. Epilepsy Behav 2006; 8:267–271

Performed a retrospective chart review on 889 patients with autism and no history of seizures or anticonvulsant medications. They found EEG abnormalities during sleep (but not waking) in 61% with no difference in frequency between those who had and had not regressed between 12 and 18 months of age. Valproic acid improved or normalized the EEG in 64% of treated patients.

Reprinted from Hurley RA, Lewine JD, Jones GM, et al: "Application of Magnetoencephalography to the Study of Autism." *Journal of Neuropsychiatry and Clinical Neurosciences* 12:1–3, 2000. Used with permission.

This work was supported by grants from the Cure Autism Now Foundation (G.M.J.), the March of Dimes Birth Defects Foundation (J.D.L.), the National Alliance for Research in Schizophrenia and Depression (J.D.L.), and Picker International (J.D.L. and W.W.O.).

Chapter 7

APPLICATIONS OF XENON COMPUTED TOMOGRAPHY IN CLINICAL PRACTICE

Detection of Hidden Lesions

KATHERINE H. TABER, PH.D.
JANA G. ZIMMERMAN, PH.D.
HOWARD YONAS, M.D.
WILLIAM HART, B.S.R.S., R.T.
ROBIN A. HURLEY, M.D.

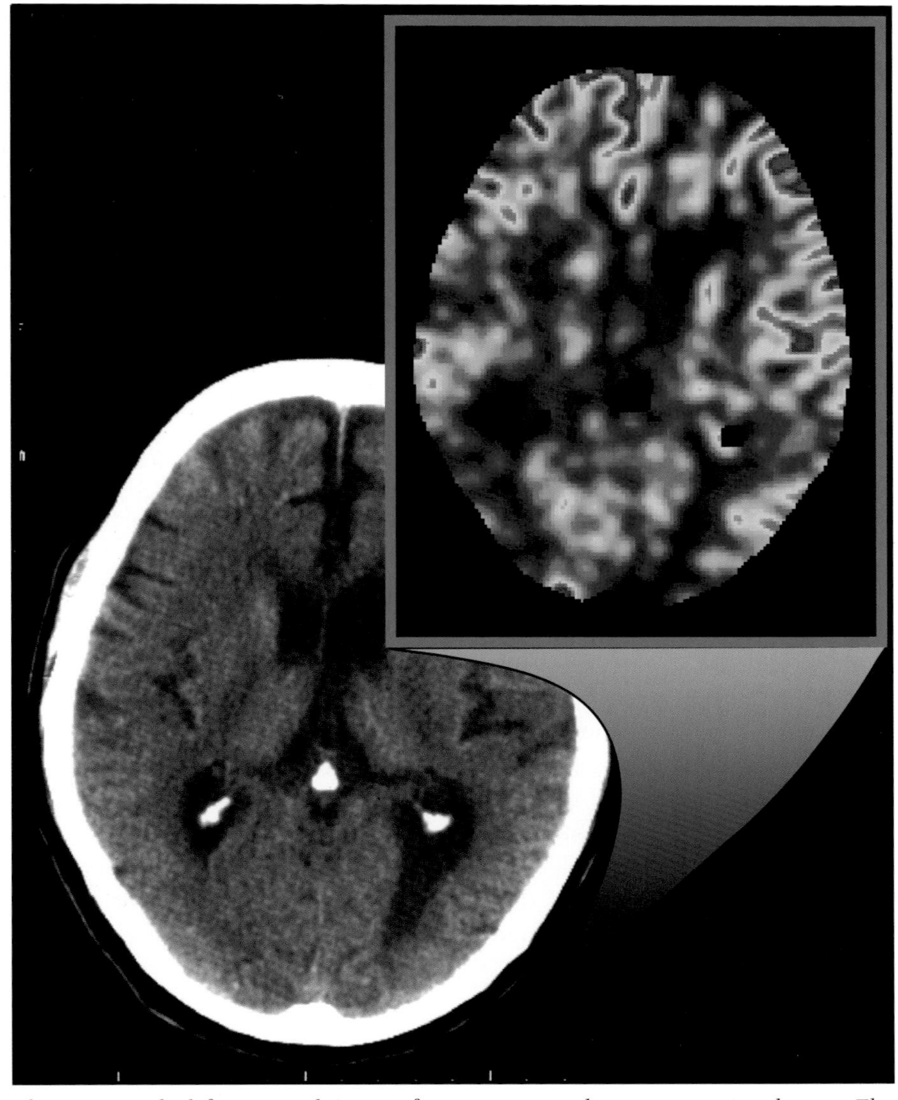

The image on the left is an axial CT scan from a patient with severe cognitive changes. The image on the right is a xenon-enhanced CT scan, showing reduced cerebral blood flow in the posterior temporal lobe.

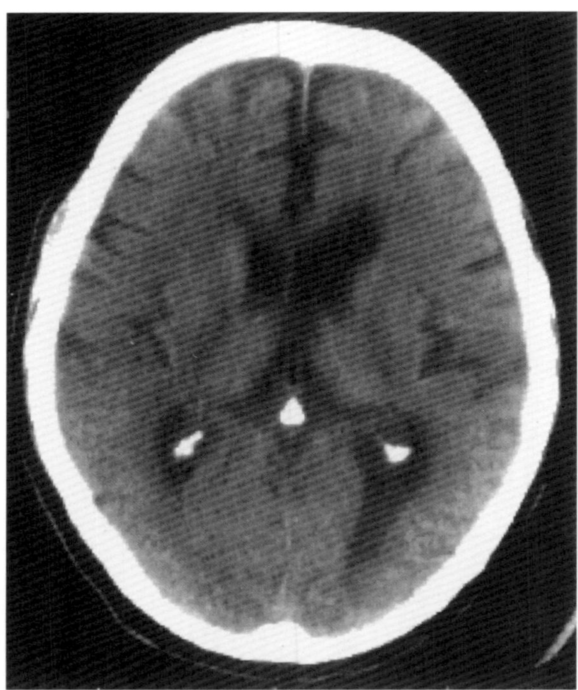

FIGURE 7–1. Axial CT image from a 78-year-old male who presented with a 2-year history of alterations in cognition and behavior, including difficulty with short-term memory, oral comprehension, oral expression, and concentration, in addition to apathy, social withdrawal, decreased initiative, and episodic confusion. His medical history included persistent headaches following a motor vehicle accident 10 years earlier, worsening 2 years ago. Neurological evaluation that included EEG, CT, and MR imaging was negative (except for mild enlargement of the left lateral ventricle compared with the right). Neuropsychological testing found a severe constructional dyspraxia, particularly significant in that premorbidly the patient was noted for his ability to work from blueprints and build anything from measurements.

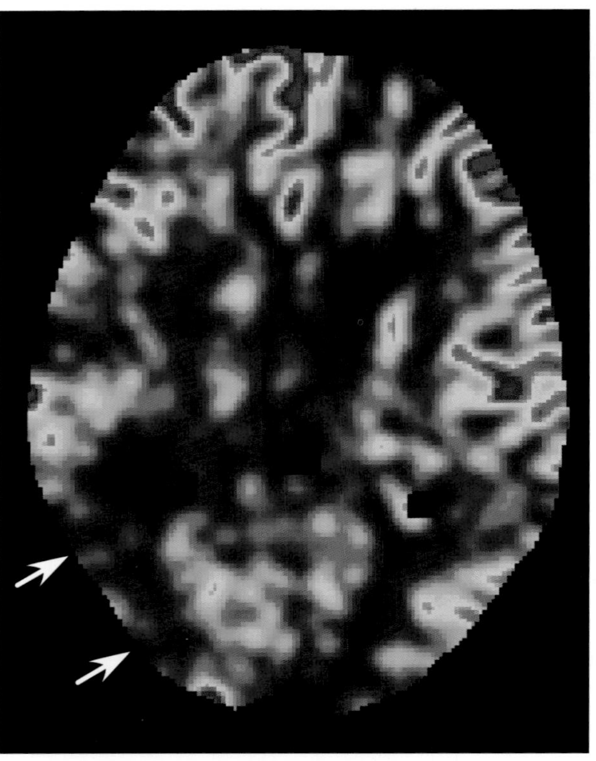

FIGURE 7–2. Companion axial xenon-enhanced CT image showing reduced cerebral blood flow in the right posterior temporal lobe (arrows, inferior parietal lobule) consistent with the patient's severe constructional dyspraxia. The color scale directly represents cerebral blood flow (mL/100 g brain/min). Normal cortical gray matter has a mean flow of about 80 mL/100 g/min (high flow rates displayed as *light yellow* and *orange*), and white matter has a mean flow of about 20 mL/100 g/min (low flow rates displayed as *dark blue* and *purple*). Areas containing both gray and white matter have a mean flow of 40–60 mL/100 g/min (moderate flow rates displayed as *green* and *blue*).[1]

Structural neuroimaging is becoming increasingly important for neuropsychiatry.[2,3] However, it is not uncommon for patients to present with neuropsychiatric symptoms consistent with brain pathology yet without clearly identifiable lesions on either computed tomographic (CT) or magnetic resonance (MR) structural images. There are no reliable estimates of how frequently this apparent absence of lesions in the presence of symptoms is likely to occur. Stroke may be missed (false negative) in 5%–30% of cases.[4–6] A study of primary progressive aphasia found CT imaging was normal in 50% and MR imaging in 17% of the cases.[7] Similarly, systemic lupus erythematosus may present with extensive neuropsychiatric symptoms but without MR-visible abnormalities.[8] It has been suggested that many types of pathology may be difficult to visualize because they are small or diffuse in nature.[9]

Adding a method of functional neuroimaging to the clinical examination may provide a way to identify such abnormalities (Figure 7–1). A recent study at a neuropsychiatric tertiary referral center found that 40% of the study population had normal MR or CT studies. Most of these (77% of patients with normal structural neuroimaging) had abnormal cerebral blood flow (CBF) images.[10] Even when structural brain imaging shows lesions are present, functional neuroimaging may provide a better assessment of brain dysfunction. Changes in cognitive symptoms closely correlated with changes on functional neuroimaging (CBF and cerebral glucose uptake), but not necessarily with changes on structural neuroimaging, in recent studies of vascular dementia.[11,12] Thus, functional neuroimaging may provide useful information for clinical management.

Until recently, functional neuroimaging techniques were available only in a research-oriented environment and were quite expensive to perform. Now, with the maturation of xenon-enhanced computed tomography (XeCT), the imaging of CBF has the potential to become widely available and may become a valuable diagnostic tool (Figure 7–2). XeCT is based on the use of stable xenon gas as an inhaled contrast agent for CT imaging, possible because it is radiodense and lipid-soluble. When inhaled, it dissolves into the blood and passes into the brain parenchyma. The patient inhales a mixture of xenon (usually 26%–33%) and oxygen for several minutes via a face mask. CT scans are acquired prior to inhalation (providing a baseline) and during this inhalation time (a "wash-in" study). More scans may be acquired following inhalation, as well (a "wash-in/washout" study). Standard CT scanners can acquire 3–4 brain slices per XeCT study. The new spiral CT systems, which are rapidly replacing the standard scanners, can acquire 8–10 slices. This is sufficient for reasonable coverage of the brain. Several sets of scans are acquired at each brain level, allowing calculation of a xenon arrival curve for each pixel of each slice. This information, along with the concentration of xenon in the expired air (an indirect measure of arterial concentration), is required to calculate CBF for each pixel.[13–15]

Initial XeCT studies were limited by the side effects of xenon gas and the time required to acquire and compute the CBF images. Advances in technology have brought the time to compute the images down from hours to seconds. Xenon is a narcotic gas, more potent than nitrous oxide. Inhalation of 71% xenon is sufficient for anesthetic effect in 50% of patients. Present studies use much lower doses than this, as noted above, but some euphoric or dysphoric side effects are seen (which may cause a temporary exacerbation of neuropsychiatric symptoms), as is somnolence. Mild nausea can also occur; thus the patient must take nothing by mouth for 4 hours prior to scanning to reduce the risks of emesis and aspiration. Very rarely, patients experience apnea, reversible by an instruction to breathe. Like other narcotic gases, xenon also causes mild cerebral vasodilation. Overall, approximately 10% of patients experience unpleasant side effects, all of them transient.[15–17]

As with any imaging examination, the patient must remain still. In some cases sedation will be required to achieve this. Bone artifacts, which impair CT imaging of areas very near bone, can be reduced by correct angulation of the patient's head.

There are several advantages of this technique over other methods of imaging CBF. Stable xenon gas is not radioactive, so the only radiation exposure is that required for the CT scan itself. This means radiation exposure is limited to the most radiation-resistant areas of the body. With other methods, a radioactive tracer is injected, so the entire body is exposed. The image resolution is good, and there is direct anatomic correlation with the baseline CT scan. The study can be repeated in 15 minutes, after xenon gas is eliminated from the body by breathing room air. Thus, it is possible to perform sequential studies with the patient in different states (i.e., after administration of a drug challenge). It is important also to note that the technique is inexpensive (the additional cost per study is less than $100), fast (it adds only 10–15 minutes to a routine CT exam), and a billable procedure when considered medically necessary.[15,18]

In the case presented here, the patient failed to respond to therapy based on working diagnoses of Alzheimer's disease and major depression. Neuropsychological testing was done, leading to the suspicion of cerebrovascular disease or stroke with bilateral hemispheric involvement. Neither CT nor MR imaging of the brain could explain the clinical deficits. The finding of decreased CBF on the XeCT examination was consistent with a cerebrovascular accident (CVA). As a result of this finding, the diagnoses changed from probable Alzheimer's disease and major depression to dementia secondary to CVA. The psychiatric day treatment program and donepezil administration were discontinued. Patient and family education focusing on poststroke management was initiated. In a study by Velakoulis and Lloyd,[10] the functional imaging finding of altered CBF changed the clinical management in almost 10% of the patients. Thus, availability of CBF imaging can have an impact on clinical management in a significant number of patients presenting with neuropsychiatric symptoms.

References

1. Yonas H, Darby JM, Marks EC, et al: CBF measured by Xe-CT: approach to analysis and normal values. J Cereb Blood Flow Metab 1991; 11:716–725
2. Weight DG, Bigler ED: Neuroimaging in psychiatry. Psychiatr Clin North Am 1998; 21:725–759
3. Wahlund LO, Agartz I, Saaf J, et al: MRI in psychiatry: 731 cases. Psychiatry Res 1992; 45:139–140
4. Bryan RN, Levy LM, Whitlow WD, et al: Diagnosis of acute cerebral infarction: comparison of CT and MR imaging. Am J Neuroradiol 1991; 12:611–620
5. Lindgren A, Norrving B, Rudling O, et al: Comparison of clinical and neuroradiological findings in first-ever stroke: a population-based study. Stroke 1994; 25:1371–1377
6. Mohr JP, Biller J, Hilal SK, et al: Magnetic resonance versus computed tomographic imaging in acute stroke. Stroke 1995; 26:807–812
7. Sinnatamby R, Antoun NA, Freer CE, et al: Neuroradiological findings in primary progressive aphasia: CT, MRI and cerebral perfusion SPECT. Neuroradiology 1996; 38:232–238
8. Kao CH, Ho YJ, Lan JL, et al: Discrepancy between regional cerebral blood flow and glucose metabolism of the brain in systemic lupus erythematosus patients with normal brain magnetic resonance imaging findings. Arthritis Rheum 1999; 42:61–68
9. Alberts MJ, Faulstich ME, Gray L: Stroke with negative brain magnetic resonance imaging. Stroke 1992; 23:663–667
10. Velakoulis D, Lloyd JH: The role of SPECT scanning in a neuropsychiatry unit. Aust N Z J Psychiatry 1998; 32:511–522

11. Meyer JS, Muramatsu K, Mortel KF, et al: Prospective CT confirms differences between vascular and Alzheimer's dementia. Stroke 1995; 26:735–742
12. Sabri O, Ringelstein EB, Hellwig D, et al: Neuropsychological impairment correlates with hypoperfusion and hypometabolism but not with severity of white matter lesions on MRI in patients with cerebral microangiopathy. Stroke 1999; 30:556–566
13. Kashiwagi S, Nagamitsu T, Yamashita T: Current status and controversies in the inhalation protocols for the xenon CT CBF method. Acta Neurol Scand Suppl 1996; 166:51–53
14. Yonas H, Johnson DW, Pindzola R: Xenon-enhanced CT of cerebral blood flow. Sci Am 1995; 2:58–67
15. Yonas H, Pindzola RP, Johnson DW: Xenon/computed tomography cerebral blood flow and its use in clinical management. Neurosurg Clin N Am 1996; 7:605–616
16. Fang H, Xu J-X, Zhang Z-M: Adverse reaction to xenon-enhanced CT cerebral blood flow measurement (abstract). Acta Neurol Scand Suppl 1996; 166:50
17. Holl K, Becker H, Haubitz B: Effect of xenon. Acta Neurol Scand Suppl 1996; 166:38–41
18. Pindzola RR, Yonas H: The xenon-enhanced computed tomography cerebral blood flow method. Neurosurgery 1998; 43:1488–1492

Recent Publications of Interest

Mullins ME: Stroke imaging with xenon-CT. Semin Ultrasound CT MR 2006; 27:219–220
Provides a brief overview of this technique.

Sase S, Honda M, Machida K, et al: Comparison of cerebral blood flow between perfusion computed tomography and xenon-enhanced computed tomography for normal subjects: territorial analysis. J Comput Assist Tomogr 2005; 29:270–277
Compares regional cerebral blood flow measurements made by perfusion CT and xenon CT in normal individuals. The authors conclude that the observed differences between the two techniques for the major cerebral artery territories result from factors that are intrinsic to the perfusion CT method.

Latchaw RE: Cerebral perfusion imaging in acute stroke. J Vasc Interv Radiol 2004; 15:S29-S46
Reviews the physiological changes that occur when cerebral perfusion is impaired and the methods available for perfusion imaging, including strengths and weaknesses of each technique.

Casey SO, McKinney A, Teksam M, et al: CT perfusion imaging in the management of posterior reversible encephalopathy. Neuroradiology 2004; 46:272–276
Is an interesting case report illustrating the value of xenon CT for monitoring cerebral blood flow changes in response to antihypertensive therapy.

Reprinted from Taber KH, Zimmerman JG, Yonas H, et al: "Applications of Xenon CT in Clinical Practice: Detection of Hidden Lesions." *Journal of Neuropsychiatry and Clinical Neurosciences* 11:423–425, 1999. Used with permission.

Chapter 8

New Techniques for Understanding Huntington's Disease

Robin A. Hurley, M.D.
Edward F. Jackson, Ph.D.
Ronald E. Fisher, M.D., Ph.D.
Katherine H. Taber, Ph.D.

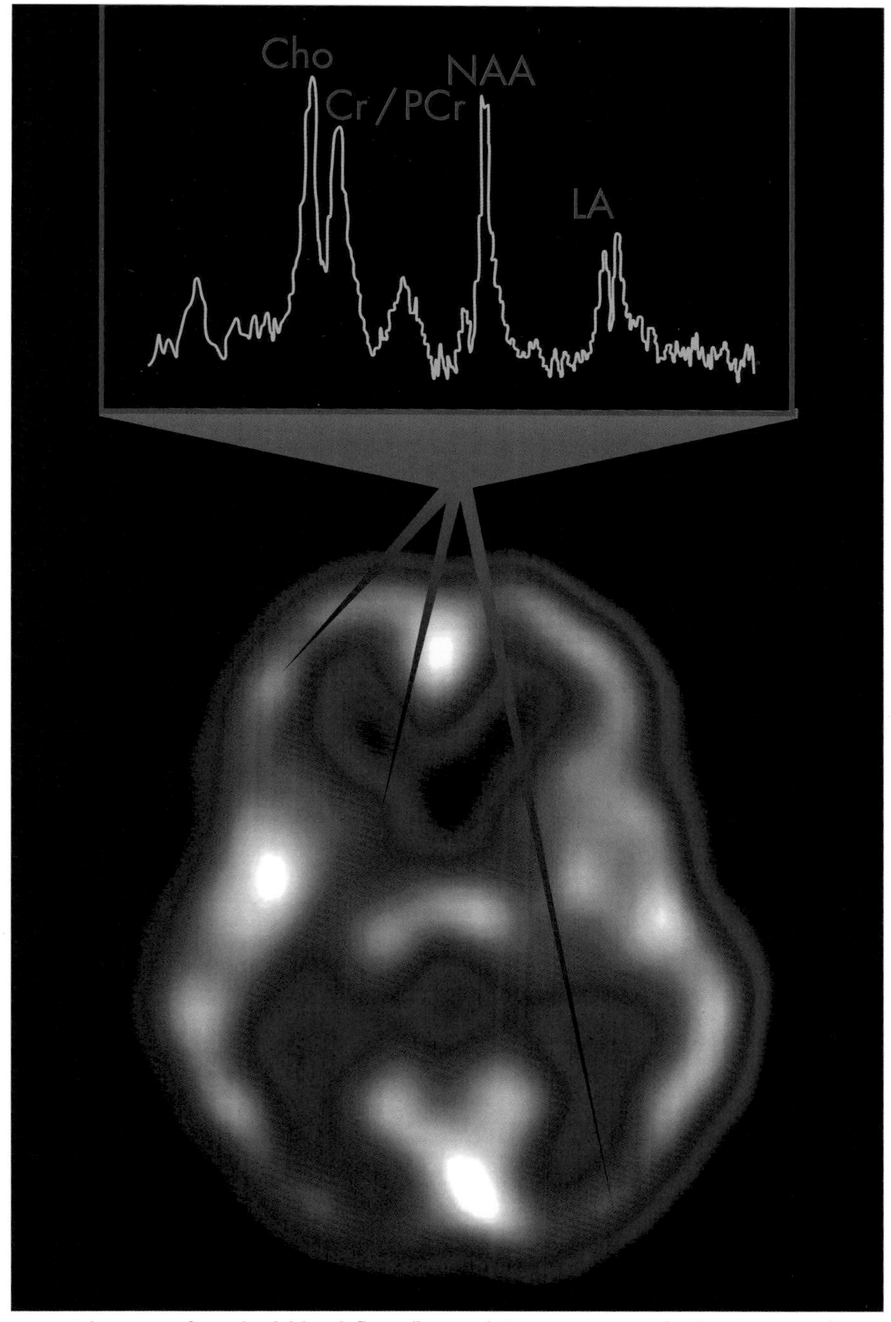

An axial image of cerebral blood flow (bottom) in a patient with Huntington's disease shows reduced flow in the caudate nuclei. A representation of a proton magnetic resonance spectrum (top) from similar patients shows alterations indicating tissue abnormalities.

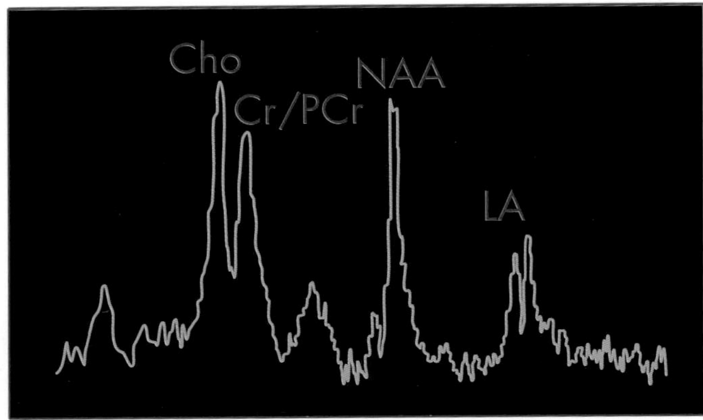

FIGURE 8–1. Schematic drawing of a short-echo-time proton magnetic resonance spectrum illustrating the most common findings in symptomatic gene-positive Huntington's disease patients, particularly from regions in the left striatum and occipital cortex. The lactic acid (LA) peak, which is not detectable in normal subjects, is typically elevated, and the *N*-acetylaspartate (NAA) peak is typically substantially decreased. (At this echo time, the NAA peak should be approximately a factor of 1.6 times that shown.) Normal peaks labeled for orientation in the spectrum include the mixed creatine/phosphocreatine peak (Cr/PCr) and choline (Cho).

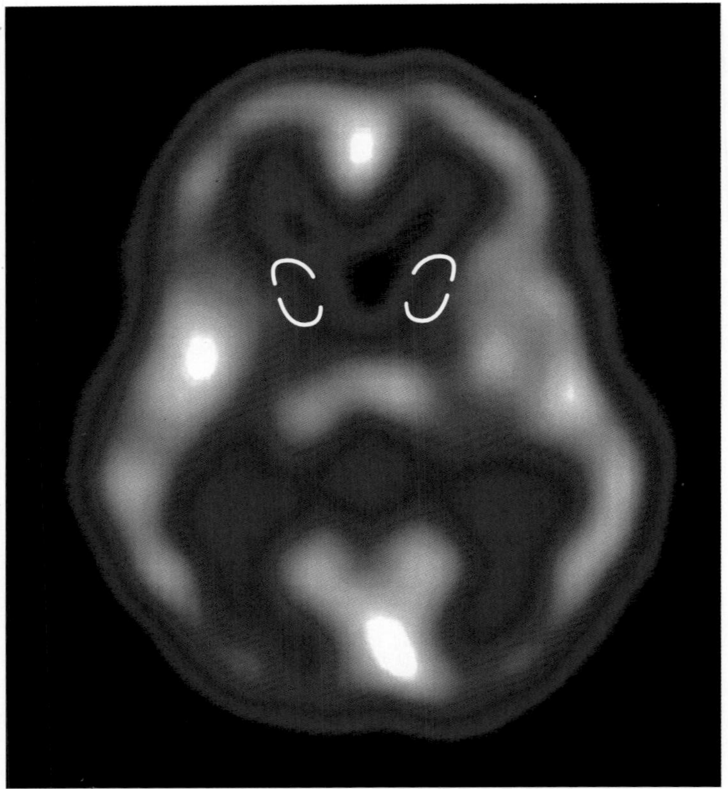

FIGURE 8–2. Transaxial slice of a SPECT brain perfusion scan from a 23-year-old male with juvenile-onset, genetically proven Huntington's disease. The patient was placed in a darkened, quiet room, where he received 25 mCi of technetium-99m hexamethylpropylenamine oxime intravenously prior to SPECT imaging of the brain. Areas of highest tracer uptake appear *white/orange* (high blood flow); lowest uptake is *blue/black* (low blood flow). Note the markedly reduced uptake in the caudate nuclei bilaterally (outlined by *white dashed lines*). The adjacent thalami are normal. Activity in the cortex is essentially normal in this patient, but it typically becomes abnormal (reduced perfusion) as the disease progresses. High activity in the visual cortex is secondary to visual stimulation the patient received in the partially darkened room. This patient presented with a history of progressive dyskinetic and choreiform movements, hyperkinesia, dysarthria, anger dyscontrol, very inappropriate speech, depressed mood, and episodic crying. The dyskinesias first appeared at age 16.

Huntington's disease (HD) is a progressive neurodegenerative disorder that is inherited in an autosomal dominant fashion. It occurs in approximately 3–8 per 100,000 population in the United States. HD has been reported in all races and cultures, but it occurs less in individuals of African or Japanese descent. HD was first formally described by George Huntington in 1872 and has been studied as a classic neurodegenerative disorder since that time. An excellent recent review summarizes historical, diagnostic, and clinical aspects of the disease.[1] Folstein's text provides a more comprehensive treatment of this subject.[2] In brief, HD presents with either an adult or a juvenile onset. The adult form is more common, with onset between 35 and 45 years of age and progression to death within 15–20 years. The juvenile form (usually paternally transmitted) presents before age 20 and has a more rapid progression. Although most clinicians are aware of the classic motor findings in HD (involuntary choreiform movements, dysarthrias, dystonias, and rigidity), the psychiatric and cognitive findings, almost always present, are often overlooked.

All patients with HD develop a progressive subcortical dementia that is characterized by frontal lobe executive dysfunction and memory deficits. Neuropsychological testing reveals deficits in recent and remote memory; impaired visuospatial function; difficulty with shifting sets, planning, and organization; and overall decreasing IQ. Psychiatric syndromes (present in up to 79% of patients) most commonly include impulse control disorders, depression, personality changes, and, more rarely, psychosis or mania. Symptoms include disinhibition, irritability, aggression, apathy, and neurovegetative markers of depression. The suicide rate has been reported to be up to 20 times that of the general population over age 50.[1] Increased criminal behavior and hypersexuality have often been reported in HD patients. A recent Danish study found that there is a statistically significant increase in nonviolent crime in male HD patients compared with their nonaffected relatives and control subjects.[3] These criminal behaviors, as well as the psychiatric syndromes, are felt to be related to the destruction of the medial caudate, which disrupts the memory and emotion tracts descending from the frontal lobes.[1,4]

In 1993, the Huntington's Disease Collaborative Research Group discovered the genetic defect responsible for HD. It is a long repetition of the trinucleotide CAG (cytosine-adenosine-guanosine) sequence in the first exon of a gene on chromosome 4. This repeating sequence leads to the production of a protein called *huntingtin*. Accumulation of this protein is theorized to lead to nuclear inclusions and cell death in medium spiny GABAergic neurons of the caudate.[5] Currently, probability studies are under way to coordinate the number of CAG repeats with expected age at onset, symptoms, and length of survival.[6]

Several methods of studying brain functioning, including magnetic resonance spectroscopy (MRS), single-photon emission computed tomography (SPECT), and positron emission tomography (PET), have been applied to HD. MRS provides a relative measure of certain brain metabolites, most commonly presented as the spectrum of the amount of signal produced by the metabolites being measured rather than as an image. MRS uses the same scanners and magnets as traditional magnetic resonance imaging (MRI), but with special hardware and software that allow substances other than water to be studied. Using ^{1}H (proton) MRS, several groups have found decreased levels of *N*-acetylaspartate (NAA, a neuronal marker) in the cerebrum of symptomatic gene-positive patients.[7–12] This change was particularly common in the occipital cortex and striatum (Figure 8–1).[7,9,11,12] Some have also reported increased levels of lactate (LA; an indication of metabolic distress), although this is still controversial.[13] Increased LA was asymmetric in the striatum, with levels in the left hemisphere exceeding levels in the right.[7] The degree of decrease in NAA and increase in LA in the striatum has been shown to correlate with the duration of symptoms.[7] Experimental treatment with coenzyme Q10 resulted in significant decreases in cortical LA in symptomatic patients,[11] indicating a possible defect in energy metabolism. Asymptomatic carriers typically are characterized by normal ^{1}H MRS spectra, although elevated LA has been reported in some.[7,8] A study using ^{31}P (phosphorus) MRS found a decrease in the phosphocreatine (PCr) to inorganic phosphate (P_i) ratio in the resting calf muscle of symptomatic patients, another indication of a defect in energy metabolism.

In both SPECT and PET, radioactive tracers are used to measure quantities such as cerebral blood flow, glucose metabolism, and receptor density. It has been known since the 1980s that these methods can demonstrate reductions in caudate glucose metabolism (by PET scanning) and caudate blood flow (by PET and SPECT scanning) in patients with HD prior to clear evidence of structural changes on MRI or computed tomography (CT). More recent studies have suggested that reduced putamen volume can also be seen quite early in the disease by using MRI.[14] Cortical damage can also be demonstrated earlier in the course of the disease on SPECT or PET than on MRI, as is the case with other dementias, such as Alzheimer's disease.[15] There is a good correlation between the reductions in striatal and cortical blood flow and the degree and type of neuropsychological impairment, indicating that SPECT scans may be useful in assessing the degree of neuronal damage and disease progression (Figure 8–2).[16] PET scanning with radiolabeled neuroreceptor ligands, such as the D_2 ligand carbon-11 raclopride, has revealed markedly reduced dopamine receptor density in the striatum of HD patients.[17] D_2 radioligands for SPECT imaging have shown similar results and may soon be available for routine clinical use. These results are especially interesting clinically, given that SPECT, unlike PET, is now available at nearly all medical centers.

The role that these new approaches to HD will play in clinical management is not yet clear. However, the results obtained thus far with functional brain imaging demonstrate the potential usefulness of these modalities for evaluating both asymptomatic and symptomatic HD patients, particularly in monitoring both disease progression and the effects of therapy.

To date, there is no treatment for Huntington's disease. Typical antipsychotics such as fluphenazine and haloperidol have been used to decrease the choreiform movements early in the course of the disease, but they produce significant side effects, including tardive dyskinesia and worsening cognition. There are limited reports of improvements with both clozapine and electroconvulsive therapy. However, the most innovative and potentially useful treatment is neuronal cell transplantation via stereotaxic injection.[18] This method is ethically controversial because embryonic donors provide the only viable source of stem cells for this therapy. Extensive research is currently under way to develop new strategies to grow early stem cells in the laboratory.

The techniques discussed here are certainly exciting and are leading to a new understanding of Huntington's disease and possible treatments. The potential now exists to apply these concepts to other neurodegenerative diseases.

References

1. Haddad MS, Cummings JL: Huntington's disease. Psychiatr Clin North Am 1997; 20:791–807
2. Folstein SE: Huntington's Disease: A Disorder of Families. Baltimore, MD, John Hopkins University Press, 1989
3. Jensen P, Fenger K, Bolwig TG, et al: Crime in Huntington's disease: a study of registered offenses among patients, relatives, and controls. J Neurol Neurosurg Psychiatry 1998; 65:467–471
4. Burruss JW, Hurley RA, Taber KH, et al: Functional neuroanatomy of the frontal lobe circuits. Radiology 2000; 214:227–230
5. Walling HW, Baldassare JJ, Westfall TC: Molecular aspects of Huntington's disease. J Neurosci Res 1998; 54:301–308
6. Brinkman RR, Mezei MM, Theilmann J, et al: The likelihood of being affected with Huntington disease by a particular age, for a specific CAG size. Am J Hum Genet 1997; 60:1202–1210
7. Jenkins BG, Rosas HD, Chen YC, et al: ^{1}H NMR spectroscopy studies of Huntington's disease: correlations with CAG repeat numbers. Neurology 1998; 50:1357–1365
8. Harms L, Meierkord H, Timm G, et al: Decreased *N*-acetylaspartate/choline ratio and increased lactate in the frontal lobe of patients with Huntington's disease: a proton magnetic resonance spectroscopy study. J Neurol Neurosurg Psychiatry 1997; 62:27–30
9. Taylor-Robinson SD, Weeks RA, Bryant DJ, et al: Proton magnetic resonance spectroscopy in Huntington's disease: evidence in favour of the glutamate excitotoxic theory. Mov Disord 1996; 11:167–173
10. Tsai G, Coyle JT: *N*-acetylaspartate in neuropsychiatric disorders. Prog Neurobiol 1995; 46:531–540
11. Koroshetz WJ, Jenkins BG, Rosen BR, et al: Energy metabolism defects in Huntington's disease and effects of coenzyme Q10. Ann Neurol 1997; 41:160–165
12. Jenkins BG, Koroshetz WJ, Beal MF, et al: Evidence for impairment of energy metabolism in vivo in Huntington's disease using localized ^{1}H NMR spectroscopy. Neurology 1993; 43:2689–2695
13. Hoang TQ, Bluml S, Dubowitz DJ, et al: Quantitative proton-decoupled ^{31}P MRS and ^{1}H MRS in the evaluation of Huntington's and Parkinson's diseases. Neurology 1998; 50:1033–1040
14. Harris GJ, Aylward EH, Peyser CE, et al: Single photon emission computed tomographic blood flow and magnetic resonance volume imaging of basal ganglia in Huntington's disease. Arch Neurol 1996; 53:316–324
15. Sax DS, Powsner R, Kim A, et al: Evidence of cortical metabolic dysfunction in early Huntington's disease by single-photon-emission computed tomography. Mov Disord 1996; 11:671–677
16. Rauch SL, Savage CR: Neuroimaging and neuropsychology of the striatum. Psychiatr Clin North Am 1997; 20:741–768
17. Andrews TC, Brooks DJ: Advances in the understanding of early Huntington's disease using the functional imaging techniques of PET and SPET. Mol Med Today 1998; 4:532–539
18. Dunnett SB, Kendall AL, Watts C, et al: Neuronal cell transplantation for Parkinson's and Huntington's diseases. Br Med Bull 1997; 53:757–776

Recent Publications of Interest

Handley OJ, Naji JJ, Dunnett SB, et al: Pharmaceutical, cellular and genetic therapies for Huntington's disease. Clin Sci (Lond) 2006; 110:73–88

Provides a comprehensive overview of present and future therapeutic interventions for HD. The available evidence from both preclinical (animal models) and clinical trials is presented.

Montoya A, Price BH, Menear M, et al: Brain imaging and cognitive dysfunctions in Huntington's disease. J Psychiatry Neurosci 2006; 31:21–29

Reviews the structural and functional brain imaging literature on adult HD. The emphasis is on the evidence linking specific cognitive deficits with particular structural and functional changes, particularly in the striatum and frontal cortex.

Bates GP: History of genetic disease: the molecular genetics of Huntington disease—a history. Nat Rev Genet 2005; 6:766–773

Gives an excellent summary of the history of HD, beginning with Huntington's widely acclaimed 1872 paper describing the disease in adults. A timeline of the major advances in HD research is provided. A very helpful glossary of terms is included for the reader unfamiliar with genetic terminology.

Smith R, Brundin P, Li JY: Synaptic dysfunction in Huntington's disease: a new perspective. Cell Mol Life Sci 2005; 62:1901–1912

Presents a brief review of what is known about the distribution and functions of the normal huntingtin protein, followed by a discussion of the cellular functions that may be affected by mutation of the protein, particularly effects on synaptic functions that may underlie early symptoms.

Reprinted from Hurley RA, Jackson EF, Fisher RE, et al: "New Techniques for Understanding Huntington's Disease." *Journal of Neuropsychiatry and Clinical Neurosciences* 11:173–175, 1999. Used with permission.

Part 2

SPECIFIC DISEASES

The disease-focused section is the largest in the book. The *Windows to the Brain* audience is largely practicing neuropsychiatrists and neuropsychologists. With each passing year, the neurobiology of brain disease advances and "organic" underpinnings become more widely accepted. Although the boundaries of purely neurologic, psychiatric, or those conditions belonging to rehabilitation medicine become increasingly blurred, the biology remains the same. Many of these brain diseases can now be imaged in either the clinical or research setting. This section covers a wide range of diseases/injuries across the adult life span where imaging techniques have contributed to current understanding. Included are genetic, degenerative, infectious, traumatic, and hypoxic conditions.

The imaging methods discussed in reference to a particular disease may not be the only available options to study or evaluate that condition. They are, however, techniques where exciting new advances are under way in reference to a particular illness/pathology. Each paper, although disease specific, contains information to assist in understanding brain pathology as a whole. These documents can be read in sequence or as a single reference on a disease of interest. At the conclusion of this section, the reader should have a basic understanding of how to apply a variety of imaging techniques to the study of adult neuropsychiatric disease.

Chapter 9

SUDDEN ONSET PANIC

Epileptic Aura or Panic Disorder?

ROBIN A. HURLEY, M.D.
RONALD E. FISHER, M.D., PH.D.
KATHERINE H. TABER, PH.D.

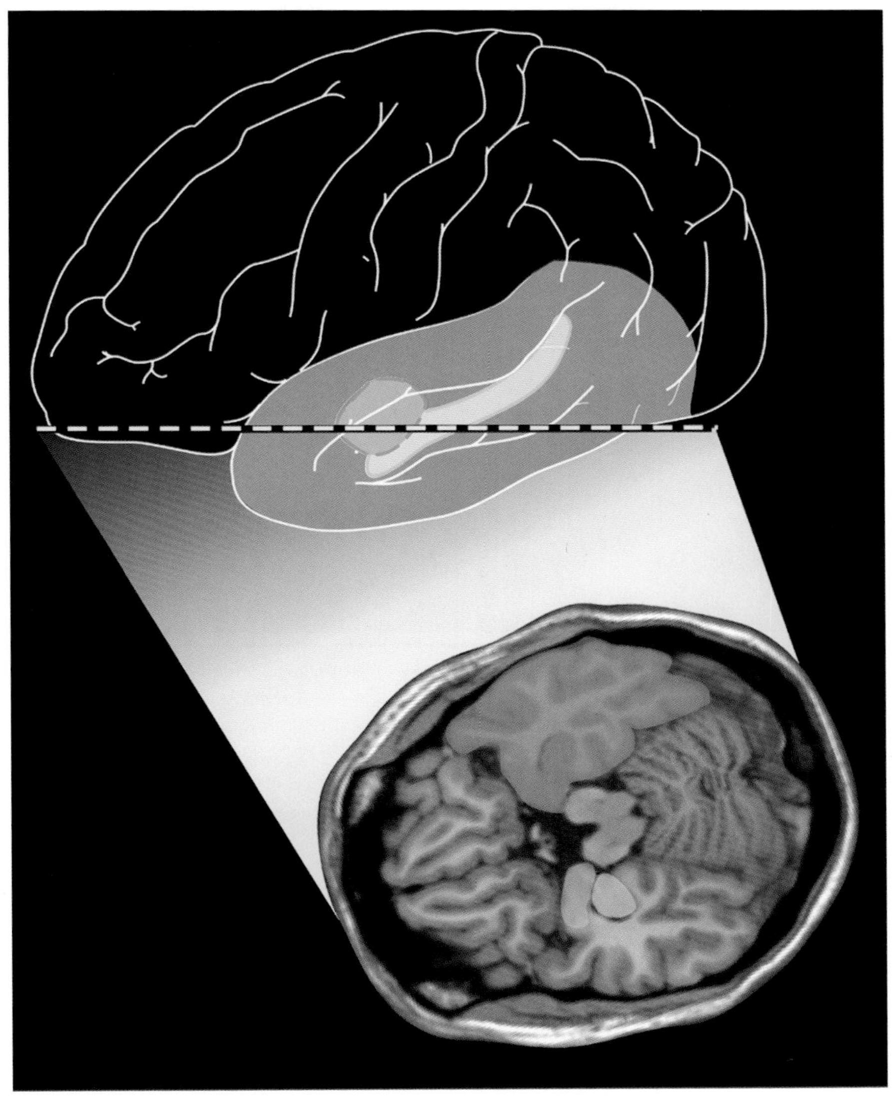

The location and extent of the temporal lobe (*pink*), the hippocampus (*green*), and the amygdala (*blue*) are color-coded onto a lateral drawing of the brain and a representative axial MR image. The dashed line on the lateral view of the brain indicates the approximate location for the axial image.

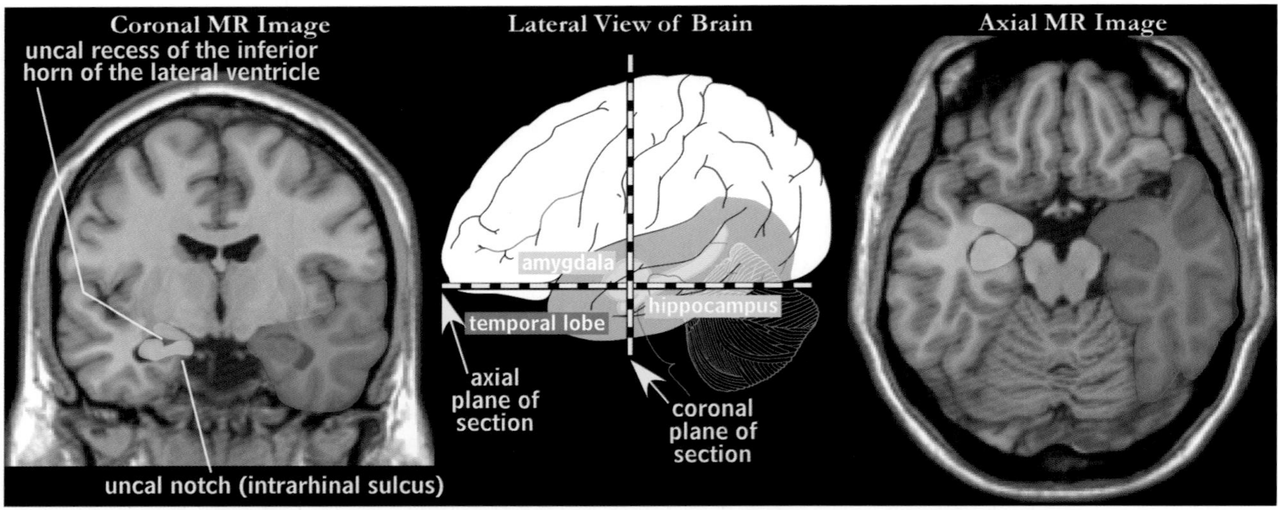

FIGURE 9–1. The location and extent of the temporal lobe (*pink*), the hippocampus (*green*), and the amygdala (*blue*) are color-coded onto a lateral drawing of the brain (middle) and representative coronal (left) and axial (right) MR images. Landmarks commonly used for identification of the boundary between the amygdala and anterior hippocampus are labeled in *yellow*.[1,2] The dashed lines on the lateral view of the brain indicate the locations and orientations for the two MR sections.

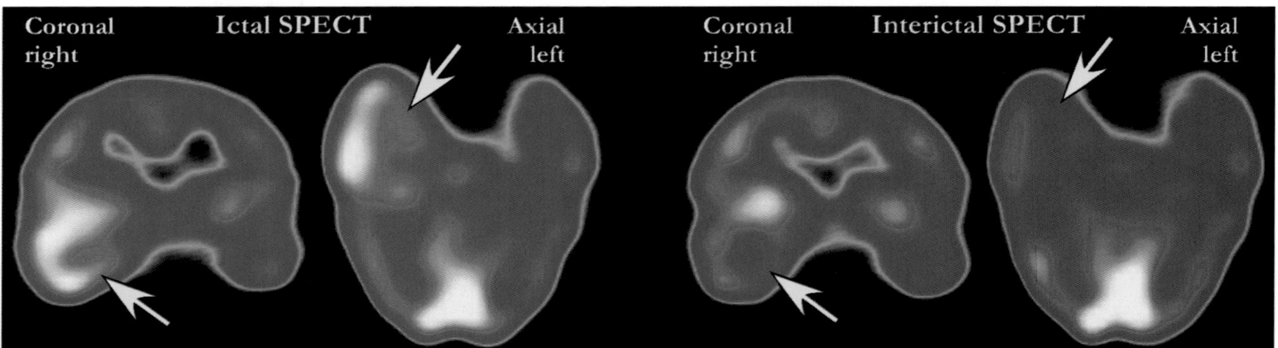

FIGURE 9–2. Nuclear medicine scans obtained during a seizure (ictal scan) will show increased perfusion or metabolism in the epileptic focus (arrows), as illustrated here with both coronal and axial single-photon emission computed tomography (SPECT) images of cerebral blood flow. Scans obtained in the absence of seizure (interictal scan) will show decreased perfusion or metabolism (arrows).

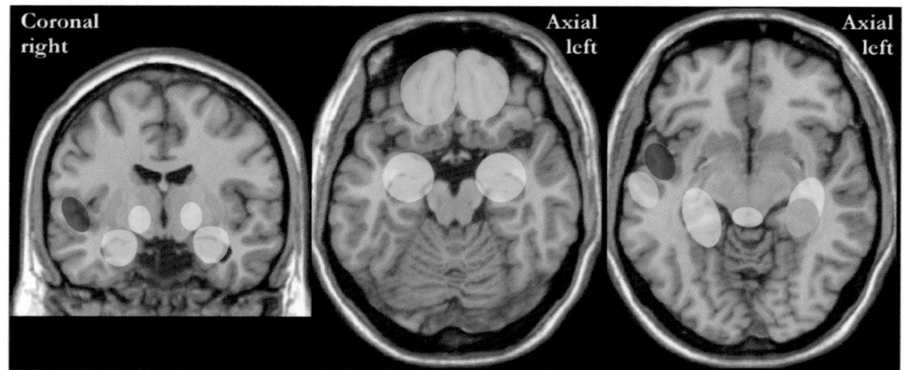

FIGURE 9–3. Nuclear medicine scans acquired under resting conditions from patients with panic disorder have areas of increased (*yellow, orange*) and decreased (*blue, green, purple*) perfusion or metabolism compared with healthy individuals.[3–6] Reported differences were in the range of 5%–10%, smaller than is typically seen in epilepsy.

The differential diagnosis of patients who experience symptoms of paresthesias, derealization, dizziness, chest pain, tremors, and palpitations can be quite challenging. These symptoms occur across a wide range of disorders, including cardiac, psychiatric, and neurological disorders. It can be particularly difficult to differentiate partial seizures without generalization of temporal lobe origin from panic disorder, as all of the above symptoms can be found in both conditions.[7,8] In fact, panic disorder has been found to be the most common condition that must be distinguished from seizure disorder.[9] The possibility that panic disorder and temporal lobe epilepsy with ictal fear can be comorbid has also been raised.[10]

Panic disorder occurs in 1%–3% of the population. Older estimates place the incidence of seizures at 0.03%, with ictal fear occurring in one-third of these patients.[11,12] New estimates place lifetime incidence of epilepsy at 3%.[13] Although a rare occurrence, multiple case reports have documented that patients initially diagnosed with panic disorder may later receive a diagnosis of temporal lobe seizures. Initial patient presentation can be quite varied.[14–18] It has been proposed that panic attacks with an onset consistent with an epileptic aura may sometimes be the result of simple partial seizures with a psychological presentation.[19] This hypothesis is supported by several lines of evidence, including concomitant symptoms, multiple cases with initial diagnosis of panic disorder but eventual electroencephalographic (EEG) documentation of seizures, comorbidity of the two conditions, nonepileptic EEG abnormalities in panic disorder, the proposed amygdala-driven kindling of the fear network, and limited clinical data suggesting successful treatment of panic attacks with antiepileptic medications.[19]

The literature does provide guidance for distinguishing between these two conditions[8,11]: panic attacks are generally longer in duration than seizures; ictal episodes are more stereotyped, whereas panic episodes are likely to vary more in presentation; although seizure disorders may initially present with fear/anxiety, they may progress to the more classic symptoms (e.g., olfactory auras, aphasias, amnestic features, motionless state, visceral automatisms); initial presentation of these classic epileptic features (i.e., before the fear/panic feelings) suggests seizures; panic disorder is more likely associated with agoraphobia (50% of cases); panic disorder has stronger familial links (25% for first-degree relatives); panic disorder can be worsened by emotional distress; presence of temporal lobe lesions on imaging can indicate epilepsy; and some treatments for panic disorder can worsen seizures (e.g., tricyclic antidepressants).[8,9] If the presentation is suggestive of epilepsy, EEG examination may be required to identify the characteristic spike/wave pattern of seizure discharge. A full evaluation for epilepsy may require 24-hour EEG and video monitoring or intracerebral depth electrodes with subdural grid arrays, as these procedures can sometimes identify abnormal electrical discharges not observed on routine EEG.[18,20,21] High resolution magnetic resonance imaging (MRI) is recommended for visualization of the deep temporal lobe structures.[2,22] This is particularly important for reliable separation of the amygdala and hippocampus in order to obtain accurate volume measurements.[23] Given the similar clinical features and divergent treatments for these two diagnoses, it is imperative for the clinician to understand the neuroanatomical features of the temporal lobe and the noninvasive imaging techniques available to assist in decision-making.

Anatomy of the Temporal Lobe

The mesial temporal lobe contains structures that are part of the limbic circuits, including the amygdala and hippocampus (Figure 9–1).[1,2,24] These structures have been implicated in the genesis of both panic disorder and seizure disorders.[8,9,18] Fear and panic have been elicited by electrical stimulation of the amygdala.[25–29] These symptoms can also occur as the initial symptoms of temporal lobe discharges.[7,14,30] Abnormal electrical activity in the frontal lobes, due either to spread from the temporal lobe or to a frontal focus, has also been found to be associated with fear or panic.[30]

Structural Imaging

Temporal Lobe Epilepsy

It is a common finding that temporal lobe structures, particularly the hippocampus and amygdala, are decreased in volume in patients with temporal lobe epilepsy.[23,31] One study reported that amygdala volume was more decreased in temporal lobe epilepsy patients who reported experiencing fear during seizure onset than in those who did not.[32] However, a later study from the same group did not confirm this association.[33]

Panic Disorder

Earlier studies compared volumetric measurement of temporal lobe structures between patients with panic disorder and healthy individuals based upon edge-tracing regions of interest.[34–36] One study reported that only the amygdala was decreased in size (bilaterally).[34] This study found no differences in the volumes of the hippocampus or the whole temporal lobe, and no anatomic measure correlated significantly with any clinical or demographic measure. In contrast, two studies found the volume of the temporal lobe (on the left in one, bilaterally in the other) was significantly decreased, but not the volume of the hippocampus or amygdala.[35,36] One study found a perplexing inverse correlation between duration of panic disorder and hippocampal volume, with a more recent onset associated with a smaller hippocampus.[35] Recently, several groups have utilized voxel-based morphometry to compare gray matter volumes of patients with panic disorder (diagnosis confirmed by a structured clinical interview [SCID], no mention made of any EEG studies) to healthy individuals.[37–39] With strict statistical criteria applied, there is little agreement, with one study reporting decreased gray matter only in the parahippocampal gyrus, the second reporting decreases only in the putamen, and the third reporting increased gray matter in several areas of the brainstem as well as ventral hippocampus. With less stringent statistical criteria, decreased gray matter volume was also found in the inferior and superior frontal and temporal gyri, and increased gray matter volume was found in the middle temporal gyrus in at least two of the three studies, although the laterality was not always the same. None reported changes in the amygdala. An inverse correlation was reported between volume of the putamen and clinical symptoms, with a lower volume associated with greater symptom severity and illness duration.[38]

The diversity of these findings may be due, at least in part, to differences in the measurement techniques employed. Edge-tracing region-of-interest analysis is based on the recognition of anatomic landmarks that are used to hand-trace regions onto magnetic resonance images. This approach has the advantage that individual differences in anatomy can be easily taken into account. It is also stronger statistically, because fewer comparisons need to be made. However, fewer areas can be assessed. Anatomic criteria and anatomic expertise vary across studies. Image resolution and section thickness also vary, a critical factor when small structures, such as the amygdala, are measured. Voxel-based morphometry provides a method of automatic analysis of the entire brain, allowing many more areas to be compared. However, this creates a statistical challenge. The likelihood of getting a false positive increases with the number of comparisons made. A mathematical correction for multiple comparisons must be performed. This approach also requires transformation of each individual's data onto an average brain template, which inevitably results in some distortion of individual anatomy, and often in some loss in image resolution, particularly if smoothing is also performed. In addition, image voxels are relatively large in terms of the size of many structures in the brain. If 1 mm sections with an in-plane resolution of 1 mm are acquired, for example, the cortical ribbon would be no more than three voxels wide. As a result, many voxels contain both gray and white matter, and partial-volume averaging is inevitable.

Finally, there is also diversity across studies including patient population and medication status. It should also be noted that EEG was not used to rule out any electrical abnormalities. As noted above, temporal lobe epilepsy has also been associated with reduced amygdala volumes as well as multiple areas of temporal lobe injuries.

Functional Imaging—Cerebral Blood Flow/Cerebral Metabolism

Given the common abnormal structural findings in both conditions, functional imaging may be needed to further inform the differential for panic disorder from temporal lobe epilepsy.

Temporal Lobe Epilepsy

During an epileptic seizure (ictus) there is an increase in both blood flow and metabolism in the seizure focus. Generally, seizures are brief, lasting only seconds to minutes. During the immediate postictal period, there is a drastic fall to a state of severe hypoperfusion. This is followed by a gradual recovery to a lessened level of hypoperfusion, which becomes the new resting state. This sequence is called the "postictal switch." Thus, interictally, there is a general hypometabolism in the abnormal area, and at times in the surrounding cortex, subcortical nuclei, or even in the contralateral temporal lobe. Comparative studies indicate that this depressed state deepens with the duration of the seizure disorder, with cerebral metabolism more affected than cerebral blood flow.[40] This mismatch between metabolism and blood flow indicates that 18-fluoro-2-deoxyglucose (FDG) positron emission tomography (PET), which provides images of cerebral metabolic rate, will more accurately delineate the seizure focus for scans acquired during the interictal period than single-photon emission computed tomography (SPECT), which provides images of cerebral blood flow.[40,41]

Both SPECT and FDG-PET are used to identify areas of seizure focus, evaluate patients for surgical resection of the affected temporal cortex, and predict clinical outcome postsurgery.[13,31] A major advantage of SPECT is the ability to capture ictal activity (i.e., hyperperfusion), due to rapid (e.g., 30–60 seconds) radiotracer uptake.[31] Ictal SPECT scans are compared with the interictal SPECT to determine the area of seizure focus (areas that are "hot" during the seizure and "cold" between seizures) (Figure 9–2). The sensitivity and accuracy of this technique are reported to be approximately 80%.[13] In clinical practice they are likely to be somewhat lower than this. Many research studies include patients for whom nuclear imaging would not be required because the seizure focus can be identified by visualization of lesions on structural images.

FDG-PET has higher image resolution, but radiotracer uptake is generally too slow for ictal imaging. The better spatial resolution of interictal FDG-PET scanning does allow for quantitative evaluation of abnormal areas that can be compared with the structural magnetic resonance (MR) images. Current FDG-PET techniques allow statistical parametric mapping that can identify abnormal areas sometimes not evident on visual interpretation. Both FDG-PET and SPECT are more valuable in conjunction with inpatient video EEG monitoring. Partial-volume averaging may cause small areas of abnormality to artificially appear healthier than they really are. Nonlimbic (nontemporal lobe) seizures are more likely to have normal interictal scans than are limbic/temporal lesions. FDG-PET and SPECT may identify patients who have two independent areas of seizure focus, not identifiable on structural imaging or by EEG data. Additionally, they can identify temporal lobe dysfunction in atypical panic/fear episodes, signaling the need for an epilepsy investigation. Two recent case reports illustrate a clinical presentation of atypical fear/panic attacks resulting from mesial temporal sclerosis. In each case, nuclear imaging identified the temporal lobe hypometabolism/hypoperfusion of the epileptic focus.[17,42]

Areas of abnormal metabolism or blood flow may be present at a distance from the epileptic focus. Statistical parametric mapping was used to assess the extent of both ictal and interictal cerebral blood flow (SPECT) alterations in patients with mesial temporal sclerosis compared with healthy individuals.[43] In addition to the expected increased perfusion in the ipsilateral temporal lobe (including the temporal stem white matter), ictal SPECT identified areas of hyperperfusion in the contralateral temporal lobe, anterior frontal lobe (left-sided focus), and parietal lobe (right-sided focus). Areas of decreased perfusion on interictal SPECT included hippocampus, thalamus, midbrain, superior paracentral lobule, insula (left-sided focus), and cingulate gyrus (right-sided focus). The authors of this study noted that these results are consistent with functional impairment of the cortico-thalamo-hippocampal circuit. A recent study compared the localization of interictal hypometabolism (FDG-PET) with the outcome of surgery.[44] Patients with hypometabolism confined to the temporal cortex containing the focus had better outcomes (78% seizure-free) than patients with hypometabolism in additional ipsilateral areas (45% seizure-free) or contralateral areas (22% seizure-free).

Panic Disorder

Two studies have used statistical parametric mapping to compare cerebral metabolic rate (FDG-PET) of patients with panic disorder (medication free) with healthy individuals (Figure 9–3).[4,6] Both found increases in hippocampus and parahippocampal structures. One also found increases in the thalamus, cerebellum, medulla, and pons.[4] The authors of this study[4] noted that these areas are part of the amygdala-based fear network. The other study found decreases in inferior parietal and superior temporal areas.[6] A third study of medication-free patients with panic disorder utilized visual and semiquantitative analysis of regional cerebral blood flow (SPECT).[5] They found significantly decreased perfusion only in the inferior frontal area (Figure 9–3). The authors commented that this might be due to an inhibitory influence from the amygdala. None of the studies mentioned above reported any correlation between functional imaging findings and clinical symptoms.

In contrast, a study that compared cerebral perfusion (SPECT) in medicated patients with panic disorder to healthy individuals found decreases only in the superior temporal lobe (Figure 9–3, right). This study reported an inverse correlation between blood flow and both duration of illness and clinical symptoms (lower perfusion with higher scores).[3] One group performed a second functional imaging examination (FDG-PET) at the conclusion of 10 sessions (over 6 months) of cognitive behavior therapy.[45] Most of the patients (11/12) were responsive to treatment. In comparison with pretreatment levels, the responsive group exhibited normalization of cerebral metabolism, with decreases in the hippocampus, cerebellum, and pons, and increases in the medial prefrontal cortex bilaterally. Overall, these results are consistent with altered reactivity in the fear circuitry that may normalize with successful treatment.

Functional Imaging—Receptor/Neurotransmitter Mapping

As radiotracers for a variety of neurotransmitter receptors become more widely available, they add yet another nuclear imaging tool that may help to clarify temporal lobe function and pathology. At the present time, ligands for the benzodiazepine-$GABA_A$ receptor, the serotonin $5\text{-}HT_{1A}$ receptor, and the muscarinic acetylcholine receptor have been evaluated for their ability to improve visualization of the epileptic focus. Only a handful of studies utilizing some of these ligands have been performed in patients with panic disorder.

Benzodiazepine-GABA$_A$ Receptor

GABA has been known to be associated with the temporal lobe, anxiety disorders, and seizures for many years.[46,47] Ligands for the central benzodiazepine-GABA$_A$ receptor suitable for both PET (^{11}C flumazenil, FMZ) and SPECT (^{123}I iomazenil, IMZ) studies are available, although neither is yet approved for clinical use in the United States.[48]

Temporal Lobe Epilepsy

Reduced benzodiazepine receptor binding has been demonstrated (by autoradiography) in surgically resected specimens from temporal lobe epilepsy patients.[49] It has not yet been proven that either of the available benzodiazepine ligands is more accurate for delineation of the seizure focus than the functional imaging techniques already in clinical use (as detailed above).[48,50–52] There are promising indications. When hippocampal sclerosis was present, the area of abnormality was often larger on FDG-PET than on FMZ-PET, which more closely matched the epileptogenic zone as determined by intracranial EEG.[50] A case was recently published in which interictal IMZ-SPECT provided correct laterality of the seizure focus (as determined by intracranial EEG) while ictal perfusion SPECT did not.[53] Timing of the examination in relation to seizure activity may be a critical factor, as a recent study found within-subject short-term changes in binding.[54] Lower values (better delineation of seizure focus) were obtained when the FMZ-PET was performed shortly after a seizure, suggesting a transient decrease in expression or availability. Given this evidence for dynamic seizure-related changes, the authors of the study recommend that benzodiazepine receptor imaging be performed within a few days following a seizure, for best results. Larger studies in which this factor is taken into account are needed to better assess the value of this technique. Other potentially confounding factors include medication status (many antiepileptic medications affect GABA), comorbid psychiatric diagnoses, and variations in imaging technology.

Panic Disorder

Both increases and decreases in regional benzodiazepine binding have been reported when patients with panic disorder were compared with healthy individuals.[55–57] Two studies included only patients with panic disorder who had never taken benzodiazepines.[55,56] One, using FMZ-PET and statistical parametric mapping, reported both globally reduced binding and regional decreases in orbital (right) and insular (right) cortices in patients compared with healthy individuals.[55] The other, using IMZ-SPECT and template-based analysis, reported increased binding in orbital cortex (right) and a trend toward increased binding in temporal cortex (right) in patients with panic disorder.[56] The third study included patients with panic disorder who had been medication-free for at least 6 weeks.[58] This IMZ-SPECT study utilized both statistical parametric mapping and region-of-interest analyses. No difference was found in global binding between the patient group and healthy individuals. Binding was decreased in the area of the hippocampus (left) and precuneus (left), and increased in caudate (right), medial frontal cortex (right), and middle temporal gyrus (left) in the patient group. Some patients experienced panic symptoms during scanning. Decreased binding in the medial frontal and superior frontal cortex (Brodmann's areas 8, 9, 10) correlated with increased symptoms. Diversity across studies may be due to methodological differences and/or variations in the patient population studied. While preliminary, these studies suggest that alterations in benzodiazepine binding in frontal areas may differentiate panic disorder patients from temporal lobe epilepsy patients. Further studies that explore the apparently dynamic relationship between symptom state and binding would be of great value.

Serotonin 5-HT$_{1A}$ Receptor

Serotonin has been implicated in the pathophysiology of both panic disorder and seizure disorders.[59,60] Ligands based on several 5-HT$_{1A}$ antagonists have been developed for PET imaging (^{11}C WAY100635; ^{18}F trans-4-fluoro-*N*-2-[4-(2-methoxyphenyl)piperazin-1-yl]ethyl]-*N*-(2-pyridyl)cyclohexanecarboxamide, FCWAY; ^{18}F4-[2′-(*N*-2-pyridinyl)-*p*-fluorobenzamido]-ethylpiperazine, MPPF).

Temporal Lobe Epilepsy

Several groups have evaluated 5-HT$_{1A}$ receptor binding in patients with temporal lobe epilepsy.[61–66] All found decreased receptor binding in the mesial temporal lobe containing the seizure focus, in areas of seizure spread, and in the area of the brainstem raphe. Localization was reported to be better than with cerebral blood flow or metabolic rate imaging in some studies.[61,62] One group found an inverse correlation between abnormal intracerebral activity and binding potential.[63] The most profound decreases in binding potential were in areas of seizure onset; moderate decreases were found in areas of seizure spread, with only mild decreases in areas of interictal activity. These results are promising, but must still be considered preliminary. The importance of correcting for partial-volume averaging and for differences in plasma binding related to antiepileptic medications has been emphasized by one group.[65,66]

Panic Disorder

One study comparing unmedicated patients with panic disorder to healthy individuals found decreased 5-HT$_{1A}$ receptor binding in the anterior and posterior cingulate cortices and the raphe area, with no differences in anterior insular, mesiotemporal, or anterior temporal cortices.[67] Another reported decreased binding principally in amygdala and orbitofrontal and temporal cortices as well as the raphe area.[68] This study compared binding in an unmedicated patient group and a patient group successfully treated with SSRIs and reported normalization of binding in all areas except the raphe.

Conclusions

In conclusion, although the current diagnostic classification defines panic disorder and simple partial seizure disorder as two separate entities, they clearly share similar features and common symptoms and may occur as comorbidities. Rarely, patients diagnosed with panic disorder later show evidence of mesial temporal sclerosis and EEG-proven seizure foci. The close clinical presentations of these two conditions call for a very thorough medical evaluation of those patients with preliminary suspicions of panic disorder and symptoms similar to a seizure aura. If possible, this should include high resolution MRI (with particular attention paid to the mesial temporal cortex) and nuclear imaging. Future studies utilizing new technologies may assist in distinguishing these two entities or in further defining their common pathological base. Nuclear imaging may prove helpful in this endeavor, as very early work may indicate divergent scan findings—especially with receptor-specific ligands.

References

1. Watson Laboratories, Andermann F, Gloor P, et al: Anatomic basis of amygdaloid and hippocampal volume measurement by MRI. Neurology 1992; 42:1743–1750
2. Watson Laboratories, Jack CR Jr, Cendes F: Volumetric MRI: clinical applications and contributions to the understanding of temporal lobe epilepsy. Arch Neurol 1997; 54:1521–1531
3. Lee YS, Hwang J, Kim SJ, et al: Decreased blood flow of temporal regions of the brain in subjects with panic disorder. J Psychiatr Res 2006; 40:828–834
4. Sakai Y, Kumano H, Nishikawa M, et al: Cerebral glucose metabolism associated with a fear network in panic disorder. Neuroreport 2005; 16:927–931
5. Eren I, Tukel R, Polat A, et al: Evaluation of regional cerebral blood flow changes in panic disorder with technetium-99m-HMPAO SPECT. Psychiatr Res 2003; 123:135–143
6. Bisaga A, Katz JL, Antonini A, et al: Cerebral glucose metabolism in women with panic disorder. Am J Psychiatry 1998; 155:1178–1183
7. Toni C, Cassano GB, Perugi G, et al: Psychosensorial and related phenomena in panic disorder and in temporal lobe epilepsy. Compr Psychiatry 1996; 37:125–133
8. Sazgar M, Carlen PL, Wennberg R: Panic attack semiology in right temporal lobe epilepsy. Epileptic Disord 2003; 5:93–100
9. Young GB, Chandarana PC, Blume WT, et al: Mesial temporal lobe seizures presenting as anxiety disorders. J Neuropsychiatry Clin Neurosci 1995; 7:352–357
10. Mintzer S, Lopez F: Comorbidity of ictal fear and panic disorder. Epilepsy Behav 2002; 3:330–337
11. Young AW, Aggleton JP, Hellawell DJ, et al: Face processing impairments after amygdalotomy. Brain 1995; 118:15–24
12. Katon WJ: Clinical practice: panic disorder. N Engl J Med 2006; 354:2360–2367
13. Henry TR, Van Heertum RL: Positron emission tomography and single photon emission computed tomography in epilepsy care. Semin Nucl Med 2003; 33:88–104
14. Scalise A, Placidi F, Diomedi M, et al: Panic disorder or epilepsy? A case report. J Neurol Sci 2006; 246:173–175
15. Saegusa S, Takahashi T, Moriya J, et al: Panic attack symptoms in a patient with left temporal lobe epilepsy. J Int Med Res 2004; 32:64–96
16. Huppertz HJ, Schulze-Bonhage A: Distinguishing between partial seizures and panic attacks: epileptic panic attacks are not limited to adults. BMJ 2001; 322:864
17. Meyer MA, Zimmerman AW, Miller CA: Temporal lobe epilepsy presenting as panic attacks: detection of interictal hypometabolism with positron emission tomography. J Neuroimaging 2000; 10:120–122
18. Alemayehu S, Bergey GK, Barry E, et al: Panic attacks as ictal manifestations of parietal lobe seizures. Epilepsia 1995; 36:824–830
19. Alvarez-Silva S, Alvarez-Rodriguez J, Perez-Echeverria MJ, et al: Panic and epilepsy. J Anxiety Disord 2006; 20:353–362
20. Huppertz HJ, Franck P, Korinthenberg R, et al: Recurrent attacks of fear and visual hallucinations in a child. J Child Neurol 2002; 17:230–233
21. Blume WT, Holloway GM, Wiebe S: Temporal epileptogenesis: localizing value of scalp and subdural interictal and ictal EEG data. Epilepsia 2001; 42:508–514
22. McBride MC, Bronstein KS, Bennett B, et al: Failure of standard MRI in patients with refractory temporal lobe epilepsy. Arch Neurol 1998; 55:346–348
23. Van Paesschen W: Qualitative and quantitative imaging of the hippocampus in mesial temporal lobe epilepsy with hippocampal sclerosis. Neuroimaging Clin N Am 2004; 14:373–400
24. Hurley RA, Hayman LA, Taber KH: Clinical imaging in neuropsychiatry, in The American Psychiatric Press Textbook of Neuropsychiatry and Clinical Neurosciences. Edited by Yudofsky SC, Hales RE. Washington, DC, American Psychiatric Publishing, 2002, pp 245–283
25. Lanteaume L, Khalfa S, Regis J, et al: Emotion induction after direct intracerebral stimulations of human amygdala. Cereb Cortex 2007; 17:1307–1313
26. Fish DR, Gloor P, Quesney FL, et al: Clinical responses to electrical brain stimulation of the temporal and frontal lobes in patients with epilepsy. Brain 1993; 116:397–414
27. Halgren E, Walter RD, Cherlow DG, et al: Mental phenomena evoked by electrical stimulation of the human hippocampal formation and amygdala. Brain 1978; 101:83–117
28. Wieser HG: Electroclinical Features of the Psychomotor Seizure. New York, Raven Press, 1983
29. Penfield W, Jasper W: Epilepsy and the Functional Anatomy of the Human Brain. Boston, Little, Brown and Company, 1954

30. Biraben A, Taussig D, Thomas P, et al: Fear as the main feature of epileptic seizures. J Neurol Neurosurg Psychiatry 2001; 70:186–191
31. Schauble B, Cascino GD: Advances in neuroimaging: management of partial epileptic syndromes. Neurosurg Rev 2003; 26:233–246
32. Cendes F, Andermann F, Gloor P, et al: Relationship between atrophy of the amygdala and ictal fear in temporal lobe epilepsy. Brain 1994; 117:739–746
33. Guerreiro C, Cendes F, Li LM, et al: Clinical patterns of patients with temporal lobe epilepsy and pure amygdalar atrophy. Epilepsia 1999; 40:453–461
34. Massana G, Serra-Grabulosa JM, Salgado-Pineda P, et al: Amygdalar atrophy in panic disorder patients detected by volumetric MRI. Neuroimage 2003; 19:80–90
35. Uchida RR, Del-Ben CM, Santos AC, et al: Decreased left temporal lobe volume of panic patients measured by MRI. Braz J Med Biol Res 2003; 36:7925–7929
36. Vythilingam M, Anderson ER, Goddard A, et al: Temporal lobe volume in panic disorder—a quantitative MRI study. Psychiatry Res 2000; 99:75–82
37. Protopopescu X, Pan H, Tuescher O, et al: Increased brainstem volume in panic disorder: a voxel-based morphometric study. Neuroreport 2006; 17:361–363
38. Yoo HK, Kim MJ, Kim SJ, et al: Putaminal gray matter volume decrease in panic disorder: an optimized voxel-based morphometry study. Eur J Neurosci 2005; 22:2089–2094
39. Massana G, Serra-Grabulosa JM, Salgado-Pineda P, et al: Parahippocampal gray matter density in panic disorder: a voxel-based morphometric study. Am J Psychiatry 2003; 160:566–568
40. Breier JI, Mullani NA, Thomas AB, et al: Effects of duration of epilepsy on the uncoupling of metabolism and blood flow in complex partial seizures. Neurology 1997; 48:1047–1053
41. Lee DS, Lee JS, Kang KW, et al: Disparity of perfusion and glucose metabolism of epileptogenic zones in temporal lobe epilepsy demonstrated by SPM/SPAM analysis on ^{15}0 water PET, [^{18}F]FDG-PET, and [^{99m}TC]-HMPAO SPECT. Epilepsia 2001; 42:1515–1522
42. Gallinat J, Stotz-Ingenlath G, Lang UE, et al: Panic attacks, spike-wave activity, and limbic dysfunction: a case report. Pharmacopsychiatry 2003; 36:123–126
43. Tae WS, Joo EY, Kim JH, et al: Cerebral perfusion changes in mesial temporal lobe epilepsy: SPM analysis of ictal and interictal SPECT. Neuroimage 2005; 24:101–110
44. Choi JY, Kim SJ, Hong SB, et al: Extratemporal hypometabolism on FDG PET in temporal lobe epilepsy as a predictor of seizure outcome after temporal lobectomy. Eur J Nucl Med Mol Imaging 2003; 30:581–587
45. Sakai Y, Kumano H, Nishikawa M, et al: Changes in cerebral glucose utilization in patients with panic disorder treated with cognitive behavior therapy. Neuroimage 2006; 33:218–226
46. Roy-Byrne PP: The GABA-benzodiazepine receptor complex: structure, function, and role in anxiety. J Clin Psychiatry 2005; 66:14–20
47. Avoli M, Lauvel J, Pumain R, et al: Cellular and molecular mechanisms of epilepsy in the human brain. Prog Neurobiol 2005; 77:166–200
48. Goethals I, Van de Wiele C, Boon P, et al: Is central benzodiazepine receptor imaging useful for the identification of epileptogenic foci in localization-related epilepsies? Eur J Nucl Med Mol Imaging 2003; 30:325–328
49. Sata Y, Matsuda K, Mihara T, et al: Quantitative analysis of benzodiazepine receptor in temporal lobe epilepsy: [(125)I]iomazenil autoradiographic study of surgically resected specimens. Epilepsia 2002; 43:1039–1048
50. Ryvlin P, Bouvard S, Le Bars D, et al: Clinical utility of flumazenil-PET [fluorine-18] fluorodeoxyglucose-PET and MRI in refractory partial epilepsy: a prospective study in 100 patients. Brain 1998; 121:2067–2081
51. Cascino GD: Measurement and significance of changes in benzodiazepine receptors in temporal lobe epilepsy. Epilepsy Curr 2003; 3:33–34
52. Morimoto K, Tamagami H, Matsuda K: Central-type benzodiazepine receptors and epileptogenesis: basic mechanisms and clinical validity. Epilepsia 2005; 45:184–188
53. Shuke N, Hashizume K, Kiriyama K, et al: Correct localization of epileptogenic focus with iodine-123 iomazenil cerebral benzodiazepine receptor imaging: a case report of temporal lobe epilepsy with discordant ictal cerebral blood flow SPECT. Ann Nucl Med 2004; 18:541–545
54. Bouvard S, Costes N, Bonnefoi F, et al: Seizure-related short-term plasticity of benzodiazepine receptor in partial epilepsy: a [carbon-11] fumazenil-PET study. Brain 2005; 128:1330–1343
55. Malizia AL, Cunningham VJ, Bell CJ, et al: Decreased brain GABAA-benzodiazepine receptor binding in panic disorder: preliminary results from a quantitative PET study. Arch Gen Psychiatry 1998; 55:715–720
56. Brandt CA, Meller J, Keweloh L, et al: Increased benzodiazepine receptor density in the prefrontal cortex in patients with panic disorder. J Neural Transm 1998; 105:1325–1333
57. Bremner JD, Innis RB, White T, et al: SPECT[iodine-123] iomazenil measurement of the benzodiazepine receptor in panic disorder. Biol Psychiatry 2000; 47:96–106
58. Bremner JD, Narayan M, Anderson ER, et al: Hippocampal volume reduction in major depression. Am J Psychiatry 2000; 157:115–117
59. Chugani HT, Chugani DC: Imaging of serotonin mechanisms in epilepsy. Epilepsy Curr 2005; 5:201–206
60. Maron E, Shlik J: Serotonin function in panic disorder: important, but why? Neuropsychopharmacology 2006; 31:1–11
61. Toczek MT, Carsons RE, Lang L, et al: PET imaging of 5-HT1A receptor binding in patients with temporal lobe epilepsy. Neurology 2003; 60:749–756
62. Savic I, Lindstrom P, Gulyas B, et al: Limbic reductions of 5-HT1A receptor binding in human temporal lobe epilepsy. Neurology 2004; 62:1343–1351
63. Merlet I, Ostrowsky K, Costes N, et al: 5-HT1A receptor binding and intracerebral activity in temporal lobe epilepsy: an [^{18}F]MPPF-PET study. Brain 2004; 127:900–913
64. Merlet I, Ryvlin P, Costes N, et al: Statistical parametric mapping of 5-HT1A receptor binding in temporal lobe epilepsy with hippocampal ictal onset on intracranial EEG. Neuroimage 2004; 22:886–896
65. Giovacchini G, Toczek MT, Bonwetsch R, et al: 5-HT1A receptors are reduced in temporal lobe epilepsy after partial-volume correction. J Nucl Med 2005; 46:1128–1135

66. Theodore WH, Giovacchini G, Bonwetsch R, et al: The effect of antiepileptic drugs on 5-HT1A-receptor binding measured by positron emission tomography. Epilepsia 2006; 47:499–503
67. Neumeister A, Bain E, Nugent AC, et al: Reduced serotonin type 1A receptor binding in panic disorder. J Neurosci 2004; 24:589–591
68. Nash JR, Sargent PA, Rabiner EA, et al: Altered 5HT1A binding in panic disorder demonstrated by positron emission tomography. Eur Neuropsychopharmacol 2004; 14:322–323

Recent Publication of Interest

Wiest G, Lehner-Baumgartner E, Baumgartner C: Panic attacks in an individual with bilateral selective lesions of the amygdala. Arch Neurol 2006; 63:1798–1801
An interesting report of a patient diagnosed with Urbach-Wiethe disease at age 4 who developed panic attacks and depressed mood at age 38, both of which were responsive to antidepressive treatment. Imaging indicated calcifications of the whole amygdaloid complex bilaterally.

Reprinted from Hurley RA, Fisher R, Taber KH: "Sudden Onset Panic: Epileptic Aura or Panic Disorder?" *Journal of Neuropsychiatry and Clinical Neurosciences* 18:436–443, 2006. Used with permission.

Chapter 10

BIPOLAR DISORDER
Imaging State Versus Trait

JACQUELINE N.W. FRIEDMAN, PH.D.
ROBIN A. HURLEY, M.D.
KATHERINE H. TABER, PH.D.

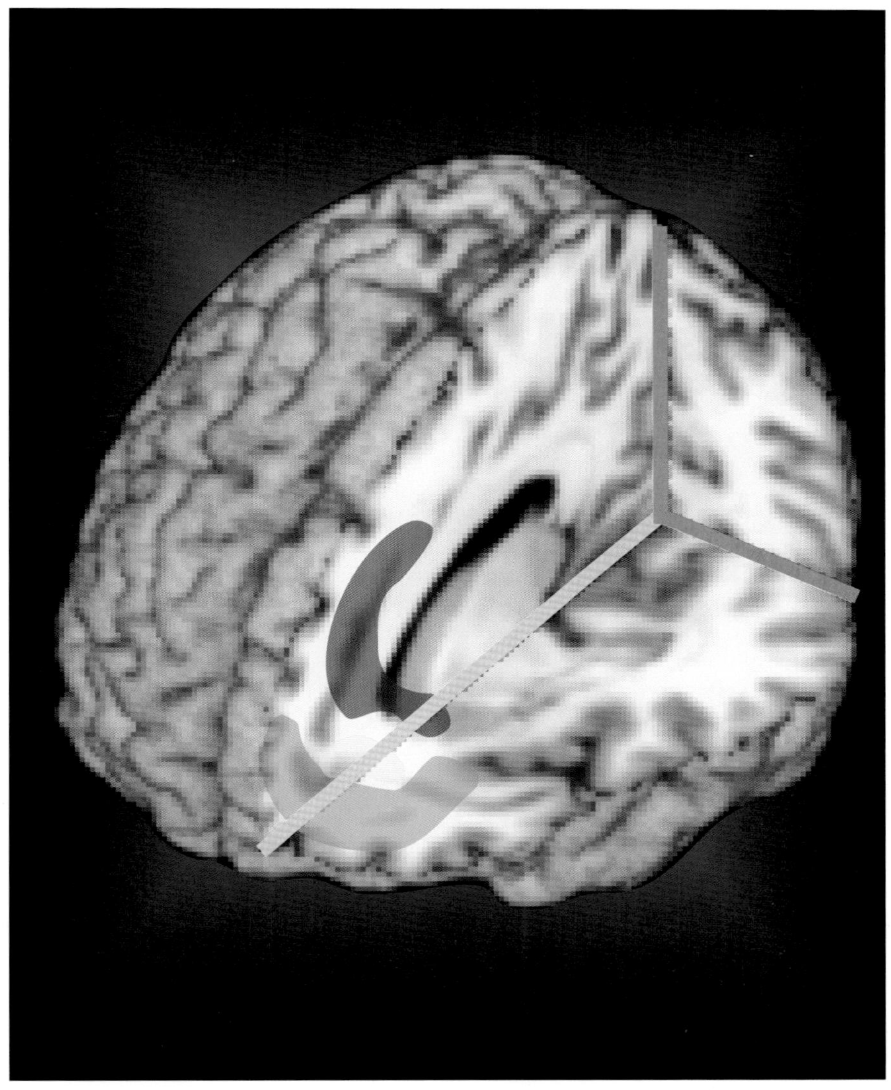

The image is of a three-dimensional reconstruction of an MR data set from a normal individual that has been cut in order to display internal structures. The approximate locations of areas in which rCBF was modulated by state in patients with bipolar disorder are indicated: dorsal anterior cingulate cortex and caudate (*pink*); subgenual cortex (*yellow*); orbitofrontal cortex (*blue*).

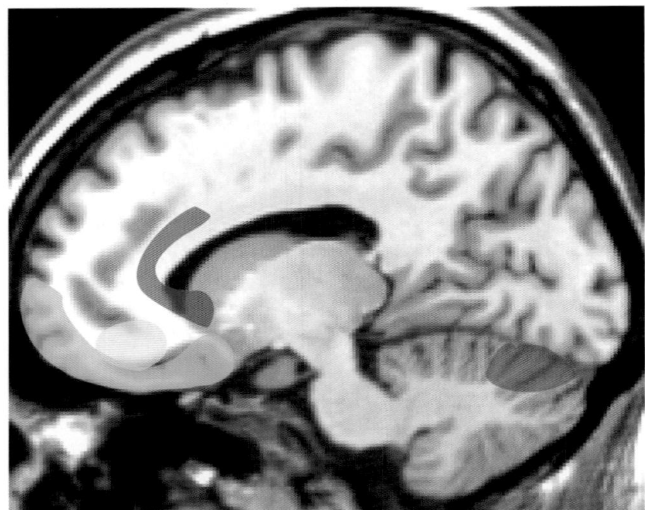

FIGURE 10-1 The approximate locations of areas in which regional cerebral blood flow (rCBF) was modulated by state in patients with bipolar disorder are indicated on a sagittal magnetic resonance image from a normal individual. Resting rCBF was higher in dorsal anterior cingulate cortex and caudate (*pink*) in patients with bipolar disorder in the manic state compared with the euthymic state.[1] In the manic state it was also higher in the subgenual cortex (*yellow*) and lower in the orbitofrontal cortex (*blue*) compared with normal.[2,3] In all three states (depressed, manic, euthymic), bipolar disorder patients had reduced activity in prefrontal (*blue*) and parietal cortices, and increased activity in cerebellum (*orange*), compared with healthy individuals.[2–5]

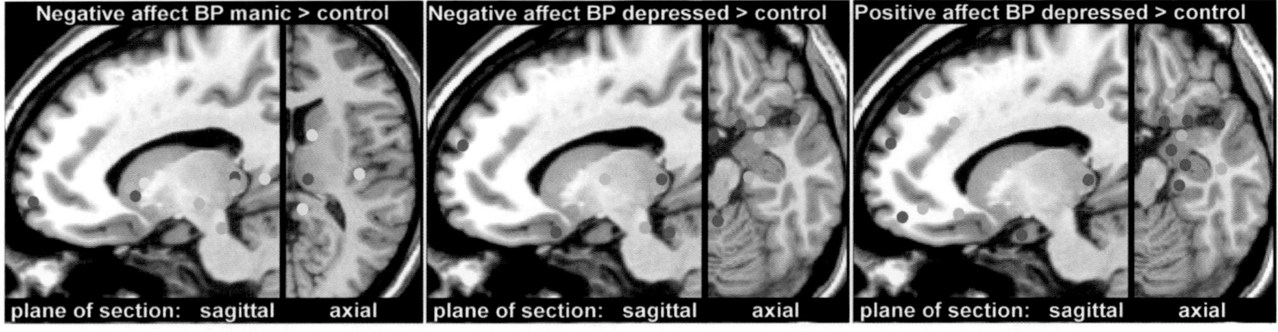

FIGURE 10–2. Regional brain activation in subjects with bipolar disorder during a facial affect recognition task varies with the valence of emotion (positive, negative) and the state (manic, depressed) of the subjects. Approximate locations where bipolar disorder groups had greater activation than normal from several studies are color-coded (each study was assigned a color) onto representative sagittal and axial magnetic resonance images.[6–9] Note that negative affect evoked greater than normal activation, primarily in subcortical regions, in both the manic and depressed states. Positive affect evoked greater than normal activation in prefrontal regions only in the depressed state.

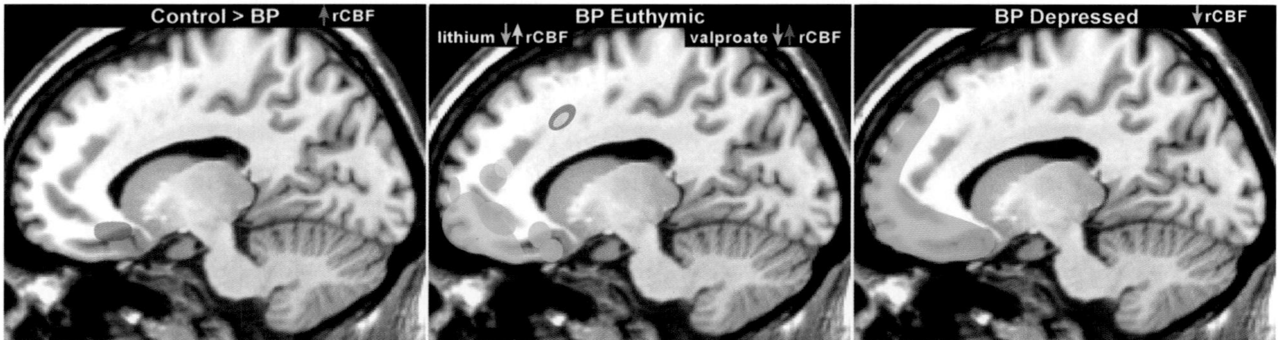

FIGURE 10–3. rCBF changes in subjects with bipolar disorder during induction of sadness differ from healthy individuals and also vary with state (euthymic, depressed) and medication.[4,10,11] Patterns of change in the medial prefrontal cortex that distinguish these groups are color-coded on a representative sagittal magnetic resonance image. Note that healthy subjects had increased rCBF in subgenual cortex (left), while all bipolar disorder groups had decreased rCBF in this area (middle, right). The euthymic bipolar disorder group stabilized on valproate had decreased rCBF in rostral anterior cingulate, while the euthymic bipolar disorder group stabilized on lithium had increased cerebral blood flow in this area (middle).

Bipolar disorder is a chronic and severe mental illness with worldwide effects. It includes both the more severe bipolar disorder type I (BD I, requiring a manic or mixed episode) and the less severe bipolar disorder type II (BD II, requiring presence of a hypomanic episode).[12] While BD I affects men and women in equal numbers, BD II, like major depressive disorder, affects women in greater numbers. Estimates of lifetime prevalence of bipolar disorder in the general population range from 2.8% to 6.5%.[13,14]

Understanding and clarifying the diagnosis of bipolar disorder requires comparison to major depressive disorder since both include major depressive episodes.[15] Previous research has focused on categorical differences between the two without considering that depressive episodes in major depressive disorder may or may not be the same clinically as depressive episodes that occur within the context of bipolar disorder.[16] Additionally, differences may exist in the functional brain systems that underlie these disorders. Thus, it is important to examine both trait and state.

In medicine, *trait* generally refers to the formal diagnosis (major depressive disorder or bipolar disorder), which is relatively stable. *State* is the status of the patient at a given point in time (e.g., manic, depressed, euthymic). Thus, it is fluid and changeable. Recent advances in neuroimaging that utilize functional imaging techniques can contribute to our knowledge base of how manic and depressive states differ. This may help develop a better understanding of etiological and treatment differences between the two disorders.

Structural Imaging

Neuroimaging studies of bipolar disorder have found conflicting results in regard to structural abnormalities. General areas of focus include limbic structures and the prefrontal cortical pathways associated with the limbic system.[17] The decision to focus on these areas seems, in part, motivated by research documenting abnormalities in the amygdala and prefrontal areas in major depressive disorder.[18,19] In general, structural studies have found abnormalities in amygdala size in bipolar disorder patients.[20] However, some studies have found amygdala enlargement and others have found reduced amygdala volume.[21,22] The sex of research subjects may also be a complicating factor, as activation studies have found male/female differences in anterior cingulate and dorsolateral prefrontal cortices as well as in the amygdala.[23] Since the proportion of men to women varies considerably across studies, this confounding factor may contribute to contradictory findings.

Some studies have focused on abnormalities in gray and white matter. A recent magnetic resonance imaging (MRI) study found abnormal gray matter density in the cingulate cortex and fronto-limbic cortex of patients with bipolar disorder who had poor outcomes on traditional treatment measures.[24] Reduced gray matter density in prefrontal regions and increased gray matter in temporal regions, including the amygdala, have also been documented.[25] Magnetization transfer imaging and voxel-based morphometry have shown small white matter density abnormalities in the anterior cingulate and subgyrus of bipolar disorder patients.[26] Diffusion tensor imaging has shown abnormal frontal white matter tracts in the prefrontal regions of bipolar disorder patients.[27] Gray matter volume was reduced in unmedicated bipolar disorder subjects in the posterior cingulate/retrosplenial cortex in a voxel-based morphometry MRI study.[28] Though specific findings are inconsistent, limbic and prefrontal regions are of interest in terms of understanding the neuropathology of mood disorders.

Role of the Limbic System in Mood Disorders

It is unclear whether the structural differences in the limbic and prefrontal areas in bipolar disorder have been highlighted because of unique differences in those areas or as a secondary function of the limbic system's theoretical role in emotional processing. Theories regarding the limbic system (e.g., amygdala, thalamus, hippocampus) and emotional processing predate imaging advances in neuroscience. While perception of and reaction to fear have been clearly linked to the amygdala, other emotions have shown activation in various aspects of the limbic system as currently defined.[29] Discussion of the controversial definition of and role of the limbic system is beyond the scope of this article.

Functional Imaging

Several factors need to be considered prior to examining bipolar disorder imaging findings. Comparison of imaging studies of bipolar disorder is complicated by the different methodological techniques employed and by individual differences within the bipolar disorder population. Imaging studies of any cohort can involve some loss of accuracy when data are averaged across the groups. There is an additional complicating factor of patient state in mood disorders at the time of the scan. It is difficult to capture and maintain a manic state during functional imaging. There is both individual variance and variance between studies in how patient state is defined and measured. Brain function during a major depressive episode may differ from brain function when not depressed (i.e., euthymic), and both may be different from brain function in a healthy individual. In addition, patients with bipolar disorder who are in a euthymic state may be experiencing manic or depressive symptoms at a subclinical level.[30,31] Functional imaging studies controlling for these state differences in bipolar disorder will serve an important role in clarifying diagnosis and pathophysiology of bipolar disorder compared to major depressive disorder.[7,32]

Medication differences within and between participant subgroups are another source of complexity for functional imaging studies. For example, the introduction of an 8-week trial of antidepressant medication has been shown to significantly reduce limbic activation in major depressive disorder patients compared to healthy subjects.[33] Many studies, especially of bipolar disorder populations, include patients on a variety of psychotropic medications. This limits comparability both within and between groups. A few studies have avoided this complication by focusing on unmedicated populations. This limits applicability to a clinical setting, where the majority of bipolar disorder and severe major depressive disorder patients would likely be medicated. Medication factors should be considered when reviewing results across studies.

Functional Neuroimaging Studies of Mania and Depression

The Resting State

With the above caveats in mind, a few recent positron emission tomography (PET) studies have provided state and trait comparisons in bipolar disorder patients (Figure 10–1). One study compared regional cerebral blood flow (rCBF) between medicated BD I patients in euthymic and manic states.[1] The only significant differences were higher rCBF on the left in dorsal anterior cingulate cortex and caudate (head) in mania. Two studies (one measuring rCBF, the other measuring regional cerebral metabolic rate, rCMR) have compared bipolar disorder patients in euthymic and depressed states.[4,5] In both studies, the patient groups were not significantly different. Reduced activity (greater reductions in the depressed state) has been noted in multiple cortical areas (dorsolateral prefrontal, medial prefrontal, orbital prefrontal, parietal) when bipolar disorder patients in all three states were compared to healthy individuals.[2,4,5] Studies have reported increased activity in cerebellum in bipolar disorder patients compared to healthy individuals.[4,5] One study also reported increased subcortical activity (ventral striatum, thalamus, right amygdala) in the depressed state.[5] Subgenual cortex rCBF has also been noted to be decreased in depression (both in bipolar disorder and major depressive disorder) and increased in manic states compared to normal.[3] Euthymic bipolar disorder patients had increased rCBF in dorsal anterior cingulate cortex when compared to healthy individuals in one study.[4] Increased rCMR in the left amygdala has also been reported in bipolar disorder patients in the depressed state, and in the unmedicated euthymic state.[34] Interestingly, this was not the case for euthymic bipolar disorder patients on mood-stabilizing medications. From these studies, it appears that the manic state is associated with increased activity in anterior cingulate regions, while the depressed state is associated with decreased activity in medial, lateral, and orbital prefrontal regions and increased activity in associated subcortical structures. Studies of the euthymic state suggest a combination of increased activity in anterior cingulate regions and decreased activity in other prefrontal areas, findings consistent with the presence of mild symptoms of both mania and depression.

A few studies have compared the depressed and euthymic states in bipolar disorder with major depressive disorder in an effort to detect trait differences. In one study, increased left amygdala metabolism was found in the depressed state for both conditions.[34] Another study used principal component analysis to group symptoms on the Beck Depression Inventory (BDI) into four clusters (negative cognitions, psychomotor-anhedonia, vegetative, somatic).[35] Intercorrelations between these components and correlations between BDI total and component scores with both absolute and normalized rCMR were evaluated for both major depressive disorder and bipolar disorder patients. The components were not intercorrelated for the major depressive disorder group, suggesting that they represent separate aspects of depression. In the bipolar disorder group, the negative cognitions, psychomotor-anhedonia, and vegetative components were highly intercorrelated, suggesting a much more unified condition. Consistent with these findings, the brain areas in which both absolute and normalized rCMR correlated with each component were distinctly different in the major depressive disorder group, supporting the involvement of different neuronal networks for each symptom cluster. In contrast, for the bipolar disorder group there were no significant correlations for the negative cognitions and vegetative symptoms components using absolute rCMR. There was considerable overlap in brain areas for all components using normalized rCMR. The psychomotor-anhedonia component score had the strongest correlations with rCMR for the bipolar disorder group (stronger than any other component or the total BDI). The psychomotor-anhedonia component scores correlated with lower absolute metabolism in the insula, anteroventral basal ganglia, and temporal and inferior parietal cortices. There was higher normalized metabolism in the anterior cingulate cortex. These results suggest considerably more variability of functioning within the subgroup of individuals diagnosed with major depressive disorder than bipolar disorder, and offer further support that depressive states in bipolar disorder are likely to be neurologically different from depressive states in major depressive disorder, though both share clinical similarities.[35]

Activation Studies

Affective Tasks, Recognition

Facial expression recognition tasks have been used in conjunction with functional imaging to probe prefrontal-limbic system–related performance. Individuals with bipolar disorder have been shown to have impaired ability to discriminate the intensity and valence of emotion. The identified deficits in emotion recognition are state-specific. Subjects in the manic state had significantly impaired recognition of fear and disgust in a task requiring recognition of the six basic emotions (fear, disgust, anger, sadness, surprise, happiness). The most common errors were mislabeling of fear as surprise and disgust as anger.[36] In addition, an inverse correlation was found between the intensity of manic symptoms and recognition of sadness.[36] Other studies have also noted impaired ability to recognize and estimate the intensity of sadness in the manic state.[8,9]

Functional magnetic resonance imaging (fMRI) studies generally have utilized comparison of two emotional states (happiness, sadness or positive, negative). Individuals with bipolar disorder in the manic state have relatively normal patterns of activations to positive emotional states, but not in response to negative emotional states. Negative emotions evoke less cortical and more subcortical activation when the manic state is compared with normal, although the specific areas vary across studies (Figure 10–2).[6–9,37] Overall, these findings are consistent with the impaired ability of bipolar disorder individuals in the manic state to identify and estimate intensity of negative emotions. Future functional imaging studies designed to probe a wider range of emotional recognition, as is done in neuropsychological testing, will be needed to clarify the specific areas associated with particular impairments.

Impaired facial affect recognition has been demonstrated in euthymic individuals with bipolar disorder, although data on specific emotions were not presented.[38] Some studies focusing on the euthymic state fit nicely with those examining mania. In one, an inverse correlation was found between the severity of subclinical manic symptoms and recognition of anger and fear.[39] However, this study also found that euthymic bipolar disorder patients had significantly better than normal identification of disgust (more detected and fewer mislabeled). Another study found that euthymic BD II subjects had significantly better than normal recognition of fear, while euthymic BD I subjects were slightly impaired.[36] In contrast, the BD II subjects were slightly impaired on recognition of disgust, but the BD I subjects were not. Brain activation correlates of these differences are not yet available, as functional imaging studies have reported results on the manic and depressed states only.

Neuropsychological studies of emotion recognition in depression have concentrated on major depressive disorder. As discussed previously, the assumption that major depressive disorder and bipolar disorder depressive states are identical is not supported. Little information is available about emotion recognition by bipolar disorder individuals in the depressed state. One recent study found bipolar disorder subjects in the depressed state no different from normal on recognition of sad, fearful, or happy faces, but more research is clearly needed in this area.[9]

Functional MRI studies have utilized comparison of two or three emotional states (happiness, sadness, fear or positive, negative). Individuals with bipolar disorder in the depressed state had more cortical and subcortical activations to positive emotional states than were seen in either healthy individuals or individuals with major depressive disorder.[7,40] Specifics varied across studies, but included areas in ventral and medial prefrontal and anterior temporal cortices (Figure 10–2). Negative emotions evoked less cortical and more subcortical activation than normal (Figure 10–2). This is similar to the response seen in the manic state, and so may be trait- (rather than state-) associated.

Acute Mood Challenge

All of the above studies have focused on tasks that involve cognitive processing of experimentally selected emotional stimuli. One group has compared rCBF changes (measured by PET) in patients with bipolar disorder following induction of sadness. Sadness was induced by exposure to a personal script of negative life events.[4,10] Bipolar disorder patients (both depressed and euthymic) differed from healthy individuals in having decreased rCBF in medial and orbitofrontal cortex and in not having increased rCBF in subgenual cortex (Figure 10–3). All three groups had increased rCBF in cerebellum and insula and decreased rCBF in parietal cortex. Healthy and depressed bipolar disorder groups both had decreased rCBF in lateral prefrontal cortex. Only the euthymic bipolar disorder group had increased rCBF in dorsal anterior cingulate and premotor cortices.[4]

Patterns of rCBF change were also compared between a euthymic bipolar disorder group and their healthy siblings.[10] Overall the patterns of response were similar, with the exception of the medial frontal cortex. The healthy sibling group had increased (rather than decreased) rCBF in this area. The authors of the study suggested that the differences from the normal pattern in orbitofrontal and dorsal anterior cingulate cortices may be trait-related, as they were present in both the bipolar disorder groups and healthy siblings. Two euthymic bipolar disorder groups responsive to different mood-stabilizing medications were also compared. The lithium-responsive group had fewer areas of decreased rCBF in medial frontal cortex, and increased (rather than decreased) rCBF in rostral anterior cingulate cortex (Figure 10–3). The authors noted that decreased activity in this region may indicate more severe illness, as it is believed to be involved in detecting shifts in affect and correcting emotional responses.

Conclusions

Functional neuroimaging of bipolar disorder is still at a relatively early stage of development, compared to neuroimaging data on other mental disorders. Multiple complicating factors have likely contributed to the relative paucity of research on bipolar disorder, including diagnostic difficulties related to subtypes and differentiation between the mood disorders. Additionally, capturing and measuring state immediately prior to scan and controlling for the medication variability further complicate neuroimaging studies. Affective tasks selected to study bipolar disorder tend to generally include a cognitive processing component. Further research in this area is needed, with specific focus on emotion induction, rather than emotion recognition tasks. Studies should consider, control, and report, as much as possible, data on vital patient variables, such as state at time of scan, medication, and comorbidities.

References

1. Blumberg HP, Stern E, Martinez D, et al: Increased anterior cingulate and caudate activity in bipolar mania. Biol Psychiatry 2000; 48:1045–1052
2. Blumberg HP, Stern E, Ricketts S: Rostral and orbital perfrontal cortex dysfunction in the manic state of bipolar disorder. Am J Psychiatry 1999; 156:1986–1988
3. Drevets WC, Price JL, Simpson JR, et al: Subgenual prefrontal cortex abnormalities in mood disorders. Nature 1997; 286:824–827
4. Kruger S, Seminowicz D, Goldapple K, et al: State and trait influences on mood regulation in bipolar disorder: blood flow differences with an acute mood challenge. Biol Psychiatry 2003; 54:1274–1283
5. Ketter TA, Kimbrell TA, George MS, et al: Effects of mood and subtype on cerebral glucose metabolism in treatment-resistant bipolar disorder. Biol Psychiatry 2001; 49:97–109
6. Malhi GS, Lagopoulos J, Sachdev P, et al: Cognitive generation of affect in hypomania: an fMRI study. Bipolar Disord 2004; 6:271–285
7. Malhi GS, Lagopoulos J, Ward PB, et al: Cognitive generation of affect in bipolar depression: an fMRI study. Eur J Neurosci 2004; 19:741–754
8. Lennox BR, Jacob R, Calder AJ, et al: Behavioral and neurocognitive responses to sad facial affect are attenuated in patients with mania. Psychol Med 2004; 34:795–802
9. Chen CH, Lennox B, Jacob R, et al: Explicit and implicit facial affect recognition in manic and depressed states of bipolar disorder: a functional magnetic resonance imaging study. Biol Psychiatry 2005; 59:31–39
10. Kruger S, Alda M, Young LT, et al: Risk and resilience markers in bipolar disorder: brain responses to emotional challenge in bipolar patients and their healthy siblings. Am J Psychiatry 2006; 163:177–179
11. Liotti M, Mayberg H, Brannan S, et al: Differential limbic–cortical correlates of sadness and anxiety in healthy subjects: implications for affective disorders. Biol Psychiatry 2000; 48:30–42
12. American Psychiatric Association: Diagnostic and Statistical Manual of Mental Disorders, 4th Edition, Text Revision. Washington, DC, American Psychiatric Association, 2000
13. Bauer M, Pfennig A: Epidemiology of bipolar disorder. Epilepsia 2005; 46:8–13
14. Hirschfeld RMA, Vornik LA: Recognition and diagnosis of bipolar disorder. J Clin Psychiatry 2004; 65:5–9
15. Malhi GS, Ivanovski B, Szekeres V, et al: Bipolar disorder: it's all in your mind? The neuropsychological profile of a biological disorder. Can J Psychiatry 2004; 49:813–819
16. Cuellar AK, Johnson SL,Winters R: Distinctions between bipolar and unipolar depression. Clin Psychol Rev 2005; 25:307–339
17. Sheline YI: Neuroimaging studies of mood disorder effects on the brain. Biol Psychiatry 2003; 54:338–352
18. Drevets WC: Functional anatomical abnormalities in limbic and prefrontal cortical structures in major depression. Prog Brain Res 2000; 126:413–431
19. Drevets WC: Neuroimaging abnormalities in the amygdala in mood disorders. Ann N Y Acad Sci 2003; 985:420–444
20. Haldane M, Fangou S: New insights help define the pathophysiology of bipolar affective disorder: neuroimaging and neuropathology findings. Prog Neuropsychopharmacol Biol Psychiatry 2004; 28:943–960
21. Blumberg HP, Kaufman J, Martin A, et al: Amygdala and hippocampal volumes in adolescents and adults with bipolar disorder. Arch Gen Psychiatry 2003; 60:1201–1208
22. Altshuler LL, Bartzokis G, Grieder T, et al: An MRI study of temporal lobe structures in men with bipolar disorder or schizophrenia. Biol Psychiatry 2000; 48:147–162
23. Soares J, Kochunov P, Monkul E, et al: Structural brain changes in bipolar disorder using deformation field morphometry. Neuroreport 2005; 16:241–244
24. Doris A, Belton E, Ebraheim NA, et al: Reduction of cingulate gray matter density in poor outcome bipolar illness. Psychiatry Res 2004; 130:153–159

25. Frangou S: The Maudsley Bipolar Disorder Project. Epilepsia 2005; 46:19–25
26. Bruno SD, Barker GJ, Cercignani M, et al: A study of bipolar disorder using magnetization transfer imaging and voxel-based morphometry. Brain 2004; 127:2433–2440
27. Adler CM, Holland SK, Schmithorst V, et al: Abnormal frontal white matter tracts in bipolar disorder: a diffusion tensor imaging study. Bipolar Disord 2004; 6:197–203
28. Nugent AC, Milham MP, Bain EE: Cortical abnormalities in bipolar disorder investigated with MRI and voxel-based morphometry. Neuroimage 2006; 30:485–497
29. LeDoux JE: Emotion circuits in the brain. Annu Rev Neurosci 2000; 23:155–184
30. Yurgelun-Todd DA, Gruber SA, Kanayama G, et al: fMRI during affect discrimination in bipolar affective disorder. Bipolar Disord 2000; 2:237–248
31. Olley A, Malhi GS, Mitchell PB, et al: When euthymia is just not enough: the neuropsychology of bipolar disorder. J Nerv Ment Dis 2005; 193:323–330
32. Malhi GS, Lagopoulos J, Owen AM, et al: Bipolaroids: functional imaging in bipolar disorder. Acta Psychiatr Scand Suppl 2004; 422:46–54
33. Fu CY, Williams SCR, Clear AJ, et al: Attenuation of the neural response to sad faces in major depression by antidepressant treatment. Arch Gen Psychiatry 2004; 61:877–889
34. Drevets WC, Price JL, Bardgett ME, et al: Glucose metabolism in the amygdala in depression: relationship to diagnostic subtype and plasma cortisol levels. Pharmacol Biochem Behav 2002; 71:431–447
35. Dunn RT, Kimbrell TA, Ketter TA, et al: Principal components of the Beck Depression Inventory and regional cerebral metabolism in unipolar and bipolar depression. Biol Psychiatry 2002; 51:387–399
36. Lembke A, Ketters TA: Impaired recognition of facial emotion in mania. Am J Psychiatry 2002; 159:302–304
37. Altshuler L, Bookheimer S, Proenza MA, et al: Increased amygdala activation during mania: a functional magnetic resonance imaging study. Am J Psychiatry 2005; 162:1211–1213
38. Addington J, Addington D: Facial affect recognition and information processing in schizophrenia and bipolar disorder. Schizophr Res 1998; 32:171–181
39. Harmer CJ, Grayson L, Goodwin GM: Enhanced recognition of disgust in bipolar illness. Biol Psychiatry 2002; 51:298–304
40. Lawrence NS, Williams AM, Surguladze S, et al: Subcortical and ventral prefrontal cortical neural responses to facial expressions distinguish patients with bipolar disorder and major depression. Biol Psychiatry 2004; 55:578–587

Recent Publications of Interest

Malhi GS, Lagopoulos J, Owen AM, et al: Reduced activation to implicit affect induction in euthymic bipolar patients: an fMRI study. J Affect Disord 2007; 97(1–3):109–122
Found diminished prefrontal, cingulate, limbic, and subcortical neural activity in euthymic bipolar patients as compared to healthy subjects during implicit induction of negative and positive affect. The authors provide an extensive discussion of the possible functional significance, organized by word valence and brain region.

Wessa M, Houenou J, Paillere-Martinot ML, et al: Fronto-striatal overactivation in euthymic bipolar patients during an emotional go/nogo task. Am J Psychiatry 2007; 164:638–646
Compared activation patterns induced by emotional and nonemotional versions of a go/nogo task. They reported increased activation in ventral-limbic, temporal, and dorsal brain areas during the emotional go/nogo task in euthymic bipolar patients compared to healthy subjects, suggesting altered emotional modulation of cognitive processing.

Mah L, Zarate CA Jr, Singh J, et al: Regional cerebral glucose metabolic abnormalities in bipolar II depression. Biol Psychiatry 2007; 61:765–775
Measured regional cerebral metabolic rate in medicated bipolar patients and healthy comparison subjects. They found increased metabolism in both cortical and subcortical areas in depressed bipolar patients, similar to what has been reported for the unmedicated state.

Reprinted from Friedman JNW, Hurley RA, Taber KH: "Bipolar Disorder: Imaging State Versus Trait." *Journal of Neuropsychiatry and Clinical Neurosciences* 18:296–301, 2006. Used with permission.

Chapter 11

BLAST-RELATED TRAUMATIC BRAIN INJURY

What Is Known?

KATHERINE H. TABER, PH.D.
DEBORAH L. WARDEN, M.D.
ROBIN A. HURLEY, M.D.

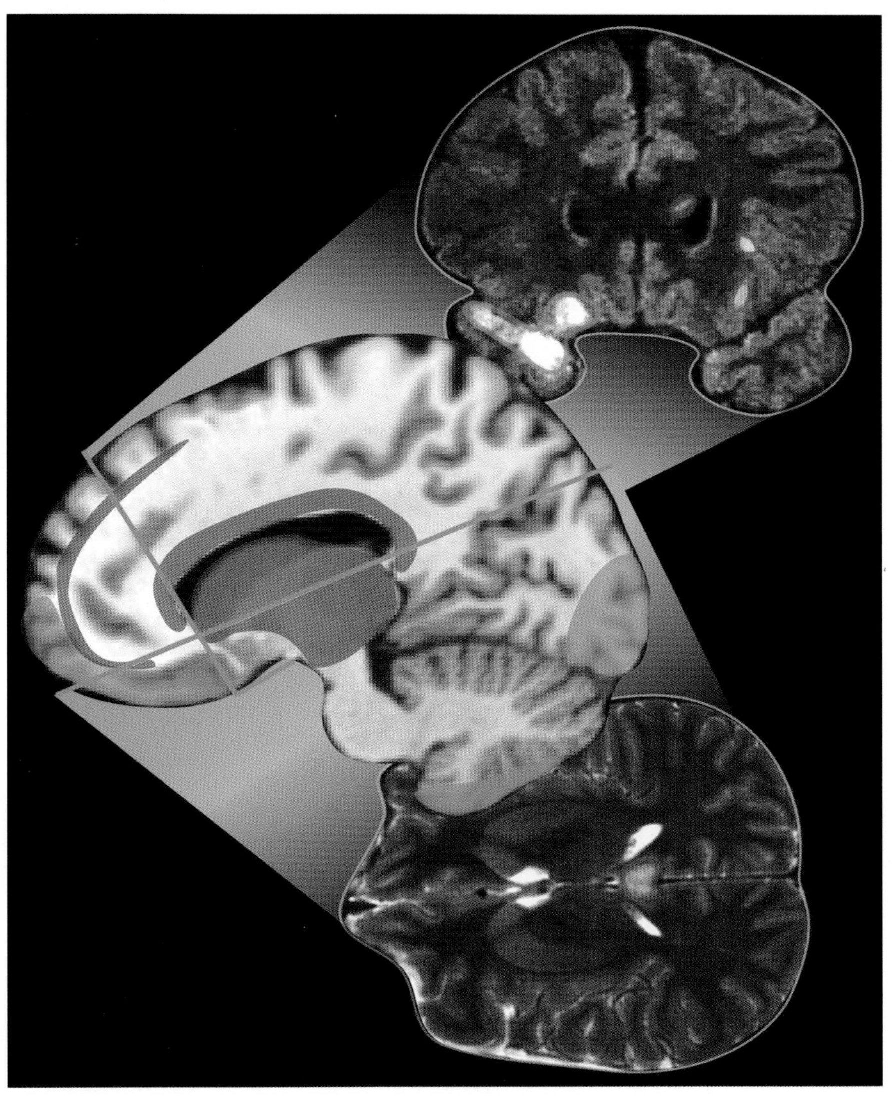

Common types and locations of traumatic brain injury are illustrated on coronal (top), sagittal (middle), and axial (bottom) magnetic resonance images of a young male with neuropsychiatric symptomatology following a combat-related blast exposure (see Figure 11–2 for color-coding).

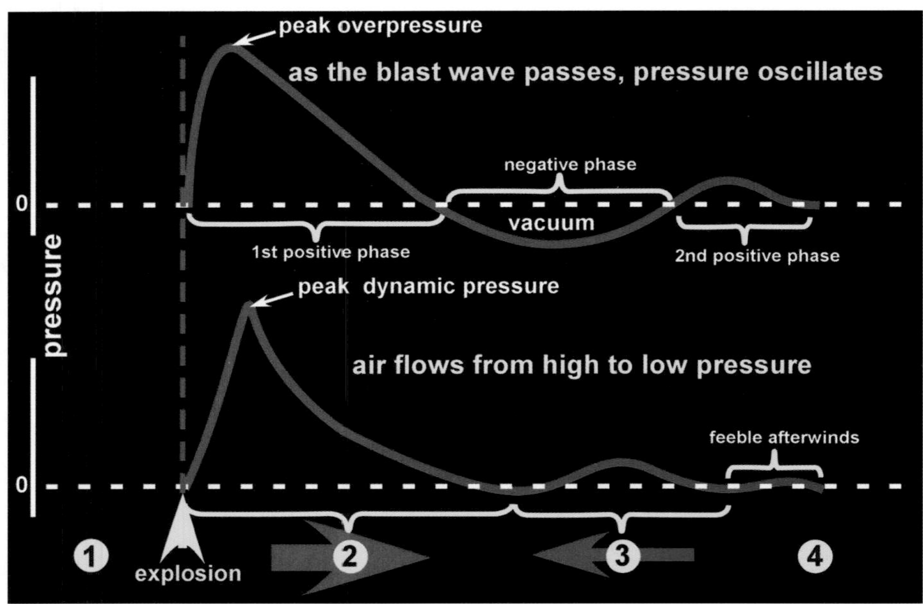

FIGURE 11–1. The sequence of changes in atmospheric pressure following an explosion make up the blast wave. Prior to the explosion (1), pressure is normal. With the passage of the shock front (2), the blast forces are maximal and the wind flows away from the explosion (2, arrow). This is followed by a drop in atmospheric pressure to below normal (3), resulting in the reversed blast wind (3, arrow). Atmospheric pressure returns to normal after the blast wave subsides (4).

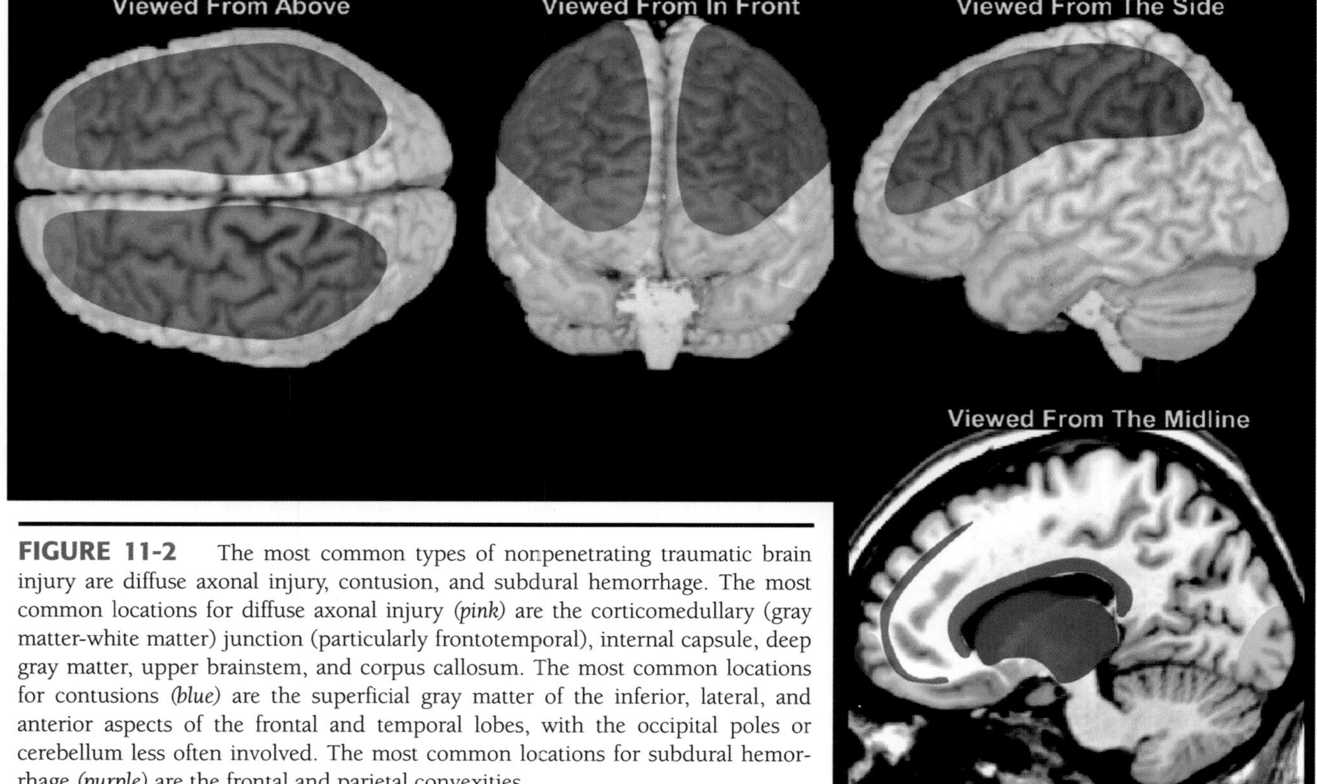

FIGURE 11-2 The most common types of nonpenetrating traumatic brain injury are diffuse axonal injury, contusion, and subdural hemorrhage. The most common locations for diffuse axonal injury *(pink)* are the corticomedullary (gray matter-white matter) junction (particularly frontotemporal), internal capsule, deep gray matter, upper brainstem, and corpus callosum. The most common locations for contusions *(blue)* are the superficial gray matter of the inferior, lateral, and anterior aspects of the frontal and temporal lobes, with the occipital poles or cerebellum less often involved. The most common locations for subdural hemorrhage *(purple)* are the frontal and parietal convexities.

There is an increasing use of improvised explosive devices (IEDs) in terrorist and insurgent activities. Exposure to blast is becoming more frequent. Injuries occur as a direct result of blast wave–induced changes in atmospheric pressure (primary blast injury), from objects put in motion by the blast hitting people (secondary blast injury), and by people being forcefully put in motion by the blast (tertiary blast injury).[1–3] Blast-related injury during war is now very common. A recent study found that 88% of military personnel treated at an echelon II medical unit in Iraq had been injured by IEDs or mortar.[4] Many (47%) of these injuries involved the head. Similarly, 97% of the injuries to one Marine unit in Iraq were due to explosions (65% IEDs, 32% mines).[5] The majority of these (53%) involved the head or neck. The authors noted the importance of prompt evaluation of central nervous system (CNS) symptoms indicative of concussion. Most (82%) returned to duty following an average of 3 (range = 0–30) light duty days.

Historical accounts note that as more powerful explosives came into general use in warfare, a condition was described in which soldiers were rendered dazed or unconscious by an explosion that caused no external visible injury. Retrograde and anterograde amnesia were commonly present upon regaining consciousness or awareness, as were severe headache, tinnitus, hypersensitivity to noise, and tremors.[6–9]

During World War I, there was significant interest in studying and reporting about cases of soldiers who survived blast exposure and developed neuropsychiatric symptoms. Drs. Fred Mott and Gordon Holmes, two famous physicians with the British Army, wrote in great detail about their battlefront hospital experiences.[6,7,10,11] They attempted to describe the neurological/psychiatric status of soldiers postcombat. A variety of names were used for this condition, including *commotio cerebri*, shell shock, and functional neurosis. These early authors had difficulty differentiating physical injury to the brain from emotional trauma. Thus, these terms were often used loosely to describe what would in the year 2006 be diagnosed as posttraumatic delirium or agitation, concussion, acute stress syndrome, posttraumatic stress disorder, psychosis, or conversion disorders. Mott separated these into two groups. For those who were buried by the explosion, he believed the overriding injury to the brain was carbon monoxide poisoning. In the absence of burial or external injury, Mott believed that the condition was purely due to "psychic trauma" or emotional distress.[6,7,10,12] The controversy regarding physical versus emotional cause for "shell shock" (often in this time referred to as cerebral blast syndrome and cerebral blast concussion) continued into World War II. While some physicians were convinced that there was no "organic" injury to the brain, others reported electroencephalographic (EEG) changes similar to those from confirmed closed head injury.[8,9]

Blast-Related Forces

The changes in atmospheric pressure that cause primary blast injuries arise because a high-explosive detonation results from the nearly instantaneous conversion of a solid or liquid into gases.[1–3] Momentarily these gases occupy the same volume as the parent solid or liquid and thus they are under extremely high pressure. The gases expand rapidly, causing compression in the surrounding air, forming a pulse of pressure (blast overpressure, positive phase of the blast wave) (Figure 11–1). As the gases continue to expand the pressure drops, creating a relative vacuum (blast underpressure, negative phase of the blast wave). Extreme pressure differences occur as the blast wave reaches the body, resulting in both stress and shear waves.

Primary blast injury results from blast wave–induced changes in atmospheric pressure (*barotrauma*). Organs and tissues of different densities are accelerated at different relative rates, resulting in displacement, stretching, and shearing forces. The most vulnerable parts of the body to primary blast injury are considered to be those with air–fluid interfaces, particularly the lungs, bowel, and middle ear. Rupture of the tympanic membrane is the most frequent injury. Both the blast wave and blast wind can propel objects with considerable force, causing secondary and tertiary blast injuries. Secondary blast injury results from objects put in motion by the blast wind impacting a person (ballistic trauma). This category includes both injuries due to flying debris and those due to collapse of structures. Tertiary blast injury results from a person being blown into solid objects by the blast wind.

Blast-Related Brain Injury

The brain is clearly vulnerable to both secondary and tertiary blast injury. A still unresolved controversy is whether primary blast forces directly injure the brain. Shear and stress waves from the primary blast could potentially cause traumatic brain injury (TBI) directly (e.g., concussion, hemorrhage, edema, diffuse axonal injury). The primary blast can also cause formation of gas emboli, leading to infarction.[13]

Clinical data for brain injury due to primary blast forces are quite limited. Most studies involve war-related injuries, although blast-related injury due to air blast and firecrackers has also been reported. In a battlefield situation, it can be extremely difficult to confidently identify cases in which *only* primary blast injury is present. In addition, neuropathological information was only occasionally available. Almost a century of medical literature provides a handful of cases in which brain injuries were likely to have resulted from primary blast forces.[9,12,14–17] Reported neuropathological changes have included small hemorrhages within white matter, chromatolytic changes in neurons (due to degeneration of Nissl bodies, an indication of neuronal damage), diffuse brain injury, and subdural hemorrhage. Mott wrote in detail about a few cases where primary blast was the proposed cause of death.[12] He noted a variety of microscopic findings, including an "extremely congested" cortex, perivascular space enlargement, subpial hemorrhages, venous engorgement, white matter hemorrhage into the myelin sheath and perivascular spaces, and chromatolysis. Although Mott believed that most cases of "shell-shock" resulted from "psychic trauma," he was aware that available methods for examining the brain were quite limited.

> So complex is the structure of the human CNS, and so subtile the chemical and physical changes underlying its functions, that because our gross methods of investigating dead material do not enable us to say that the living matter is altered...[6]

The truth of this caution today, though written more than 90 years ago, has recently been reinforced by findings from experimental (animal) studies of TBI.[18] It has been shown that severely injured axons do not necessarily swell. The presence of focal axonal swellings, the most commonly used neuropathological marker for TBI, may therefore seriously underestimate the magnitude of injury present. The authors also noted that the insensitivity of presently used neuropathological markers to the unmyelinated fine caliber axons that make up 30% of corpus callosum may also contribute to inaccurate injury evaluation. Thus, the search for better methods of delineating the microscopic aspects of brain injury continues.

The vulnerability of the brain to primary blast forces is supported by recent animal studies. One group examined the effects of exposure to pure primary blast forces by enclosing their subjects (rats) within a concrete bunker to prevent injury by other mechanisms. They reported widespread microglial activation (a hallmark of neural degeneration), particularly in the superficial layers of the cerebral and cerebellar cortices.[19] Other areas, such as the pineal gland, were also affected.[20] In a later study, performance on tests of coordination, balance, and strength was significantly impaired by exposure to a 20 kPa (kPa is a measure of pressure) explosion but not by exposure to a 2.8 kPa explosion.[21] More degenerating neurons were seen in cerebral cortex following the larger explosion.

Another group (utilizing rabbits and rats) studied the effect on the brain of exposure to primary blast (delivered by a shock tube) sufficient to cause a moderate level of lung injury.[22–24] Special holders were used to prevent occurrence of secondary and tertiary blast injuries. In some cases, the effect of exposing the whole body was compared to exposing only the thoracic region (with the head protected by a steel plate).[23] Both types of blast exposure resulted in ultrastructural evidence of neuronal injury (expanded perineuronal spaces, cytoplasmic vacuoles, myelin deformation, axoplasmic shrinkage) in the areas examined (hippocampus, brainstem reticular formation). The authors noted that the pattern of neuronal abnormalities was similar to those seen in diffuse axonal injury. Biochemical changes indicative of oxidative stress were also present. The degree of neuronal damage correlated with impaired performance on an active avoidance task.

Other groups have reported the effects of exposure to blast forces at levels designed to be below the threshold for induction of macroscopic lung injury.[25,26] One reported a change in localization of neurofilament protein staining from axons and dendrites to the cell body in cortical neurons following exposure (of rats).[25] The authors noted that these changes were likely the result of disturbed anterograde axonal transport. Another group used an open air exposure (utilizing pigs oriented with their hindquarters closest to the explosive) just below the threshold for induction of macroscopic lung injury.[26] Depression of EEG activity was reported in one-half the animals immediately following the blast exposure. EEG amplitude was reduced by about 50% for a short time (5–15 seconds), with a return of normal activity within 1–2 minutes.

Traumatic Brain Injury

The most common types of TBI are diffuse axonal injury, contusion, and subdural hemorrhage (Figure 11–2).[27] Diffuse axonal injuries are very common following closed head injuries. They result when shearing, stretching, and/or angular forces pull on axons and small vessels.[28] Impaired axonal transport leads to focal axonal swelling and (after several hours) may result in axonal disconnection.[29] The most common locations are the corticomedullary (gray matter-white matter) junction (particularly in the frontal and temporal areas), internal capsule, deep gray matter, upper brainstem, and corpus callosum (Figure 11–2, *pink*).[27] Magnetic resonance imaging (MRI) is more sensitive than computed tomography (CT) in detecting diffuse axonal injury.[27,29] T_2-weighted magnetic resonance (MR) images, especially fluid attenuated inversion recovery (FLAIR) images, are best for visualizing nonhemorrhagic lesions. Some studies indicate that diffusion-weighted MRI may be even more sensitive than T_2- weighted for identifying edema.[30] Gradient echo MR images are more sensitive to areas of hemorrhage.[30,31]

Contusions occur when the brain moves within the skull enough to impact bone, causing bruising of the brain parenchyma (hemorrhage and edema). The most common locations are the superficial gray matter of the inferior, lateral, and anterior aspects of the frontal and temporal lobes, with the occipital poles or cerebellum less often involved (Figure 11–2, *blue*).[27] The imaging appearance of contusion is variable.[27] Edema has lower signal intensity than brain on CT. In the absence of hemorrhage, CT may initially be only minimally abnormal. If hemorrhage is present, there are commonly multiple bright areas of variable size. Edema appears bright on T_2-weighted or FLAIR MRI. The most common sequence in the appearance of hemorrhage on T_2-weighted MRI is from bright initially, to mildly strongly dark within the first 2–3 days, to bright again by 2–3 weeks.[32] Small areas of hemorrhage may be most easily identified with gradient echo MRI. Progression is common, with 25% demonstrating delayed hemorrhage over the initial 48 hours.[33]

Traumatic subdural hemorrhage occurs when the brain moves within the skull enough to tear the tributary surface veins that bridge from the brain surface to the dural venous sinus.[32] The most common locations are the frontal and parietal convexities on the same side as the injury (Figure 11–2, *purple*).[27] The usual imaging appearance of subdural hemorrhage is an extraaxial, crescent- shaped, homogeneous fluid collection that conforms to the cerebral surface.[27,32] Its spread is limited by the dural reflections, and it rarely crosses the midline. Collections greater than 5 mm are easily recognized. Smaller collections may be missed due to partial volume effects with adjacent bone. Acute subdural hemorrhage is usually hyperintense on CT, the preferred imaging modality to evaluate for hemorrhage. It may be of mixed intensity or isointense to gray matter in patients with anemia. In these cases, it can be identified by its mass effects, including sulcal effacement, inward buckling of the gray-white interface, and presence of midline shift.

Conclusion

The potential neuropsychiatric implications of such widespread exposure to blast are still uncertain. However, the Defense and Veterans Brain Injury Center (DVBIC) has reported that 59% of an "at risk" group of injured soldiers returning from Afghanistan or Iraq to Walter Reed (2003–2004) suffered at least a mild TBI while in combat.[34,35] Further characterization of 433 war fighters revealed that the TBI was moderate or severe in more than half the group. The TBI was due to a closed head injury in 88%. Similarly, a study of patients with explosive injury only to the lower extremities found that 51% (665/1303) had neurological symptoms (e.g., headache, insomnia, psychomotor agitation, vertigo) consistent with TBI.[36] Of these, 36% had EEG alterations during the acute stage (most commonly hypersynchronous, discontinuous, or irregular brain activity). Both neurological and EEG abnormalities persisted into the chronic stage for 30% of this group. An earlier study found that veterans with posttraumatic stress disorder who had been exposed to blast had EEG abnormalities and attentional difficulties consistent with mild TBI.[37] Thus, the limited clinical evidence to date suggests a similar range of neuropsychiatric impairments as seen with other traumas (e.g., accidents, assaults). In many cases, TBI clearly resulted from secondary and/or tertiary blast injuries. The vulnerability of the human brain to primary blast injury is controversial and an area of active research.[38]

References

1. Mayorga MA: The pathology of primary blast overpressure injury. Toxicology 1997; 121:17–28
2. Wightman JM, Gladish SL: Explosions and blast injuries. Ann Emerg Med 2001; 37:664–678
3. DePalma RG, Burris DG, Champion HR, et al: Blast injuries. N Engl J Med 2005; 352:1335–1342
4. Murray CK, Reynolds JC, Schroeder JM, et al: Spectrum of care provided at an echelon II medical unit during Operation Iraqi Freedom. Mil Med 2005; 170:516–520
5. Gondusky JS, Reiter MP: Protecting military convoys in Iraq: an examination of battle injuries sustained by a mechanized battalion during Operation Iraqi Freedom II. Mil Med 2005; 170:546–549
6. Mott FW: The effects of high explosives upon the CNS. Lecture I. Lancet 1916; 4824:331–338
7. Mott FW: The effects of high explosives upon the CNS. Lecture III. Lancet 1916; 4828:545–553
8. Fabing HD: Cerebral blast syndrome in combat soldiers. Arch Neurol Psychiatry 1947; 57:14–57
9. Cramer F, Paster S, Stephenson C: Cerebral injuries due to explosion waves—"cerebral blast concussion." Arch Neurol Psychiatry 1949; 61:1–20
10. Mott FW: The effects of high explosives upon the CNS. Lecture II. Lancet 1916; 4826:441–449
11. Macleod AD: Shell shock, Gordon Holmes and the Great War. J R Soc Med 2004; 97:86–89
12. Mott FW: The microscopic examination of the brains of two men dead of *commotio cerebri* (shell shock) without visible external injury. J R Army Med Corps 1917; 29:662–677

13. Guy RJ, Glover MA, Cripps NP: Primary blast injury: pathophysiology and implications for treatment. Part III: Injury to the central nervous system and the limbs. J R Nav Med Serv 2000; 86:27–31
14. Sylvia FR, Drake AI, Wester DC: Transient vestibular balance dysfunction after primary blast injury. Mil Med 2001; 66:918–920
15. Murthy JMK, Chopra JS, Gulati DR, et al: Subdural hematoma in an adult following a blast injury. J Neurosurg 1979; 50:260–261
16. Hirsch AE, Ommaya AK: Head injury caused by underwater explosion of a firecracker. J Neurosurg 1972; 37:95–99
17. Levi L, Borovich B, Guilburd JN, et al: Wartime neurosurgical experience in Lebanon, 1982–85. II. Closed craniocerebral injuries. Isr J Med Sci 1990; 26:555–558
18. Povlishock JT, Katz DI: Update of neuropathology and neurological recovery after traumatic brain injury. J Head Trauma Rehabil 2005; 20:76–94
19. Kaur C, Singh J, Lim MK, et al: The response of neurons and microglia to blast injury in the rat brain. Neuropathol Appl Neurobiol 1995; 21:369–377
20. Kaur C, Singh J, Lim MK, et al: Macrophages/microglia as 'sensors' of injury in the pineal gland of rats following a non-penetrative blast. Neurosci Res 1997; 27:317–322
21. Moochhala SM, Md S, Lu J, et al: Neuroprotective role of aminoguanidine in behavioral changes after blast injury. J Trauma 2004; 56:393–403
22. Cernak I, Savic J, Malicevic Z, et al: Involvement of the CNS in the general response to pulmonary blast injury. J Trauma 1996; 40:100–104
23. Cernak I, Wang Z, Jiang J, et al: Ultrastructural and functional characteristics of blast injury-induced neurotrauma. J Trauma 2001; 50:695–706
24. Cernak I,Wang Z, Jiang J, et al: Cognitive deficits following blast injury-induced neurotrauma: possible involvement of nitric oxide. Brain Inj 2001; 15:593–612
25. Saljo A, Bao F, Haglid KG, et al: Blast exposure causes redistribution of phosphorylated neurofilament subunits in neurons of the adult rat brain. J Neurotrauma 2000; 17:719–726
26. Axelsson H, Hjelmqvist H, Medin A, et al: Physiological changes in pigs exposed to a blast wave from a detonating high-explosive charge. Mil Med 2000; 165:119–126
27. Gutierrez-Cadavid JE: Imaging of head trauma, in Imaging of the Nervous System. Edited by Latchaw RE, Kucharczyk J, Moseley ME. Philadelphia, PA, Elsevier Mosby, 2005, pp 869–904
28. Mendez CV, Hurley RA, Lassonde M, et al: Mild traumatic brain injury: Neuroimaging of sports-related concussion. J Neuropsychiatry Clin Neurosci 2005; 17:297–303
29. Hurley RA, McGowan JC, Arfanakis K, et al: Traumatic axonal injury: Novel insights into evolution and identification. J Neuropsychiatry Clin Neurosci 2004; 16:1–7
30. Huisman TAGM, Sorensen AG, Hergan K, et al: Diffusion-weighted imaging for the evaluation of diffuse axonal injury in closed head injury. J Comput Assist Tomogr 2003; 27:5–11
31. Tong KA, Ashwal S, Shutter LA, et al: Hemorrhagic shearing lesions in children and adolescents with posttraumatic diffuse axonal injury: improved detection and initial results. Radiology 2003; 227:332–339
32. Taber KH, Hayman LA, Diaz-Marchan PJ, et al: Imaging of intracranial blood, in Imaging of the Nervous System. Edited by Latchaw RE, Kucharczyk J, Moseley ME. Philadelphia, PA, Elsevier Mosby, 2005, pp 555–575
33. Orrison WW, Moore KR: Neuroimaging and head trauma, in Neuroimaging. Edited by Orrison WW. WB Philadelphia, PA, Saunders Company, 2000, pp 885–915
34. Okie S: Traumatic brain injury in the war zone. N Engl J Med 2005; 352:2043–2047
35. Warden DL, Ryan LM, Helmick KM, et al: War neurotrauma: the Defense and Veterans Brain Injury Center (DVBIC) experience at Walter Reed Army Medical Center (WRAMC)(abstract). J Neurotrauma 2005; 22:1178
36. Cernak I, Savic J, Ignjatovic D, et al: Blast injury from explosive munitions. J Trauma 1999; 47:96–103
37. Trudeau DL, Anderson J, Hansen LM, et al: Findings of mild traumatic brain injury in combat veterans with PTSD and a history of blast concussion. J Neuropsychiatry Clin Neurosci 1998; 10:308–313
38. Cernak I: Blast (explosion)-induced neurotrauma: A myth becomes reality. Restorative Neurology and Neuroscience 2005; 23:139–140

Recent Publications of Interest

Kato K, Fujimura M, Nakagawa A, et al: Pressure-dependent effect of shock waves on rat brain: induction of neuronal apoptosis mediated by a caspase-dependent pathway. J Neurosurg 2007; 106:667–676

Examined the brains (of rats) for evidence of hemorrhage, contusion, and apoptosis at 4, 24, or 72 hours after exposure to a single explosion-generated shock wave. While only the higher level of shock wave resulted in hemorrhage and contusion, neuronal changes were present at the lower level. The authors speculate that the threshold for shock wave–induced brain injury may be lower than for other organs.

Chavko M, Koller WA, Prusaczyk WK, et al: Measurement of blast waves by a miniature fiber optic pressure transducer in the rat brain. J Neurosci Methods 2007; 159:277–281

Measured the pressure wave within the 3rd ventricle (of rats) following exposure to a low level blast wave generated by a pneumatic pressure–driven shock tube. They found that only a small part of the blast wave was absorbed by the skull, and noted that the changes in wave shape inside the brain suggest differences in wave propagation velocity as a result of reflection from boundaries between tissues of different densities.

Yilmaz S, Pekdemir M: An unusual primary blast injury? Traumatic brain injury due to primary blast injury. Am J Emerg Med 2007; 25:97–98

Presents a clinical case in which a steam boiler explosion resulted in fatal brain injury apparently due to primary blast forces, as there was no evidence of blunt or penetrat-

ing injuries to the head and neck or neurological deficits during the initial examination in the emergency room.

Finkel MF: The neurological consequences of explosives. J Neurol Sci 2006; 249:63–67
Reviews the physics, mechanics, and consequences of explosive blasts, the evolution of nervous system injury, and treatment strategies.

Warden D: Military TBI during the Iraq and Afghanistan wars. J Head Trauma Rehabil 2006; 21:398–402
Provides a brief overview of the epidemiology of combat-related traumatic brain injury, types and mechanisms of blast-related brain injuries, and posttraumatic stress disorder following TBI.

Chapter 12

MILD TRAUMATIC BRAIN INJURY

Neuroimaging of Sports-Related Concussion

CECILIA V. MENDEZ, M.D.
ROBIN A. HURLEY, M.D.
MARYSE LASSONDE, PH.D.
LIYING ZHANG, PH.D.
KATHERINE H. TABER, PH.D.

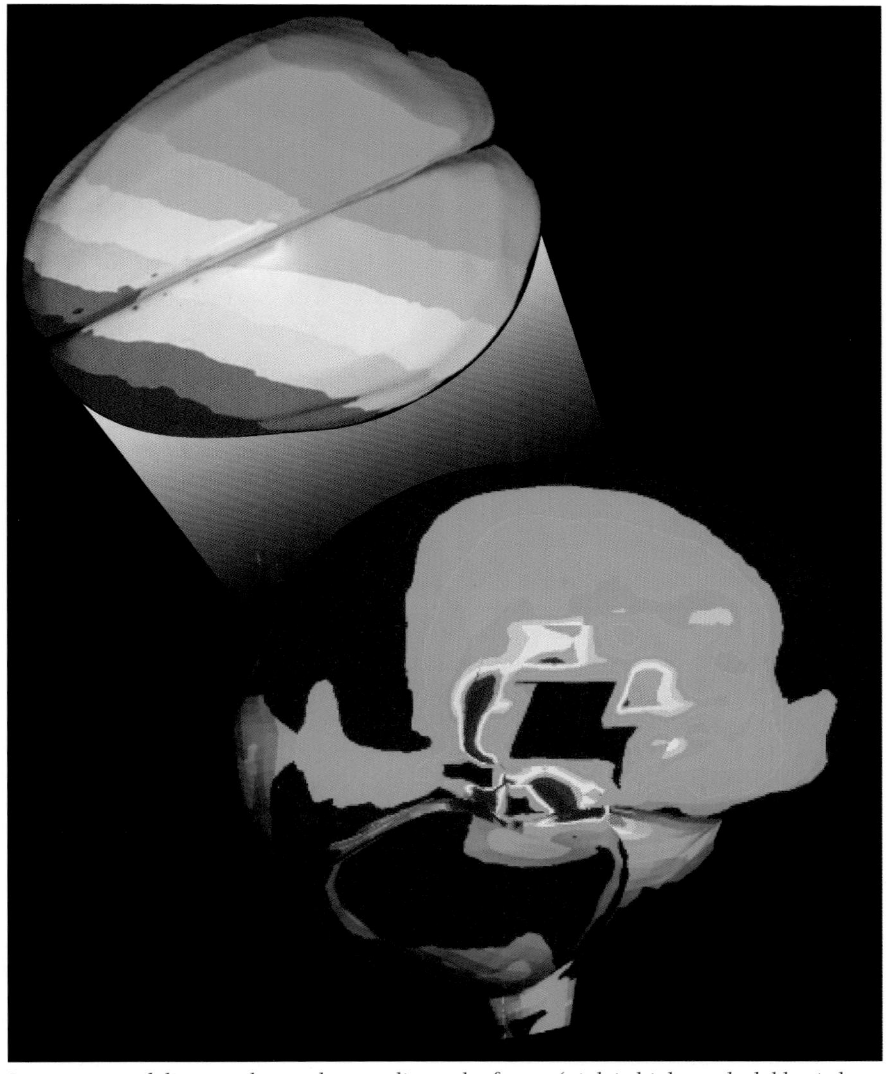

Computer modeling can be used to predicate the forces (*pink* is highest, *dark blue* is lowest) within the brain following a strong blow to the head. The upper image is a view from above of the predicted intracranial pressure. The lower image is a view from the side of the predicted shear stress.

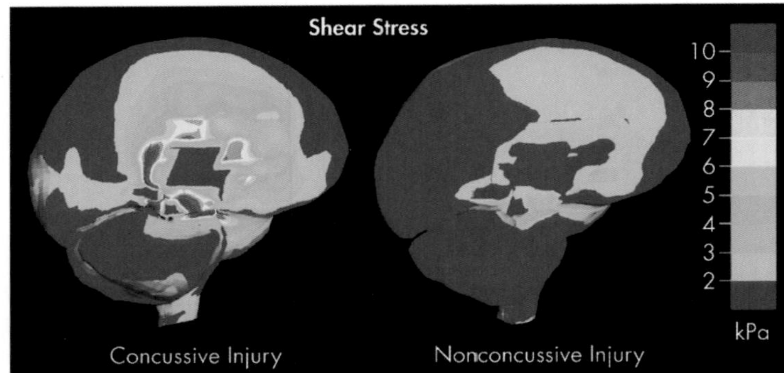

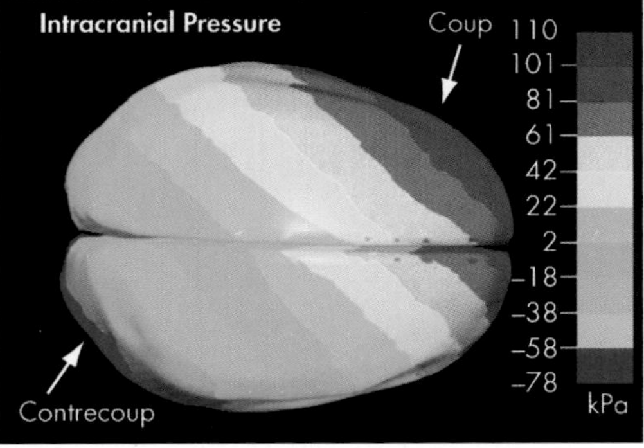

FIGURE 12–1. Computer modeling of forces (expressed as pressure, kPa) can be used to predicate the forces within the brain following a strong blow to the head. The predicted shear stresses (left panel) differentiate concussive from nonconcussive injury. Note the high shear stress (*pink*) in the central core of the brain. The predicted intracranial pressure wave following a concussive blow is shown in the right panel. Note the drastic change from positive pressure (*pink*, coup) to negative pressure (*blue*, contrecoup) across the brain.

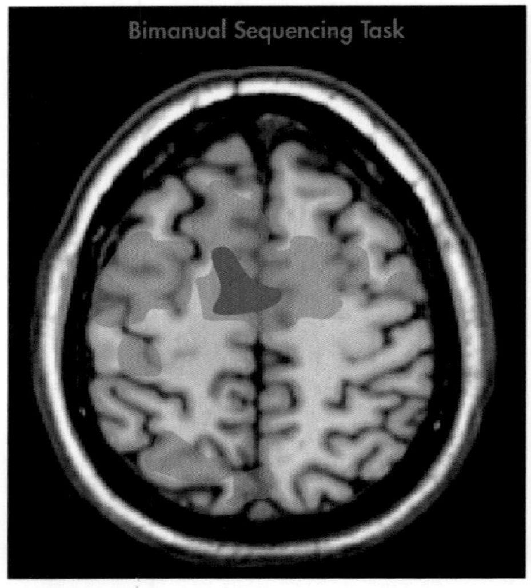

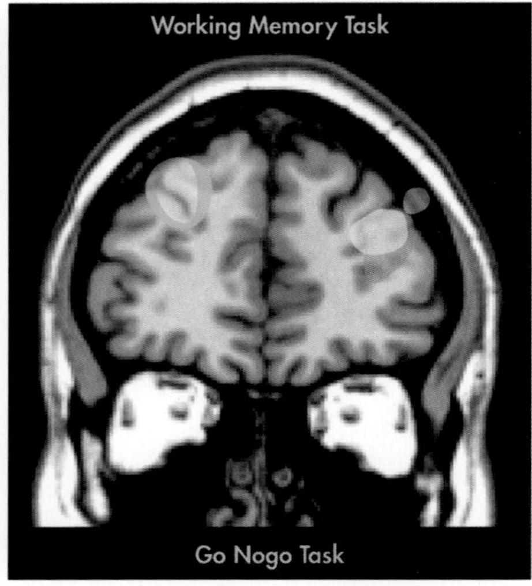

FIGURE 12–2. Task-related brain activation on fMRI may be changed postconcussion.[1–3] Athletes with concussions (shown in light shades) have many more regions of activation than those without (shown in dark shades) during a bimanual sequencing task (*pink*, left) or working memory task (*blue*, right).[1,2] In addition, concussion may be associated with decreased activation in areas critical for task performance. Athletes with concussion had reduced activation in right dorsolateral prefrontal cortex during a working memory task (*light blue*, right).[2] In another study, comparison subjects showed more activation in left dorsolateral prefrontal cortex (*gold*, right) than athletes with concussion during a Go-NoGo task.[3]

Public awareness of sports-related head injuries came to the forefront in the early twentieth century. Between 1869 and 1905, there were 18 deaths and 159 documented serious injuries attributed to the game of football. In response to these alarming numbers, President Theodore Roosevelt convened representatives from the academic institutions governing football to discuss reforming the game. The American Football Rules Committee arose from these conferences.[5–8]

In 1962, the American Medical Association's Committee on Medical Aspects of Sports organized a conference addressing head protection in athletes and associated matters in sports medicine.[5] A greater understanding of the need to determine patterns of injury in order to reduce morbidity in the professional and recreational athletic arenas resulted. Although football was the main focus on the American front, emphasis was placed on head protection in other sports arenas elsewhere. In Sweden, for example, the use of hockey helmets became mandatory in 1963. This was subsequent to an insurance survey that found over 100 closed head injuries, including 1 death, 22 mild traumatic brain injuries (MTBIs), and 3 facial fractures as a result of hockey participation.[9]

Today, multiple sports are associated with concussive events. In excess of 1.5 million people participate in football (i.e., recreational, high school, collegiate, and profes-

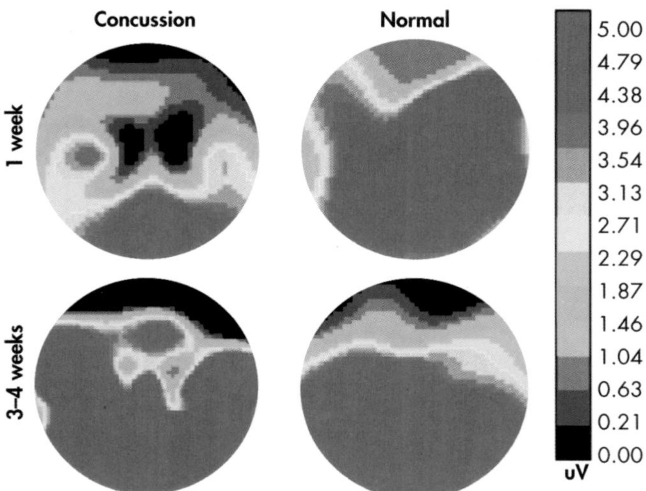

FIGURE 12–3. Bidimensional view of the scalp distribution of the P300 component of the event-related potential associated with the oddball effect (obtained by subtracting the P300 component elicited by the frequent stimulus from that elicited by the rare stimulus) in an athlete who suffered a mild (grade 1) concussion. At 1 week, when the subject was clearly displaying postconcussive symptoms, the oddball effect was quite small. By 4 weeks the patient's symptoms had resolved and a strong oddball effect was seen, very similar to that exhibited by the comparison athlete (matched for age, sex, education) tested at the same time intervals. The color bar presents level of activation from greatest (*orange*) to least (*black*). Used with permission.[4]

sional) annually. The estimated annual incidence of MTBIs in football is 4%–20%.[5] A systematic review of the literature from 1985 to 2000 found ice hockey and rugby to have the highest incidence of concussion for high school, college, and amateur athletes, while soccer had the lowest.[10] At the recreational level, female taekwondo participants and male boxers had the highest frequency of concussion.[10] Of the injuries, 6.2% were concussive in a three-year prospective study among intercollegiate athletes.[11] According to a survey of 1,659 children participating in contact sports, 3% suffered concussions.[12] In addition, an epidemiologic study of collegiate and high school football players found that players who sustain one concussion are three times more likely to sustain a second one in the same season.[13]

Concussion and Postconcussive Syndrome

The term "concussion" is derived from the Latin word *concutere* (to strike together).[14] Another synonymous term, *commotio cerebri*, was introduced in the 16th century by the French military surgeon Pare.[15] Although the symptoms associated with concussion have been recognized for centuries, the term "postconcussion syndrome" was first used in 1934 to describe the "subjective posttraumatic syndrome . . . due directly to the blow on the head."[16,17] Symptoms associated with postconcussion syndrome may include persistent headache, irritability, inability to concentrate, memory impairment, generalized fatigue, dizziness, or a generalized loss of well-being. Commonly, the course is self-limited, resolving usually within 6–8 weeks of the incident.[5]

Most recently, it has been recognized that MTBI may occur as a result of concussion. The Centers for Disease Control and Prevention (CDC) Mild Traumatic Injury Workgroup conceptually defined MTBI as "an injury to the head as a result of blunt trauma or acceleration or deceleration forces that result in one or more of the following conditions: (1) Any period of observed or self-reported transient confusion, disorientation, impaired consciousness, dysfunction of memory around the time of injury, or loss of consciousness lasting less than 30 minutes. (2) Observed signs of neurological or neuropsychological dysfunction, headache, dizziness, irritability, fatigue or poor concentration."[18] According to the CDC (based on the 1991 National Health Interview Survey), the incidence of athletic traumatic brain injuries was approximately 300,000, with only 12% of those injuries requiring hospitalization.[19] The remaining 88% most likely include many MTBIs based on currently accepted definitions.[19] It is important to note that this survey included weighted data collected from 46,761 households where the main outcome measure was the occurrence of one or more incidences of head injury with loss of consciousness. As many concussions in athletics do not result in loss of consciousness, actual occurrence of MTBIs in the athletic arena is likely much higher. A survey of high school football players found that only

47.3% of the athletes who sustained a concussion had reported it at the time of injury.[20] The most common reason for not reporting was the belief that the injury was not serious enough to need medical attention (66.4%). Other cited reasons included not wanting to leave the game (41%), not recognizing that a concussion had occurred (36.3%), and not wanting to disappoint their teammates (22.1%).

The large numbers of athletic-related MTBIs raise concerns about possible short- and long-term sequelae of repetitive injury.[9] Dementia pugilistica in boxers results from repetitive head injury and leads to chronic disability.[5,21] Second impact syndrome (SIS) is rare and potentially fatal. SIS occurs when ". . . an athlete who has sustained an initial head injury, most often a concussion, sustains a second head injury before symptoms associated with the first have fully cleared."[22,23] SIS may result from increased vascular congestion creating cerebral swelling resulting in transtentorial herniation and subsequent death. There were 35 probable cases of SIS in football between 1980 and 1993.[5] There are reports of possible SIS in other sports, including field hockey and skiing. The existence of SIS is controversial, as not all cases fully satisfy diagnostic criteria.[22]

Postconcussive symptoms can also contribute to performance limitations and overall decreased functionality. Athletes who do not exhibit on field mental status changes or report any postconcussive symptoms may still be impaired on neuropsychological testing.[24] A National Collegiate Athletic Association (NCAA) Concussion Study found that college football players with a history of concussion are likely to have future concussive injuries with a 7–10 day window of increased susceptibility. Repetitive concussions may be associated with slower recovery of neurological function.[9] Another study found a prolonged course of recovery in high school as compared to college athletes. Significant memory impairment was present up to 7 days after injury in high school athletes but for only 1 day in college athletes.[25,26] Thus, the age of the athlete must be considered when addressing MTBI management.

Concussion is characterized by a disturbance in neural function that can be profound, causing brief loss of consciousness. Early studies utilizing animal models of concussion indicated that loss of consciousness occurred when the head was unrestrained and hit by an angular acceleration/deceleration process.[27] Recently, finite element (FE) modeling based on professional football head-to-head field collisions has found that rotational acceleration produced maximum shear stress (Figure 12–1).[28] No significant relationship was found between translational acceleration and shear stress. This theoretical analysis is supported by multiple sports studies. A six-year investigation of National Football League players demonstrated that the most susceptible to concussion were quarterbacks, wide receivers, and defensive secondaries who received a face mask impact at an oblique angle.[29] Concussion in hockey is commonly associated with an eccentric blow to the head, a strike to the face or jaw, or a hit directed to the chin.[30] In taekwondo, concussion is primarily due to a roundhouse kick (i.e., angular kick) to the temporal region of the head.[31] Additional proposed biomechanical mechanisms of injury include: sudden movement of the head about the axis of the neck severely stressing the craniospinal junction; hemisphere movement causing stretch of brainstem neurons; rotational loading causing violent impact between the skull and brain; and propagation of intracranial pressure waves deforming brain tissue and depressing skull bone.[32]

Several theories of concussion have been developed to explain the immediate loss of consciousness.[27] Reticular theory is based on the premise that a concussive blow temporarily paralyzes the brainstem reticular formation. Centripetal hypothesis attributes concussion to mechanically induced strains disrupting brain function. Activation of cholinergic neurons resulting in suppression of behavioral responses is central to pontine cholinergic system theory. Convulsive hypothesis attributes concussion to generalized neuronal firing. This theory is supported by the sequence of cerebral hyperexcitability followed by a longer period of depression acutely after head injury.[32–34]

A neurochemical cascade develops immediately following biomechanical insult to the brain, bringing a multitude of cellular changes.[32] Disruption of neuronal membranes and axonal stretching leads to an increase in extracellular potassium and subsequent depolarization and release of excitatory neurotransmitters. This has been termed *neurotransmitter storm*. Thereafter, neuronal suppression occurs diffusely throughout the brain, activating membrane pumps and increasing glucose utilization. Increased lactate production follows. The resultant accumulation may leave neurons more susceptible to further injury.[32] Cerebral blood flow also decreases. *N*-methyl-D-aspartate (NMDA) receptors are activated. There is an influx of calcium into the cell with accumulation in the mitochondria. This impairs oxidative metabolism, leading to energy failure and the possibility of microtubule breakdown. Other neurochemical changes may include: a decrease in γ-aminobutyric acid (GABA) and other inhibitory neurotransmitters, possibly lowering the seizure threshold; decreased magnesium, leading to impaired energy production and neurologic deficits; and loss of forebrain cholinergic neurons, resulting in impaired neurotransmission with possible learning and memory difficulties.[32]

Neuropsychological Testing

Neuropsychological testing is increasingly used in initial assessment of concussion, both on and off the field. In the late 1980s, the University of Virginia completed the first large-scale research study on MTBI in athletes.[35] Neuropsychological testing was utilized to assess cognitive function prior to and following concussion. The Pittsburgh Steelers began using neuropsychological testing in the 1990s to determine return to play decisions. It is now used in other areas of professional athletics, including ice hockey and auto racing.[36] Neuropsychological batteries are also utilized for assessment of short- and long-term postconcussive symptoms. Several return to play guidelines have been developed, based on the degree of symptomatology experienced by the athlete. These guidelines have slight differences in their definitions of grades of concussion and recommendations. At present, all are based on expert opinion rather than prospective studies.[15,37–39] Ideally, baseline testing is obtained at the beginning of the season. At the time of injury, testing is repeated. The choice of specific neuropsychological tests varies, but a battery is chosen to assess cognitive skills, including immediate and delayed recall, orientation, verbal memory, attention span, word fluency, visual scanning, and coordination.[36] Methods of testing range from sideline assessment to computer-based inventories (e.g., Immediate Post Concussion Assessment and Cognitive Testing [ImPACT]).[40]

Imaging

Imaging of diffuse axonal injury was recently reviewed.[41] In brief, computed tomography (CT) is the initial method of choice to evaluate and exclude hemorrhage. T_2-weighted magnetic resonance imaging (MRI), particularly fluid attenuated inversion recovery (FLAIR) MRI, is more sensitive to traumatic lesions.[42,43] Gradient echo MRI is better at detecting hemorrhagic change. However, studies have not been able to correlate abnormal findings on MRI with either postconcussive symptoms or long-term outcome.[42] Diffusion-weighted imaging (DWI) has been shown to identify shearing injuries not evident on T_2/FLAIR or gradient echo sequences, thus making it valuable in evaluating closed head injuries.[44] Diffusion tensor imaging (DTI) examines the integrity of the white matter tracts by measuring the degree and direction of water diffusion, providing a potential marker for white matter injury.[45,46]

Studies utilizing positron emission tomography (PET) and single-photon emission computed tomography (SPECT) have demonstrated frontal and/or temporal hypometabolism following MTBI at rest and during working memory tasks.[47,48] This has been hypothesized to correlate with decreased memory function. Several recent studies have assessed the potential of functional MRI (fMRI) to provide more thorough assessment following concussion. fMRI provides information regarding neural function during task performance and is noninvasive.[1–3] Tasks can be tailored to obtain information regarding specific neurological functions. A small prospective study of college football players compared individual brain activation patterns prior to and following concussive injury.[1] Brain activation was more widespread following concussion compared to both preinjury levels and uninjured subjects during the performance of various memory and sensorimotor tasks (Figure 12–2). Performance was unchanged compared to baseline measures. The motor sequencing tasks were the most sensitive to concussion. The authors note that these results are consistent with cognitive load–induced recruitment of neural resources. Another fMRI study evaluated working memory in adult athletes who had sustained a concussion (1–14 months prior to study) and were experiencing postconcussive symptoms.[2] Athletes with concussions had less task-related activation in the mid-dorsolateral prefrontal cortex (important for working memory) than comparison subjects (Figure 12–2). There was an inverse correlation between right dorsolateral prefrontal cortex activation and severity of symptoms. None of the symptomatic athletes had evidence of axonal injury on structural MRI. Thus, functional impairment may be present in the absence of abnormalities on clinical imaging. In addition, concussed athletes had widespread activations in areas not activated in comparison subjects. In one subject, a follow-up study showed that resolution of symptoms was accompanied by normalization of the activation pattern. Finally, less than normal activation was found in dorsolateral prefrontal cortex in a task requiring response inhibition (Figure 12–2).[3] These studies provide the framework for the possible clinical utility of fMRI in concussive injury in athletes.

Standard electroencephalographic (EEG) techniques have had limited value in the assessment of MTBI.[49,50] One study utilized EEG patterns in isolation and during postural tasks in comparison subjects versus asymptomatic athletes postinjury (mean of 89.4 days) to evaluate any residual effects of concussion on global cortical function.[51] The authors reported an overall decrease in EEG power in all bandwidths studied, an effect most prominent during standing postures. This suggests a possible explanation for the reduced functional capabilities, such as postural instability, observed in athletes subsequent to concussive injury.[52,53]

Studies utilizing evoked potentials (EPs) and event-related potentials (ERPs) in the evaluation of MTBI have shown more promising results. Both EPs and ERPs represent the averaged EEG signal in response to a given stimulus. EPs are thought to represent processing in the primary sensory pathways, whereas ERPs are associated with cognitive processes. EP studies have consistently found the cortical waveform to be briefly extinguished immediately after concussion in animal models.[54] The brainstem auditory evoked potential (BAEP) has been primarily utilized as it is a marker of brainstem function. There have been reports of change in BAEP latency subsequent to concussion, as well as studies that report no change.[50,54] Thus, to date, results are mixed.

ERPs may be more useful. One study examined ERPs evoked following MTBI in college athletes.[4] Concussed athletes demonstrated a significant decrease in the waveform around 300 msec (P300), which was related to the severity of postconcussive symptoms (Figure 12–3). Another study compared the effects of concussion on attention and ERPs in athletes based on their symptomatology.[55] Longer reaction times were exhibited by symptomatic athletes compared to asymptomatic ones. In addition, there was an inverse relationship between severity of postconcussion symptoms and P300 amplitude. This effect was not influenced by the length of time since injury. This suggests that concussive symptomatology affects attentional capacities. As ERPs are resistant to practice effects, this approach is promising as a possible diagnostic tool in MTBI.

A relatively new approach to evaluation of MTBI is magnetic source imaging (MSI). MSI integrates anatomic data from MRI with electrophysiology data from magnetoencephalography (MEG).[56] MEG measures the neuromagnetic field of the dendrites organized parallel to the skull surface (as compared to EEG that measures the potential gradients of dendrites perpendicular to the skull surface). It allows tracking of real-time brain activity without distortions by differences in conductivity between the brain, skull, and scalp.[57] One study compared MRI and resting EEG with resting MSI in postconcussive subjects versus comparison subjects.[56] Results indicated that MSI detected more patients with postconcussive symptoms than either EEG or MRI alone. All patients with abnormal EEG or MRI also had abnormal MSI. To date, there are no published studies evaluating MTBI with MSI in athletes.

Conclusion

Recognition of the high incidence of sports-related concussions has increased interest in MTBI assessment and prognosis. Neuropsychological testing is beginning to play a more integral role in the evaluation of the concussed athlete. Functional imaging studies allow comparison pre- and postinjury. In this context, fMRI, ERPs, and MSI are promising tools in the evaluative process. It is critical to find a means of detecting possible neurological consequences of MTBI, however subtle, and identifying the neuropsychological and neurophysiological impairments caused by a sports-related concussion. Specifically, assessing recovery for several brain functions and their underlying neuronal mechanisms will permit development of tools for rapid and efficient diagnosis. Further, a better understanding of recovery will guide return to play decisions as well as special measures and accommodations that need to be taken to carry out daily activities.

References

1. Jantzen KJ, Anderson B, Steinberg FL, et al: A prospective functional MR imaging study of mild traumatic brain injury in college football players. Am J Neuroradiol 2004; 25:738–745
2. Chen JK, Johnston KM, Frey S, et al: Functional abnormalities in symptomatic concussed athletes: an fMRI study. Neuroimage 2004; 22:68–82
3. Easdon C, Levine B, O'Connor C, et al: Neural activity associated with response inhibition following traumatic brain injury: an event-related fMRI investigation. Brain Cogn 2004; 54:136–138
4. Dupuis F, Johnston KM, Lavoie M, et al: Concussions in athletes produce brain dysfunction as revealed by event-related potentials. Neuroreport 2000; 11:4087–4092
5. Bailes JE, Cantu RC: Head injury in athletes. Neurosurgery 2001; 48:26–46
6. Kay Hawes, National Collegiate Athletic Association: The NCAA Century Series Part I: 1900–1939. http://www.ncaa.org/about/ncaacenturyseries.html
7. The Roosevelt Rough Writer: The Newsletter for Volunteers in Part at Sagamore Hill. 2005; 1
8. Levy ML, Ozgur BM, Berry C, et al: Birth and evolution of the football helmet. Neurosurgery 2004; 55:656–661
9. Guskiewicz KM, McCrea M, Marshall SW, et al: Cumulative effects associated with recurrent concussion in collegiate football players. JAMA 2003; 290:2549–2555
10. Koh JO, Cassidy JD, Watkinson EJ: The incidence of concussion in contact sports: a systematic review of the evidence. Brain Inj 2005; 17:901–917
11. Covassin T, Swanik CB, Sachs ML: Epidemiological considerations of concussions among intercollegiate athletes. Appl Neuropsychol 2003; 10:12–22
12. Radelet MA, Lephart SM, Rubinstein EN, et al: Survey of the injury rate for children in community sports. Pediatrics 2002; 110:e28
13. Guskiewicz KM, Weaver NL, Padua DA, et al: Epidemiology of concussion in collegiate and high school football players. The American Journal of Sports Medicine 2000; 28:643–650
14. The American Heritage Dictionary of the English Language, 4th edition. Boston, MA, Houghton Mifflin, 2000

15. Maroon JC, Lovell MR, Norwig J, et al: Cerebral concussion in athletes: evaluation and neuropsychological testing. Neurosurgery 2000; 47:659–669
16. Pellman EJ, Viano DC, Casson IR, et al: Concussion in professional football: injuries involving 7 or more days out—part 5. Neurosurgery 2004; 55:1100–1119
17. Strauss I, Savitsky N: Head injury: neurologic and psychiatric aspects. Arch Neurol Psychiatry 1934; 31:893–955
18. Gerberding JL, Binder S: Report to Congress on mild traumatic brain injury in the United States: steps to prevent a serious public health problem. 2003
19. Sosin DM, Sniezek JE, Thurman DJ: Incidence of mild and moderate brain injury in the United States, 1991. Brain Inj 1996; 10:47–54
20. McCrea M, Hammeke T, Olsen G, et al: Unreported concussion in high school football players: implications for prevention. Clin J Sport Med 2004; 14:13–17
21. Rabadi MH, Jordan BD: The cumulative effect of repetitive concussion in sports. Clin J Sport Med 2001; 11:194–198
22. McCrory P: Does second impact syndrome exist? Clin J Sport Med 2001; 11:144–149
23. Cantu RC, Voy R: Second impact syndrome: a risk in any contact sport. Phys Sportsmed 1995; 23:27–34
24. Lovell MR, Collins MW, Iverson GL, et al: Grade 1 or "ding" concussions in high school athletes. Am J Sports Med 2004; 32:47–54
25. Lovell MR, Collins MW, Iverson GL, et al: Recovery from mild concussion in high school athletes. J Neurosurg 2003; 98:296–301
26. Field M, Collins MW, Lovell MR, et al: Does age play a role in recovery from sports-related concussion? A comparison of high school and collegiate athletes. J Pediatr 2003; 142:546–553
27. Shaw N: The neurophysiology of concussion. Prog Neurobiol 2002; 67:281–344
28. Zhang L, Yang KH, King AI: A proposed injury threshold for mild traumatic brain injury. J Biomech Eng 2004; 126:226–236
29. Pellman EJ, Viano DC, Tucker AM, et al: Concussion in professional football: location and direction of helmet impacts—part 2. Neurosurgery 2003; 53:1328–1340
30. Biasca N, Wirth S, Tegner Y: The avoidability of head and neck injuries in ice hockey: an historical review. Br J Sports Med 2002; 36:410–427
31. Roh JO, Watkinson EJ: Video analysis of blows to the head and face at the World Taekwondo Championships. J Sports Med Phys Fitness 2002; 42:348–353
32. Giza CC, Hovda DA: The neurometabolic cascade of concussion. J Athl Train 2001; 36:228–235
33. Hayes RL, Dixon CE: Neurochemical changes in mild head injury. Semin Neurol 2005; 14:25–31
34. Regner A, Alves LB, Chemale I, et al: Neurochemical characterization of traumatic brain injury in humans. J Neurotrauma 2005; 18:783–792
35. Alves WM, Rimel RW, Nelson WE: University of Virginia prospective study of football-induced minor head injury: status report. Clin Sports Med 1987; 6:211–218
36. Pellman EJ, Lovell MR, Viano DC, et al: Concussion in professional football: neuropsychological testing—part 6. Neurosurgery 2004; 55:1290–1305
37. Cantu RC: Return to play guidelines after a head injury. Clin Sports Med 1998; 17:45–60
38. Fick DS: Management of concussion in collision sports. Guidelines for the sidelines. Postgrad Med 1995; 97:53–60
39. Kelly JP, Rosenberg JH: The development of guidelines for the management of concussion in sports. J Head Trauma Rehabil 1998; 13:53–65
40. Iverson GL, Lovell MR, Collins MW: Interpreting changes on ImPACT following sports concussion. Clin Neuropsychol 2005; 17:460–467
41. Hurley RA, McGowan JC, Arfanakis K, et al: Traumatic axonal injury: Novel insights into evolution and identification. J Neuropsychiatry Clin Neurosci 2004; 16:1–7
42. Hughes DG, Jackson A, Mason DL, et al: Abnormalities on magnetic resonance imaging seen acutely following mild traumatic brain injury: correlation with neuropsychological tests and delayed recovery. Neuroradiology 2004; 46:550–558
43. Kelly AB, Zimmerman RD, Snow RB, et al: Head trauma: comparison of MR and CT—experience in 100 patients. Am J Neuroradiol 1988; 9:699–708
44. Huisman TAGM, Sorensen AG, Hergan K, et al: Diffusion-weighted imaging for the evaluation of diffuse axonal injury in closed head injury. J Comput Assist Tomogr 2003; 27:5–11
45. Huisman TA, Schwamm LH, Schaefer PW, et al: Diffusion tensor imaging as potential biomarker of white matter injury in diffuse axonal injury. Am J Neuroradiol 2004; 25:370–376
46. Arfanakis K, Haughton VM, Carew JD, et al: Diffusion tensor MR imaging in diffuse axonal injury. Am J Neuroradiol 2002; 23:794–802
47. Chen SHA, Kareken DA, Fastenau PS, et al: A study of persistent post-concussion symptoms in mild head trauma using positron emission tomography. J Neurol Neurosurg Psychiatry 2003; 74:326–332
48. Umile EM, Sandel ME, Alavi A, et al: Dynamic imaging in mild traumatic brain injury: Support for the theory of medial temporal vulnerability. Arch Phys Med Rehabil 2002; 83:1506–1513
49. Pointinger H, Sarahrudi K, Poeschl G, et al: Electroencephalography in primary diagnosis of mild head trauma. Brain Inj 2002; 16:799–805
50. Gaetz M, Bernstein DM: The current status of electrophysiologic procedures for the assessment of mild traumatic brain injury. J Head Trauma Rehabil 2001; 16:386–405
51. Thompson J, Sebastianelli W, Slobounov S: EEG and postural correlates of mild traumatic brain injury in athletes. Neurosci Lett 2005; 377:158–163
52. Bleiberg J, Cernich AN, Cameron K, et al: Duration of cognitive impairment after sports concussion. Neurosurgery 2005; 54:1073–1078
53. Echemendia RJ, Putukian M, Mackin RS, et al: Neuropsychological test performance prior to and following sports-related mild traumatic brain injury. Clin J Sport Med 2001; 11:23–31
54. Noseworthy JH, Miller J, Murray TJ, et al: Auditory brainstem responses in postconcussive syndrome. Arch Neurol 1981; 38:275–278
55. Lavoie ME, Dupuis F, Johnston KM, et al: Visual p300 effects beyond symptoms in concussed college athletes. J Clin Exp Neuropsychol 2004; 26:55–73
56. Lewine JD, Davis JT, Sloan JH, et al: Neuromagnetic assessment of pathophysiologic brain activity induced by minor head trauma. Am J Neuroradiol 1999; 20:857–866
57. Wheless JW, Castillo E, Maggio V, et al: Magnetoencephalography (MEG) and magnetic source imaging (MSI). Neurologist 2004; 10:138–153

Recent Publications of Interest

Kirkwood MW, Yeates KO, Wilson PE: Pediatric sport-related concussion: a review of the clinical management of an oft-neglected population. Pediatrics 2006; 117:1359–1371

Reviews the literature related to postconcussion clinical care for young athletes, including how younger and older athletes may differ.

Gosselin N, Theriault M, Leclerc S, et al: Neurophysiological anomalies in symptomatic and asymptomatic concussed athletes. Neurosurgery 2006; 58:1151–1161

Compared event-related potentials in athletes still symptomatic following a concussion, asymptomatic athletes, and nonconcussed athletes. Both symptomatic and asymptomatic athletes exhibited deficits in auditory information processing, suggesting impaired brain function in both groups.

Wall SE, Williams WH, Cartwright-Hatton S, et al: Neuropsychological dysfunction following repeat concussion in jockeys. J Neurol Neurosurg Psychiatry 2006; 77:518–520

Compared neurological and neuropsychological functioning in jockeys reporting multiple versus single concussions. They found greater impairment in response inhibition and divided attention associated with a history of multiple injuries, with younger individuals more vulnerable than older.

Reprinted from Mendez CV, Hurley RA, Lassonde M, et al: "Mild Traumatic Brain Injury: Neuroimaging of Sports-Related Concussion." *Journal of Neuropsychiatry and Clinical Neurosciences* 17:297–303, 2005. Used with permission.

Chapter 13

TRAUMATIC AXONAL INJURY

Novel Insights Into Evolution and Identification

ROBIN A. HURLEY, M.D.
JOSEPH C. MCGOWAN, PH.D.
KONSTANTINOS ARFANAKIS, PH.D.
KATHERINE H. TABER, PH.D.

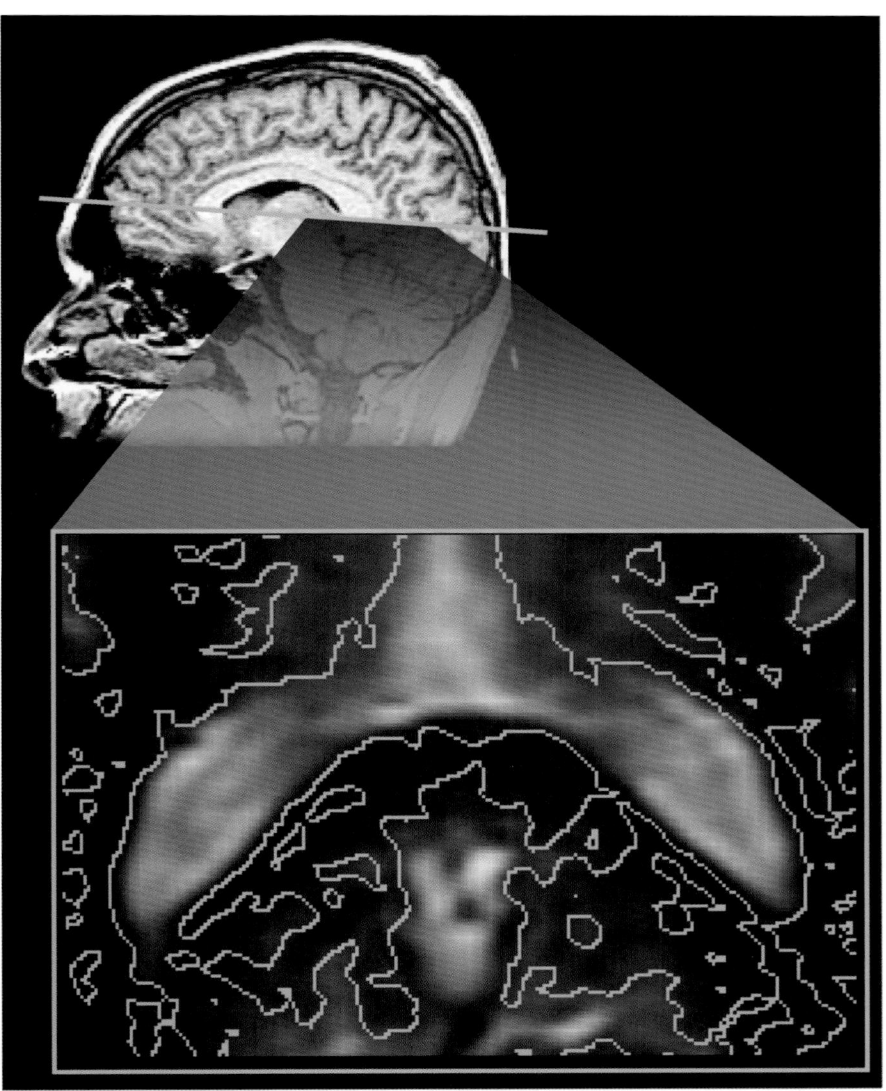

(Bottom) An axial contour map (*irregular green lines*) of areas that are more than 2 standard deviations below normal white matter magnetization transfer ratio in the region of the splenium of the corpus callosum in a patient with traumatic brain injury. (Top) The approximate axial section is indicated (*straight green line*) on a normal sagittal T_1-weighted MR scan.

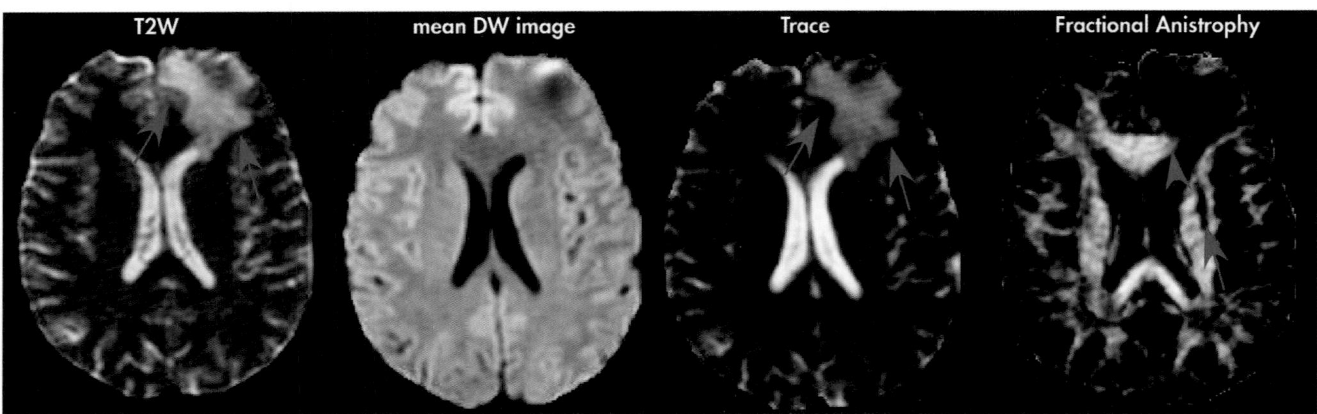

FIGURE 13–1. Axial diffusion tensor imaging. An area with vasogenic edema is visible in the left frontal lobe on the T_2-weighted image (arrows). It is much less evident on the mean diffusion-weighted (DW) map of the same section, produced by averaging the diffusion-weighted images obtained in all 23 noncolinear directions of the diffusion gradients. The corresponding trace map shows increased diffusivity in the left frontal lobe (arrows). In the fractional anisotropy map of the same section, decreased anisotropy is visible in the left anterior portion of the corpus callosum due to the presence of vasogenic edema (arrowhead). Diffusion anisotropy is also decreased in the anterior portion of the left internal and external capsules (arrow), although these regions are characterized by normal T_2 and trace values.

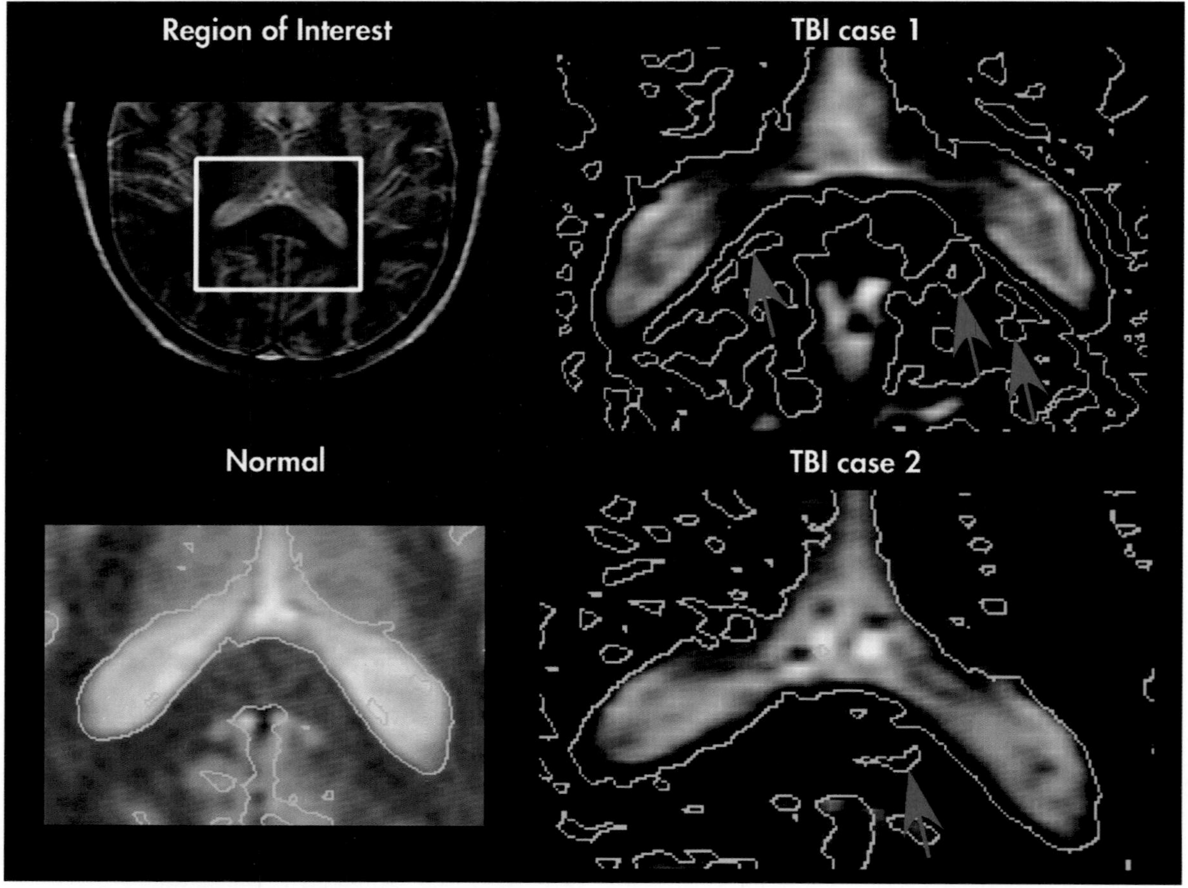

FIGURE 13–2. Axial magnetization transfer imaging. A box indicates the region of the splenium of the corpus callosum in which a detailed analysis was performed by overlaying contours that correspond to 2 standard deviations (SD) below normal white matter magnetization transfer ratio (MTR). Arrows indicate regions in which the MTR was more than 2 SD below normal in these two traumatic brain injury (TBI) cases. Both patients had cognitive impairments consistent with TBI.

Traumatic brain injury (TBI) is an often devastating and common problem that affects today's society. Only rough estimates of incidence and sequelae can be obtained, as many of the milder injuries go initially unreported. Current estimates note an incidence of 1.5–2 million a year in the United States, most commonly from motor vehicle accidents.[1] It occurs bimodally in age groups from the teens through the twenties and after age 70. 80% are mild injury; 10%–13% moderate; and 7%–10% severe.[2] A large portion of these surviving patients will have cognitive or emotional sequelae and will need neuropsychiatric interventions years after the injury. For example, 10%–75% of these patients have been reported to have depression.[3] It is therefore essential to try to understand the pathophysiology of brain injury, be able to perform adequate diagnostic evaluations, and intervene as early as possible, in hopes of limiting continual injury processes.

In the last 20 years, improved clinical management has significantly reduced mortality, and for those who survive, new research has identified secondary injury processes that continue in the first hours and days postinjury that may be amenable to therapeutic intervention. Much of the current work in TBI focuses on these processes and their therapeutic management potential. An excellent review of the history of research in acute brain injury was recently written.[4] Beginning with a review of the anatomy of the neuron, its subcellular structure, and normal function, the authors discuss the biomechanics of the forces of TBI (rotational and translational), the implications of injury impact location, and the microscopic sequelae of the initial impact. Primary, secondary, and tertiary processes of injury to axons are emphasized. Difficulties in creating laboratory models of acceleration/deceleration injury, the problems associated with current research strategies, and how the theories of axonal injury have changed over the years are also addressed. The review closes with a consideration of imaging techniques for the acute TBI patient as well as potential interventions that may be on the horizon.[4] This current communication focuses on three new concepts—new information regarding microscopic pathophysiology of secondary axonal injury; new diagnostic tests to quantify injury; and new imaging techniques that better identify axonal injury in TBI patients.

Diffuse Axonal Injury—Microscopic Evaluation

Diffuse axonal injury (DAI) is a term applied to TBI-induced scattered destruction of white matter tracts. It was first described in 1955 by Lindenberg in patients with posttraumatic hemorrhage of the corpus callosum.[5] DAI can only be definitively diagnosed postmortem. DAI, as detected via histological assessment, is generally associated with shearing injuries, especially those involving acceleration/deceleration. Typically, these patients show significant morbidity without evidence of mass lesions on early imaging. Correlation between axonal injury and the presence of neuropsychological abnormalities, even years after injury, has been described [for review see[6]].

Recent research has determined that initial axonal injury is an ongoing process, evolving over several hours to days. When first identified almost 50 years ago in postmortem analysis using silver salts, the finding of grossly swollen axonal bulbs in humans suggested that the axons were mechanically torn at the moment of injury, with an expulsion of their axoplasm to form the axonal bulb.[4] Experimental studies in animals as well as humans, by Povlishock and colleagues in the early eighties, rejected this premise, showing that the forces of injury focally perturbed the axon, leading to impaired axonal transport that then led to focal axonal swelling, followed over several hours by axonal disconnection.[7] These findings have been confirmed by multiple laboratories, leading to universal acceptance of the phenomenon that diffuse axonal injury involves progressive/evolving change and ultimately leads to axonal disconnection many hours postinjury.

In addition to the recognition of the evolving changes associated with DAI, Povlishock and colleagues have also followed the downstream consequences of the axonal disconnection, showing that the diffuse axonal injury translates into diffuse synaptic terminal loss that then sets the stage for either adaptive or maladaptive neuroplasticity, perhaps explaining some of the morbidity found in these patients.[7] Recognizing the evolving nature of diffuse axonal injury and its linkage to focally impaired axonal transport, more contemporary studies seeking to identify DAI in both the laboratory and forensic setting have relied on antibodies targeting amyloid precursor protein (APP), which is known to be delivered by axonal transport. Its anterograde passage is impeded by axonal injury, with subsequent accumulation in the axonal swelling. At present, antibodies to APP are the gold standard in both the experimental and forensic setting as well as in the evaluation of many preclinical drug studies focusing on the ability of various drugs to attenuate APP-positive swellings.[4]

While members of the research and clinical community have agreed that axonal swellings and disconnection are the consequence of injury and, as such, contribute to the adverse consequences of traumatic injury, new information arising from the experimental setting suggests that not all traumatically injured axons may go on to swell.[8] This suggests that studies focusing on APP-positive swellings may underestimate the total number of axons injured by the traumatic event. This potential was first recognized by Povlishock and colleagues in studies seeking to better understand the subcellular mechanisms initiating traumatically induced axonal injury and swelling. Previous studies had shown that the traumatic episode perturbed the interaxonal cytoskeleton and impaired axonal transport. The assumption was advanced that these events were casually interrelated within the same axon. Recently, however, more critical assessment of these issues, using double label immunofluorescent approaches, suggested that this premise was overly simplistic, underestimating the complexity of the pathobiology of DAI.[9] Specifically, via double label approaches, some axons were recognized to demonstrate cytoskeletal alteration and detachment, without the subsequent formation of an axonal swelling. In contrast, in other axons, axonal swelling occurred, sometimes independent of overt cytoskeletal damage. These studies have been subsequently confirmed via other approaches, collectively illustrating the complexity of the pathobiology of traumatically induced axonal change and the danger of relying on one individual marker of axonal injury to estimate the degree and extent of the traumatically induced axonal change.[9,10] Preliminary studies conducted by Stone and colleagues in humans suggest that these same events described in animals are also ongoing in man, thereby suggesting the need for caution in human postmortem and forensic analyses that rely exclusively on markers targeting axonal swelling as the sole endpoint.[9]

Clinical Interventions

Serum Markers

As novel discoveries are occurring on the pathological level, newer laboratory and imaging techniques are also finding use in the acute TBI setting. Recently two serum and cerebrospinal fluid (CSF) markers of central nervous system (CNS) injury have been studied in Europe. S-100B is an acidic calcium-binding protein found in glial and Schwann cells with high specificity for CNS white matter. Neuron-specific enolase (NSE) is an isoenzyme located in neurons, neuroendocrine cells, smooth muscle fibers, and adipose tissue. Both markers have been tentatively linked to the severity of the TBI and outcome predictability, particularly with severe injuries.

The evidence for S-100B is considerably stronger than for NSE. Most authors agree that initial levels should be measured within 6 hours of the injury, certainly within the first day. Levels fall rapidly over the next few days. Levels have been measured both in CSF and, most commonly, in serum. A recent study suggests that to be strictly relevant to TBI, levels in CSF must be measured, as serum levels are affected by nonnervous system sources.[11] In addition, another study has shown that serum levels of S-100B peak 2 days after CSF levels.[12] As with most new research areas in medicine, the initial work has been with small groups of patients, study designs differ, studies have not controlled for the same preexisting factors, and outcome has generally been measured within 6 months of injury. Additionally, the primary outcome measure has been the Glasgow Outcome Scale (GOS), an 8-point scale that marks global states such as vegetative, dependency on others for activities of daily living, return to work, and minor deficits. It does not include in-depth neuropsychological or psychiatric testing.[13]

A recent comparison was done of CSF and serum S-100B and NSE levels to two immunological markers (sICAM-1 and IL-6; associated with CNS inflammatory response) and to clinical outcome and initial computed tomographic (CT) contusion size in 13 patients with Glasgow Coma Scale (GCS) scores of ≤8, as compared with 17 controls.[14] Levels were measured over 14 days. Both CSF S-100B and NSE strongly correlated with contusion size. With the serum markers, only S-100B correlated with clinical outcome and contusion size in all 13 patients. Serum NSE correlated with the release of the immune factors only. The authors surmised that NSE was related to immune function and that S-100B can be a marker for severity of injury. They also noted that it is unclear if S-100B is protective or detrimental—as it may stimulate repair processes such as glial growth but also has been linked to deleterious calcium uptake. They did not control for previous psychiatric or neurological histories or alcohol use. A later study examined a larger cohort, 51 patients, with GCS<9.[15] Results again indicated that S-100B levels correlated with outcome, as measured by the GOS and by a quality of life self-assessment questionnaire. The authors measured outcome over a wide time range (5–24 months) and did not control for previous psychiatric or alcohol histories. However, both these studies confirmed the results of several groups from the 1990s that proposed the predictive value of S-100B in severe brain injury.

The predictive value of these markers is more controversial in mild brain injury. Serum S-100B and NSE were sampled in 66 patients with both mild (GCS 13–15) and moderate-severe (GCS≤12) injury and compared with both volumetric CT lesions and initial GCS score.[16] Results indicated that, as in previous studies, the patients with moderate-severe injury had higher NSE and S-100B levels and had longer release of these agents than did those with mild injuries. Both groups, however, had initially higher levels than controls. The levels were measured serially over 3 days, and all levels correlated with volume of contusions on CT. Patients with previous CNS disorders were excluded. Previous history of alcohol abuse was not mentioned. The same group followed with a comparison of S-100B and NSE values in 69 patients with a median GCS of 13.[17] Twenty-nine of the subjects completed neuropsychological testing at 2 weeks and 6 months. Both markers correlated with initial GCS scores and neither correlated with CT findings. Patients with both subacute and chronic neuropsychological deficits had higher NSE and S-100B values and longer release times of both markers. However, at both 2 weeks and 6 months only the S-100B correlations reached statistical significance. The authors did control for past neurological, psychiatric, alcohol, and drug abuse histories. The conclusions were that, although both markers were elevated, S-100B was a more reliable marker of injury in mild TBI.

Two other groups have found correlations with outcome in larger cohorts of mildly injured patients (GCS 13–15). Townend found an inverse correlation between initial S-100B levels and GOS scores at 1 month postinjury in 119 patients completing the study.[13] de Kruijk et al. examined S-100B and NSE levels in 104 mild TBI patients as compared with 91 controls.[18] Median NSE levels in the patients were only slightly higher, while S-100B levels were significantly higher than in controls. Initial vomiting was also associated with higher S-100B levels. A self-assessment questionnaire of posttraumatic complaints was obtained at follow-up in 79 of the 104 subjects.[19] Within this group, a twofold increase in severity of cognitive and vegetative complaints was associated with higher initial serum levels of S-100B and NSE, respectively. Savola et al.[20] obtained serum S-100B levels within 6 hours of injury in 172 cases of mild TBI (GCS 13–15) and found that elevated levels (>0.5 μg/L) correlated with postconcussive symptoms reported at 2–6 weeks postinjury. Only 50% of the 8 patients with CT-confirmed intracranial lesions had elevated S-100B levels.

Other areas of study with S-100B included an initial comparison to magnetic resonance (MR) imaging findings and development of appropriate cut-off values for normal and pathological levels of this marker. In 1999, Ingebrigtsen and colleagues found that the proportion with higher serum S-100B levels was increased in patients with MR imaging findings of contusion and observed a trend towards positive findings on neuropsychological testing at 3 months.[21] However, only 14 of the 50 cohorts had detectable levels of S-100B and only 5 patients had MR imaging findings. Biberthaler compared 52 patients with mild injury (GCS 13–15) to 20 healthy controls and to 10 severely injured patients (GCS<8).[22] Results indicated that if 0.1 ng/mL of serum S-100B was used as a cut-off for normal, then the test sensitivity would reach 100%, with 40% specificity for intracranial injury.

Imaging Studies

Although it has been known for some time that MR imaging is more sensitive than CT in detecting axonal injury, both methods are widely used.[5,6] CT examination, still the standard for life-threatening acute hemorrhage, is robust and relatively inexpensive. In contrast, while MR imaging is much better for detection of white matter lesions, the exams take longer, are more expensive, and require special nonmagnetic ventilators, cardiac monitors, and other medical equipment. Both conventional and developing MR techniques can add value to the clinical assessment of TBI. Gradient echo (GE) images are sensitive to magnetic susceptibility (T_2*) and can demonstrate even very small areas of hemorrhage.[23–27] Such lesions are more easily visualized with this technique because the hemorrhagic blood creates a local magnetic field disturbance, causing a loss of signal. The number of small hemorrhagic lesions identified on T_2*-weighted GE images correlated with GCS score in several studies.[23,26,27] In addition, lesion locations were appropriate to explain all focal neurological signs and symptoms in the acute phase (≤ 3 weeks) in one study.[26] Nonhemorrhagic lesions are better visualized on T_2-weighted spin echo sequences, especially those obtained using fluid attenuated inversion recovery (FLAIR), a technique that incorporates suppression of the bright signal from CSF. In a prospective study, 33 patients with normal CT scan but abnormal neurologic status underwent MR examination within 48 hours of injury.[5] This group obtained T_1-weighted echo-planar, T_2*-weighted GE, T_2-weighted FLAIR, and T_2-weighted turbo spin echo images, and found that MR imaging demonstrated more nonhemorrhagic lesions than CT. The authors noted that presence of nonhemorrhagic lesions was associated with a relatively good clinical outcome. However, outcome was measured only with the GOS, a relatively insensitive measure. It does not, for instance, include in-depth neuropsychological or neuropsychiatric evaluation. In another prospective study, a group of 21 patients with DAI underwent MR imaging within 24 hours of injury, then again on days 1, 3, 7, and 14.[28] The signal intensity of the corpus callosum was measured on FLAIR images at each time point. The study found a positive correlation between the duration of unconsciousness and the maximum signal intensity of the corpus callosum, which occurred most commonly on day 7 (range 3–14). In addition, higher signal intensity was associated with an unfavorable outcome at 6 months, as determined by the GOS.

Newer types of MR imaging provide quantitative measures and show promise for increasing identification of DAI. A recent retrospective study examined 25 patients within 48 hours of TBI, comparing lesion visualization on T_2-weighted fast spin echo, FLAIR, T_2*-weighted GE, and diffusion-weighted (DW) images.[25] Of 427 lesions identified on at least one type of image, 58% were detected on T_2/FLAIR, 47% were detected on GE, and 22% were detected on both. DW imaging was the most sensitive, allowing visualization of 72%, including all nonhemorrhagic lesions. Importantly, 16% of lesions were visible only on DW imaging. All of these were hyperintense in appearance. The apparent diffusion constant (ADC) was decreased in the majority of lesions visible on DW imaging, indicating more restricted diffusion, perhaps an indication of cytotoxic edema. Approximately one-quarter displayed increased ADC, which may indicate the development of vasogenic edema. Consistent with expectation, many hemorrhagic lesions (23%) were seen only on the GE images. No follow-up data was presented, so the clinical significance of the lesions identified could not be assessed.

Three studies used diffusion tensor imaging (DTI) to evaluate DAI. One measured diffusion anisotropy of the corpus callosum (splenium, body, genu) in 10 patients, 2 weeks to 8 months after TBI (initial GCS scores ranged from 3 to 14) compared with normal individuals.[29] Diffusion anisotropy was decreased by an average of approximately 25% in at least one region of the corpus callosum in all 10 patients, indicating disruption of the normally highly ordered structure. Decreased anisotropy was found even in areas that looked normal on both FLAIR and GE images. No correlation with functional measures was provided. A case report of a child with hemiparesis subsequent to a severe TBI (comatose for 3 days) reported that abnormalities on conventional MR imaging did not correlate with clinical symptoms.[30] DTI demonstrated decreased anisotropy in the cerebral peduncle of the midbrain. A preliminary study evaluated diffusion anisotropy of areas that appeared normal on standard CT and MR imaging in 5 patients with mild TBI (initial GCS score 13–15).[31] All were imaged within the first 24 hours and 2 were imaged again at one month. There were areas of reduced anisotropy in regions that appeared normal by other imaging techniques in all 5 patients, most often in the internal capsule and corpus callosum (Figure 13–1). The authors noted that the decreased anisotropy in areas without edema or hemorrhage (which would have been seen on the other types of images gathered) indicates that diffusion parallel to the main axis of the axons has become impeded. They suggested misalignment of axonal membranes and of the cytoskeletal network as possible causes. By 30 days, some areas had returned to normal values, while others were still decreased. The authors suggested that these patterns may correspond to areas in which repair processes have been successful versus areas in which injury has progressed. All these studies indicate that various measures of water diffusion may be more sensitive to DAI than conventional MR imaging.

Magnetization transfer (MT) imaging is another quantitative MR technique that has been found to be related to tissue structure and thus can be used to assess structural integrity. In one study of DAI in an animal model, MT imaging results were found to be related to pathologically proven injury.[32] In a later study conducted by the same group, 28 patients who had experienced loss of consciousness as a result of head injury were compared to 15 controls.[33] Most were first imaged within 2 weeks of injury (range, 1–29 days). Follow-up scans were obtained in 10 patients. Magnetization transfer ratios (MTRs) were calculated for all white matter areas that were abnormal on the T_2-weighted images as well as for areas of normal appearing white matter. Outcome measures (GOS) were obtained 3 months to 3 years after injury. Decreased MTR was found in normal appearing white matter only in patients that had persistent functional deficits at follow-up. However, absence of decrease in MTR in normal appearing white matter was found in patients with outcomes that ranged from very good to poor. In a subsequent related study, 13 patients who had experienced mild TBI were examined with conventional MR imaging and MT imaging several months to several years following injury.[34] Neuropsychological testing was done in 9 patients, all of whom were found to be impaired. Most of the patients in the study (12/13) had negative conventional MR imaging but all were symptomatic. Contour mapping of the MTR revealed areas of profoundly decreased MTR in the splenium of the corpus callosum in four of these patients (Figure 13–2). A moderate correlation was found between a test of verbal learning and MTR for the splenium. Results of this study suggested that MT imaging may be sensitive to mild TBI when other modalities fail. In another study from this group, MT imaging and ^{1}H (proton) MR spectroscopy of the splenium of the corpus callosum were obtained in 30 patients with TBI.[35] Initial GCS scores ranged from 3 to 15 (mean score, 11). Assessment was done between 2 and 1129 days after injury. Outcome (GOS) was assessed a minimum of 3 months after injury. No correlation between MT imaging and outcome was found. However, a decreased *N*-acetylaspartate-to-creatine ratio (a possible indication of neuronal loss) was associated with poorer outcome. These results are consistent with prior suggestions that abnormal MR spectroscopy results may predict a poor clinical outcome.[36] Limitations of this study include the wide range of times from injury to examination and injury to assessment of outcome.

Conclusion

In summary, new research techniques are beginning to make it clear that brain injury is not static but rather an evolving process. A better understanding of the nature of these events should spur the development of more effective interventions. Earlier, more sensitive methods of identifying and categorizing degrees of brain injury have the potential to better predict outcome, and thus guide clinical management.

References

1. Consensus conference. Rehabilitation of persons with traumatic brain injury. JAMA 1999; 282:974–983
2. Arciniegas DB, Held K, Wagner P: Cognitive impairment following traumatic brain injury. Curr Treat Options Neurol 2002; 4:43–57
3. Hurley RA, Taber KH: Emotional disturbances following traumatic brain injury. Curr Treat Options Neurol 2002; 4:59–75
4. Sahuquillo J, Poca MA: Diffuse axonal injury after head trauma. A review. Adv Tech Stand Neurosurg 2002; 27:23–86
5. Paterakis K, Karantanas AH, et al: Outcome of patients with diffuse axonal injury: the significance and prognostic value of MRI in the acute phase. J Trauma 2000; 49:1071–1075
6. McAllister TW, Sparling MB, et al: Neuroimaging findings in mild traumatic brain injury. J Clin Exp Neuropsychol 2001; 23:775–791
7. Povlishock JT: Pathophysiology of neural injury: therapeutic opportunities and challenges. Clin Neurosurg 2000; 46:113–126
8. Stone JR, Walker SA, Povlishock JT: The visualization of a new class of traumatically injured axons through the use of a modified method of microwave antigen retrieval. Acta Neuropathol (Berl) 1999; 97:335–345
9. Stone JR, Singleton RH, Povlishock JT: Intra-axonal neurofilament compaction does not evoke local axonal swelling in all traumatically injured axons. Exp Neurol 2001; 172:320–331
10. Hoshino S, Kobayashi S, et al: Multiple immunostaining methods to detect traumatic axonal injury in the rat fluid-percussion brain injury model. Neurol Med Chir (Tokyo) 2003; 43:165–173
11. Kleine TO, Benes L, Zofel P: Studies of the brain specificity of S100B and neuron-specific enolase (NSE) in blood serum of acute care patients. Brain Res Bull 2003; 61:265–279
12. Petzold A, Keir G, et al: Cerebrospinal fluid (CSF) and serum S100B: release and wash-out pattern. Brain Res Bull 2003; 61:281–285
13. Townend WJ, Guy MJ, et al: Head injury outcome prediction in the emergency department: a role for protein S-100B? J Neurol Neurosurg Psychiatry 2002; 73:542–546
14. Pleines UE, Morganti-Kossmann MC, Rancan M, et al: S-100 beta reflects the extent of injury and outcome, whereas neuronal specific enolase is a better indicator of neuroinflammation in patients with severe traumatic brain injury. J Neurotrauma 2001; 18:491–498
15. Woertgen C, Rothoerl D, Brawanski A: Early S-100B serum level correlates to quality of life in patients after severe head injury. Brain Inj 2002; 16:807–816
16. Herrmann M, Jost S, et al: Temporal profile of release of neurobiochemical markers of brain damage after traumatic brain injury is associated with intracranial pathology as demonstrated in cranial computed tomography. J Neurotrauma 2000; 17:113–122
17. Herrmann M, Curio N, et al: Release of biochemical markers of damage to neuronal and glial brain tissue is associated with short and long term neuropsychological outcome after traumatic brain injury. J Neurol Neurosurg Psychiatry 2001; 70:95–100
18. de Kruijk JR, Leffers P, et al: S-100B and neuron-specific enolase in serum of mild traumatic brain injury patients. Acta Neurol Scand 2001; 103:175–179
19. de Kruijk JR, Leffers P, et al: Prediction of post-traumatic complaints after mild traumatic brain injury: early symptoms and biochemical markers. J Neurol Neurosurg Psychiatry 2002; 73:727–732
20. Savola O, Hillborn M: Early predictors of post-concussion syndrome in patients with mild head injury. Eur J Neurol 2003; 10:175–181
21. Ingebrigtsen T, Waterloo K, et al: Traumatic brain damage in minor head injury: Relation of serum S-100 protein measurements to magnetic resonance imaging and neurobehavioral outcome. Neurosurgery 1999; 45:468–475
22. Biberthaler P, Mussack T, et al: Evaluation of S-100b as a specific marker for neuronal damage due to minor head trauma. World J Surg 2001; 25:93–97
23. Tong KA, Ashwal S, et al: Hemorrhagic shearing lesions in children and adolescents with posttraumatic diffuse axonal injury: improved detection and initial results. Radiology 2003; 227:332–339
24. Kuzma BB, Goodman JM: Improved identification of axonal shear injuries with gradient echo MR technique. Surg Neurol 2000; 53:400–402
25. Huisman TAGM, Sorensen AG, et al: Diffusion-weighted imaging for the evaluation of diffuse axonal injury in closed head injury. J Comput Assist Tomogr 2003; 27:5–11
26. Yanagawa Y, Tsushima Y, et al: A quantitative analysis of head injury using T2*-weighted gradient-echo imaging. J Trauma 2000; 49:272–277
27. Scheid R, Preul G et al: Diffuse axonal injury associated with chronic traumatic brain injury: Evidence from T2*-weighted gradient-echo imaging at 3 T. Am J Neuroradiol 2003; 24:1049–1056
28. Takaoka M, Tabuse H, et al: Semiquantitative analysis of corpus callosum injury using magnetic resonance imaging indicates clinical severity in patients with diffuse axonal injury. J Neurol Neurosurg Psychiatry 2002; 73:289–293
29. Chan JH, Tsui EY, et al: Diffuse axonal injury: detection of changes in anisotropy of water diffusion by diffusion-weighted imaging. Neuroradiology 2003; 45:34–38
30. Lee ZI, Byun WM, Jang SH, et al: Diffusion tensor magnetic resonance imaging of microstructural abnormalities in children with brain injury. Am J Phys Med Rehabil 2003; 82:556–559
31. Arfanakis K, Haughton VM, et al: Diffusion tensor MR imaging in diffuse axonal injury. Am J Neuroradiol 2002; 97:568–575
32. McGowan JC, McCormack TM, et al: Diffuse axonal pathology detected with magnetization transfer imaging following brain injury in the pig. Magn Reson Med 1999; 41:727–733

33. Bagley LJ, McGowan JC, et al: Magnetization transfer imaging of traumatic brain injury. J Magn Reson Imaging 2000; 11:1–8
34. McGowan JC, Yang JH, et al: Magnetization transfer imaging in the detection of injury associated with mild head trauma. Am J Neuroradiol 2000; 21:875–880
35. Sinson G, Bagley LJ, et al: Magnetization transfer imaging and proton MR spectroscopy in the evaluation of axonal injury: Correlation with clinical outcome after traumatic brain injury. Am J Neuroradiol 2001; 22:143–151
36. Brooks WM, Friedman SD, Gasparovic C: Magnetic resonance spectroscopy in traumatic brain injury. J Head Trauma Rehabil 2001; 16:149–164

Recent Publications of Interest

Buki A, Povlishock JT: All roads lead to disconnection?—Traumatic axonal injury revisited. Acta Neurochir (Wien) 2006; 148:181–193
Reviews the present understanding of the sequence of events that leads to axonal disconnection following traumatic brain injury.

Bazarian JJ, Blyth B, Cimpello L: Bench to bedside: evidence for brain injury after concussion—looking beyond the computed tomography scan. Acad Emerg Med 2006; 13:199–214
Presents the evidence for neurologic injury as a result of concussion. Topics covered include pathology, structural imaging, functional imaging, serum biomarkers, and tests of cognition and balance. The strengths and weaknesses for each category of evidence are discussed.

Scheid R, Walther K, Guthke T, et al: Cognitive sequelae of diffuse axonal injury. Arch Neurol 2006; 63:418–424
Performed detailed neuropsychological testing on a group of patients with traumatic brain injury in which the magnetic resonance imaging results were consistent with the presence of only diffuse axonal injuries. All patients were impaired on at least one cognitive domain.

Povlishock JT, Katz DI: Update of neuropathology and neurological recovery after traumatic brain injury. J Head Trauma Rehabil 2005; 20:76–94
Provides a comprehensive overview of the present understanding of the neuropathology of traumatic brain injury, including initial focal and diffuse changes as well as subsequent consequences.

Reprinted from Hurley RA, McGowan JC, Arfanakis K, et al: "Traumatic Axonal Injury: Novel Insights Into Evolution and Identification." *Journal of Neuropsychiatry and Clinical Neurosciences* 16:1–7, 2004. Used with permission.

Chapter 14

FUNCTIONAL IMAGING AS A WINDOW TO DEMENTIA

Corticobasal Degeneration

ANDREEA L. SERITAN, M.D.
MARIO F. MENDEZ, M.D., PH.D.
DANIEL H.S. SILVERMAN, M.D., PH.D.
ROBIN A. HURLEY, M.D.
KATHERINE H. TABER, PH.D.

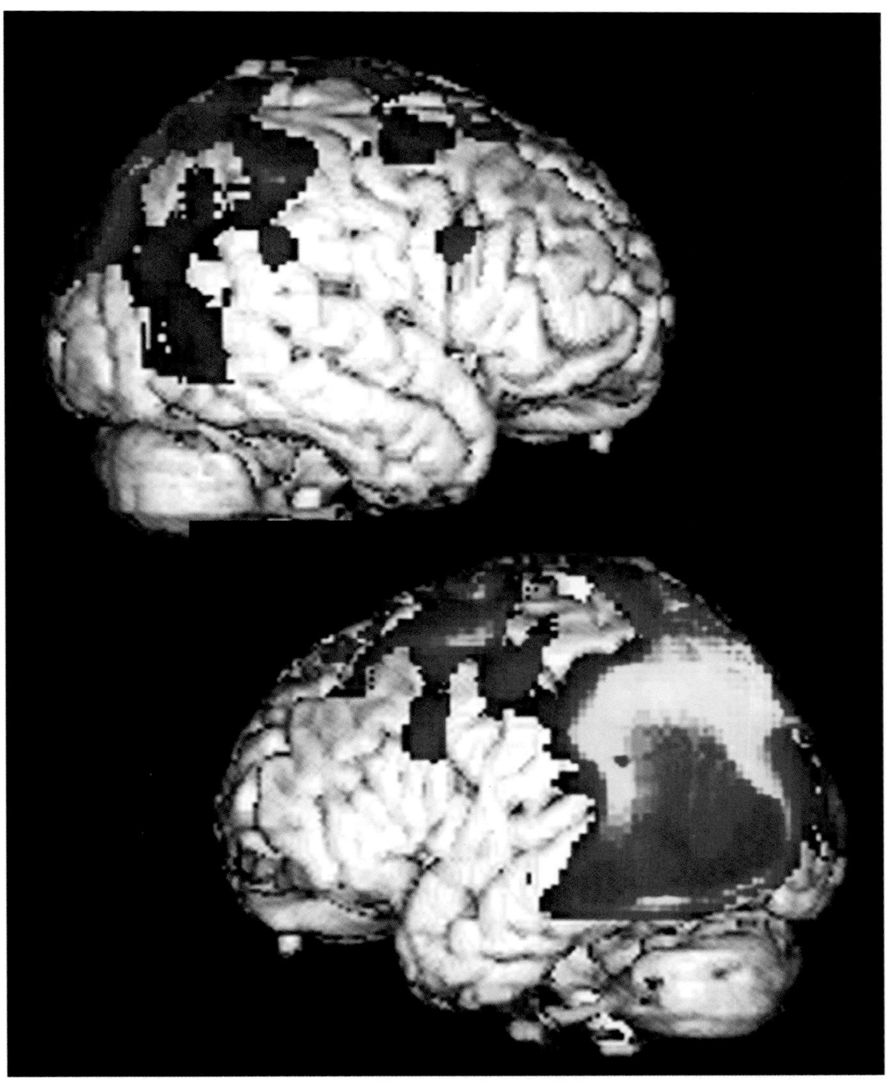

Statistical parametric maps display regions of significant hypometabolism superimposed on three-dimensional reconstructions of the magnetic resonance data set from a patient with corticobasal degeneration.

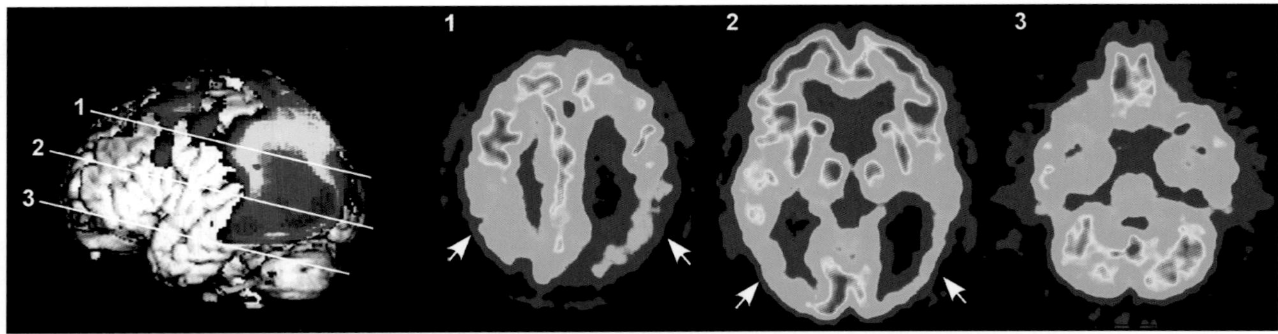

FIGURE 14–1. A statistical parametric map (left) displays regions of significant hypometabolism superimposed on a three-dimensional reconstruction of magnetic resonance images from a patient with corticobasal degeneration. Numbered lines indicate the approximate locations and angle of section for the three axial images (right) from the source positron emission tomography ^{18}F-fluorodeoxyglucose data set. The axial sections show the characteristic regional variations in cerebral metabolic rate (*red* is high, *blue* is low). Note the prominent asymmetrical metabolic decreases in the occipital and parietal lobes (arrows).

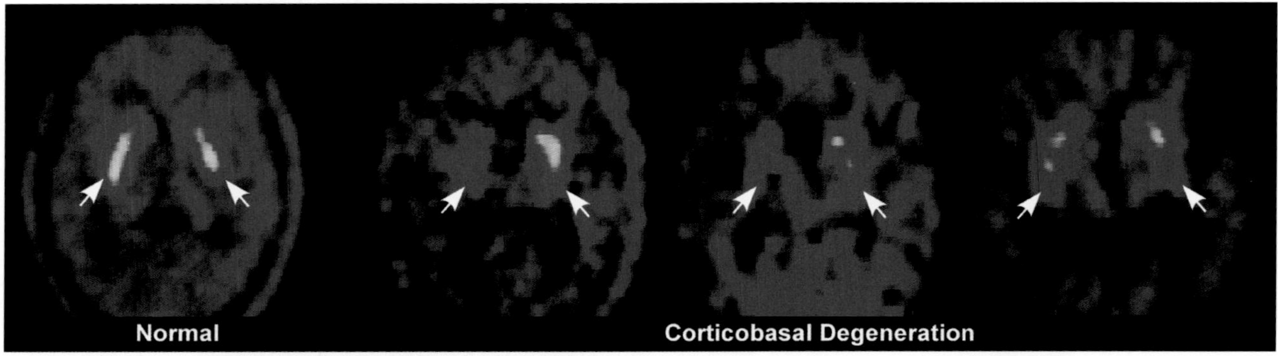

FIGURE 14–2. [^{18}F]Fluorodopa (FDOPA) positron emission tomography images in a normal subject and three patients with corticobasal degeneration show decreased uptake of FDOPA in the corticobasal degeneration group in the striatum (arrows) as well as the clearly asymmetric pattern. Used with permission.[34]

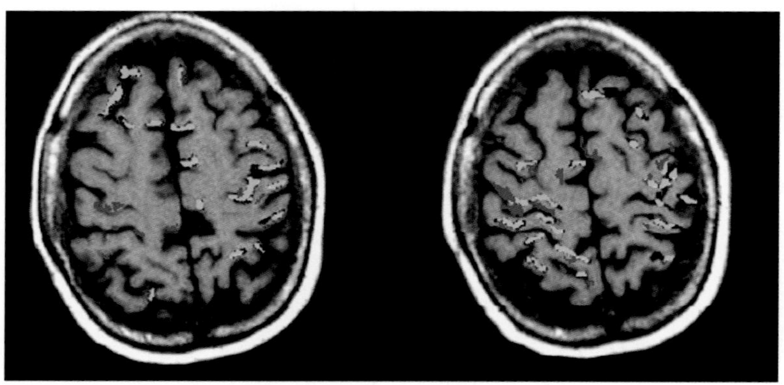

FIGURE 14-3 Functional magnetic resonance imaging results of finger opposition tasks in a patient with corticobasal degeneration are overlaid onto axial magnetic resonance images. There are clear differences in cortical activation when movement is performed with the impaired (*pink*) and the unaffected (*green*) hands. Note the decreased areas and extent of activation with the affected hand with a simple (left) and complex (right) task. Adapted with permission.[23]

Corticobasal degeneration (CBD) is a rare neurodegenerative dementia that illustrates the use of functional imaging in geriatric psychiatry. There have been numerous publications related to the more common dementias (such as Alzheimer's disease [AD]) and functional imaging. Fewer reports are available regarding CBD; functional imaging may be cardinal in differentiating this clinical entity from other dementias and/or movement disorders. Patients with CBD typically present with asymmetric parkinsonism, dystonia or focal myoclonus, and specific cognitive-behavioral changes.[1] These include one or more of the following signs: ideomotor apraxia, cortical sensory loss or alien hand phenomenon,[2,3] frontal executive deficits,[4,5] and, less often, dementia.[6] Although first described in 1968, it was not until the early 1990s that this disorder became a focus of clinical and research interest.[7] Investigators have previously referred to CBD as corticodentatonigral degeneration with neuronal achromasia, corticonigral degeneration, corticobasal ganglionic degeneration, or progressive asymmetrical rigidity and apraxia syndrome.[7] Some authors have suggested using the term *corticobasal syndrome* for the constellation of clinical features considered as defining characteristics of CBD, reserving the term *corticobasal degeneration* for the histopathological disorder.[8] CBD is now recognized as part of the spectrum of frontotemporal lobar degeneration.[2]

The prevalence of this disorder is not clear. CBD is less common than other mid- and late-life basal ganglia disorders. In an autopsy series of 226 elderly demented patients, CBD accounted for 1.3% of cases.[9] The mean age at onset is 63 years (SD = 7.7), although the disease may occur as young as 28.[2,10] The disease has an insidious onset and is steadily progressive, with a mean duration of 7.9 years (SD = 2.6).[2] The clinical diagnosis of CBD is challenging. This disorder may be markedly underdiagnosed, as one report indicates initial recognition to be as low as 35%.[11] CBD may be difficult to differentiate in its early course from Parkinson's disease (PD) or other parkinsonian disorders, like progressive supranuclear palsy (PSP) or multiple system atrophy (MSA). A lack of initial response to L-dopa therapy, although nonspecific, helps differentiate CBD from PD. Despite recommended diagnostic criteria for probable CBD, a definitive diagnosis requires neuropathological confirmation.[3]

Neuropsychiatric Features

Depression is the most common neuropsychiatric feature in CBD. The prevalence of depression may be as high as 70%, apathy 40%, and irritability 20%.[12] Less frequently described are agitation, obsessive-compulsive symptoms, anxiety, disinhibition, delusions, or aberrant motor behavior such as pacing.[12,13] The cognitive changes in CBD include a unique combination of focal parietal and frontal-subcortical deficits. Most patients with CBD develop ideomotor apraxia (inability to perform previously learned movements in the absence of weakness or sensory deficits). Frontal deficits may include psychomotor slowing, a dysexecutive syndrome, and impaired memory retrieval.[2–4] Patients with CBD often have constructional and visuospatial difficulties, acalculia, elements of Gerstmann syndrome, and nonfluent aphasia. This may indicate a possible overlap with progressive nonfluent aphasia.[14,15] The alien limb phenomenon (a "feeling that one limb is foreign or 'has a will of its own,' together with observable involuntary motor activity") is a dramatic manifestation of CBD.[16] In addition to CBD, several other disorders have been associated with the alien limb phenomenon: vascular insults (especially in the anterior cerebral artery territory), surgical lesions (corpus callosotomy or thalamotomy), tumors of the corpus callosum, Creutzfeldt-Jakob disease, and AD.[16]

Patients with CBD may have hemispatial neglect or impaired proprioception, astereognosis, and agraphesthesia in the setting of intact primary sensory modalities, indicating cortical sensory loss.[8] Balint's syndrome—a visuospatial disorder with inability to integrate complex visual scenes (simultanagnosia), inability to accurately direct hand or other movements by visual guidance (optic ataxia), and reduced voluntary eye movements to visual stimuli (oculomotor apraxia)—may also be present.[17] Alien limb sign and Balint's syndrome can co-occur.[17]

Neuropathological Findings

There are no laboratory markers for CBD. A definitive diagnosis requires neuropathology. It is a "tauopathy," diagnosed by the presence of intraneuronal tau-immunoreactive inclusions (CBD inclusions) in substantia nigra and cortical layer II.[2] Astrocytic plaques and coiled bodies in oligodendroglia are characteristic. Ballooned achromatic cells are present in the involved cortex and subcortical regions.[2] There are also cortical neuronal loss, gliosis of the frontoparietal and perirolandic cortices and caudate nuclei, as well as degeneration of the substantia nigra.

Structural Imaging Studies

Findings on magnetic resonance imaging (MRI) studies can support the clinical diagnosis of CBD. MRI typically reveals asymmetric atrophy involving the posterior frontal and parietal regions, corresponding to the clinically notable asymmetry in motor deficits.[4,5,18–20] However, a recent volumetric study did not find substantial asymmetry.[21] A longitudinal case report has demonstrated the progressive nature of the atrophy on imaging.[22] One study has reported a hyperintense appearance of the frontoparietal white matter on diffusion-weighted MRI.[20] Atrophy of the basal ganglia is present less consistently.[19,23] Increased T_2 signal intensity in the putamen ipsilateral to the cortical atrophy and decreased T_2 signal intensity bilaterally in the putamen have both been reported.[5,20] Several studies have reported atrophy of the corpus callosum, predominantly in its mid-portion.[21,24–26] In one study the degree of callosal atrophy was significantly correlated with measures of cognitive impairment.[24] The authors noted that the middle predominance is consistent with degeneration in the posterior frontal and parietal cortices and thus may reflect both the severity and location of neuronal loss.

Functional Imaging Studies

In recent years, investigators have proposed functional imaging studies as diagnostic tests to help differentiate CBD from other pathologic entities. In the last 10 years, functional imaging studies in CBD have included positron emission tomography (PET), single-photon emission computed tomography (SPECT), functional magnetic resonance imaging (fMRI), and magnetic resonance spectroscopy (MRS). Although the CBD diagnoses were rarely pathologically proven, these studies used established diagnostic criteria. Some compared CBD patients with healthy control subjects, while others contrasted them with patients with other parkinsonian or dementing disorders.

In studies utilizing ^{18}F-fluorodeoxyglucose (FDG) PET, regional cerebral metabolic rate (rCMR) was decreased most commonly in areas of frontal and parietal cortex as well as thalamus and basal ganglia (Figure 14–1).[24,27–34] Although individual patients varied considerably in the exact location and extent of deficits, primary sensorimotor cortex may be particularly affected in CBD.[30,32,34] Regional asymmetries were consistently found, with more severe hypometabolism contralateral to the more affected side of the body.[24,27–34] However, some studies have reported symmetrical hypometabolism in the presence of asymmetrical clinical deficits or a reversed asymmetry in a few patients.[27,29,32]

Two studies have compared FDG PET metabolic patterns between patients with PSP, those with CBD, and control subjects.[27,32] Both used statistical parametric mapping, an image analysis technique that allows voxel by voxel comparison of groups of images after they are normalized to a standardized space. Images from the CBD groups were mirrored when necessary so that the most affected side was always the same in order to adjust for the characteristic asymmetry, thus allowing group-wise comparisons. Both studies found that metabolic asymmetry was present in most patients with CBD but not in patients with PSP. In one study, comparison between the CBD (n=12) and PSP (n=12) groups revealed a lower metabolism in the inferior parietal lobule, precuneus, and lateral occipital cortex of the more affected hemisphere in the CBD group and a lower metabolism in the anterior cingulate and medial frontal gyri of both hemispheres and the midbrain in the PSP group.[27] In the other study, comparison between PSP (n=21) and CBD (n=22) groups indicated more metabolic impairment in sensorimotor, supplementary motor, and parietal cortices in the CBD group and lower metabolism in the midbrain, anterior cingulate, and orbitofrontal regions in the PSP group.[32] These studies suggest that FDG PET may be useful in the differential diagnosis due to the more posterior cortical findings in CBD as compared to the more anterior cortical and midbrain findings in PSP.

Regional cerebral blood flow (rCBF) has been measured by SPECT in patients with CBD using several tracers including ^{99m}Tc-hexamethylpropyleneamine oxime (HMPAO), ^{99m}Tc-ethylene cysteinate dimer, and *N*-isopropyl-p-[^{123}I]-iodoamphetamine. The most common findings have been marked perfusion asymmetry in the posterior frontal and parietal regions, with hypoperfusion contralateral to the most affected side.[22,23,35–40] Other commonly affected areas are temporal cortex, basal ganglia, thalamus, and pontocerebellar regions.[22,36–40] One study reported that CBD patients with dementia had significant reductions of relative rCBF in the inferior prefrontal region of the more affected hemisphere, compared to CBD patients without dementia.[40] Another found widespread decreases in absolute rCBF in patients with CBD (n=13), compared with control subjects (n=10), indicating that use of relative measures may not be fully informative in this group.[36]

Three studies have utilized SPECT to compare rCBF between patients with CBD and those with other parkinsonian or dementing disorders.[37–39] All three measured predetermined regions of interest. Although most regions of interest were placed in roughly similar areas (frontal, parietal, temporal, and occipital cortices, basal ganglia, thalamus, and cerebellum) in both studies comparing patients with CBD and with PSP, the results were quite different. In a study measuring absolute rCBF, values did not differ significantly between PSP (n=12) and CBD (n=12).[37] In a study measuring relative rCBF, values were significantly lower in inferior frontal, sensorimotor, and posterior parietal cortices in patients with CBD (n=6) compared with patients with PSP (n=5).[39] Technique differences as well as differences in patient samples (e.g., illness duration, clinical presentation, inclusion of cognitive deficits) may be reasons why these findings are not consistent. Both studies found significantly higher asymmetry indices in CBD, particularly in posterior frontal and parietal regions, similar to the differences in rCMR described previously. The third study found that rCBF was significantly lower in anterior cingulate cortex, sensorimotor cortex, basal ganglia, and thalamus in patients with CBD compared with patients with AD. In contrast, rCBF was significantly lower in posterior parietal cortex in patients with AD compared to patients with CBD.[38] Patients with CBD also had significantly higher asymmetry indices in inferior prefrontal and sensorimotor cortices, whereas patients with AD had significantly higher asymmetry indices in lateral and medial prefrontal cortex and posterior parietal cortex.

Several methods have been used to image the dopamine system in CBD. Two studies utilized fluorodopa (FDOPA) PET to assess functional integrity of dopaminergic neurons in the striatum.[33,34] Normally, uptake is uniform throughout caudate and putamen bilaterally. Both studies found that uptake was decreased in patients with CBD (total n=10) compared with control subjects (total n=18), particularly contralateral to the more affected side of the body (Figure 14–2). There was considerable variability in the distribution, with some individuals showing symmetrical decreases.[33] Compared with patients with PD (n= 15), patients with CBD (n=6) had more uptake (less decrease).[33] A third study utilized [^{123}I]-2β-carbomethoxy-3-β-(iodophenyl)tropane ([^{123}I]β-CIT) SPECT, a cocaine derivative with high affinity for dopamine transporters and thus another marker of presynaptic dopaminergic neurons.[41] Patients with MSA (n=18), PSP (n=8), PD (n= 48), and CBD (n=4) were compared with control subjects (n=14) and with each other. Overall β-CIT striatal binding was significantly reduced in all patient groups compared to control subjects, with the CBD group least affected. Asymmetry of striatal β-CIT binding was greatest in patients with CBD, but was found only in two of the four. The authors concluded that β-CIT SPECT was a reliable tool for visualizing presynaptic dopaminergic lesions in patients with MSA, PSP and CBD, however it was inferior to other imaging modalities in differentiating these disorders from PD. Another SPECT tracer that binds to the dopamine transporter is [2-[[2-[[[3-(4-chlorophenyl)-8-methyl-8-azabicyclo[3.2.1]oct-2-yl] methyl](2-mercaptoethyl)amino]ethyl]amino]ethanethiolato(3-)-*N2,N2′,S2,S2′*]oxo-[1R-(exo-exo]-[^{99m}Tc]technetium ([^{99m}Tc]TRODAT-1). It has been used to compare striatal function in patients with CBD (n=5) and idiopathic PD (n= 10) with that in control subjects (n=10).[42] As was found in previously discussed studies, striatal binding was significantly reduced in both patient groups compared with control subjects. In contrast to previous studies, there was no significant difference in striatal binding between the CBD and PD groups and both exhibited asymmetry. Regional analysis revealed that binding was reduced similarly in both caudate and putamen in the patients with CBD, whereas binding was relatively preserved in the caudate and decreased in the putamen in the PD patients. Postsynaptic dopaminergic D_2 receptors were measured in an individual with CBD utilizing ^{123m}I-iodobenzamide (IBZM) SPECT.[35] Tracer uptake was severely reduced in the basal ganglia contralateral to the symptoms. Overall these studies indicate that the striatal dopaminergic system is impaired in CBD, but probably less severely than in other parkinsonian disorders.

One group has used fMRI to probe cortical function in patients with CBD (total n=8).[22,23] Two finger opposition tasks of differing difficulty were used. In the simple task, each finger in order (starting with digit 2, the index finger) was touched to the thumb (digit 1). In the complex task a specified sequence was followed (1–2, 1– 4, 1–3, 1–5). Activation of the contralateral sensorimotor, supplementary motor, and parietal cortex and of the ipsilateral prefrontal cortices occurred during the execution of the simple motor task with the unaffected hand. In contrast, decreased activation of the contralateral sensorimotor and parietal cortices and supplementary motor area occurred during performance of the same task with the affected hand (Figure 14–3). During performance of the complex motor task with the unaffected hand, there was bilateral activation of the sensorimotor and parietal cortices and activation of the contralateral frontal cortex. During performance of the same task with the affected hand, there was bilateral activation of the sensorimotor cortex and supplementary motor area, but only modest bilateral activation of the parietal cortex, particularly contralaterally (Figure 14–3). These results suggest parietal lobe dysfunction contralateral to the affected hand. The authors comment that the parietal lobe participates in the motor control of movements in the intrapersonal space. There are connections between the inferior parietal lobe and inferior premotor area (which may store elementary motor programs). Thus, parietal lobe dysfunction can disconnect the supplementary motor, premotor, and sensorimotor areas. The authors propose that fMRI can provide evidence of asymmetrical disorganization of the hierarchical cortical motor program, before structural and even SPECT changes become evident.

MRS provides a relative measure of particular metabolites, most commonly presented as spectra of the amount of signal produced by each from a volume of interest (voxel) rather than as images. Three studies have utilized proton (^{1}H) MRS to examine patients with CBD and related diseases (PSP, PD, MSA, vascular parkinsonism, primary progressive aphasia, frontotemporal dementia).[43–45] With ^{1}H MRS the metabolites of interest are *N*-acetylaspartate (NAA), choline, and creatine. NAA is present almost exclusively within neurons and indicates neuronal/axonal density. Choline is mostly present within membrane constituents and can be elevated both as a result of increased synthesis and destruction. Creatine is present alone and as part of phosphocreatinine, both of which are important for energy metabolism. While this peak is normally quite stable and commonly used as a reference standard, it does change in some conditions. The only region included in all 3 studies was the basal ganglia. Although the voxel placement varied, all reported either decreased NAA/creatine or decreased NAA/choline.[43–45] Two studies found decreased NAA/creatine in frontal cortex.[44,45] Other areas reported to be affected include the centrum semiovale, parietal cortex, and perisylvian cortex. The factors that differentiated CBD from other entities (e.g., PSP, MSA, frontotemporal dementia) were marked asymmetry and perhaps involvement of parietal cortex.

In summary, the most salient findings in these functional imaging studies are asymmetrical hypoperfusion on SPECT and asymmetrical hypometabolism on PET involving the parietofrontal cortex, basal ganglia, and thalamus. These findings suggest that multiple components of neural networks related to both movement execution and production of skilled movements are disturbed in CBD.[32] The functional imaging results may confirm a clinical diagnosis of probable CBD and support the diagnosis in patients who do not fulfill sufficient clinical criteria.[46] The few reports looking at CBD using fMRI and MRS appear to support the presence of hemispheric asymmetry early in the disease.

Conclusions

In conclusion, corticobasal degeneration is a neurodegenerative dementia with abnormal movements and focal behavioral manifestations. The clinical diagnosis is difficult to make in the absence of pathological findings. Functional imaging studies may be very helpful in demonstrating asymmetrical abnormalities in frontoparietal regions, basal ganglia, and thalamus contralateral to clinical symptoms, particularly in the early stages.[46] Future studies are needed to replicate present findings. Comparison with other patient groups, such as progressive supranuclear palsy and Parkinson's disease, will be particularly important. Although an uncommon form of dementia, CBD exemplifies the future possibilities of functional imaging in the clinical evaluation of dementing illnesses.

References

1. Wenning GK, Litvan I, Jankovic J, et al: Natural history and survival of 14 patients with corticobasal degeneration confirmed at postmortem examination. J Neurol Neurosurg Psychiatry 1998; 64:184–189
2. Mendez MF, Cummings JL: Dementia. A Clinical Approach, 3rd ed. Philadelphia, PA, Butterworth Heinemann, 2003
3. Cummings JL: The Neuropsychiatry of Alzheimer's Disease and Related Dementias. London, Martin Dunitz, 2003
4. Soliveri P, Monza D, Paridi D, et al: Cognitive and magnetic resonance imaging aspects of corticobasal degeneration and progressive supranuclear palsy. Neurology 1999; 53:502–507
5. Frasson E, Moretto G, Beltramello A, et al: Neuropsychological and neuroimaging correlates in corticobasal degeneration. Ital J Neurol Sci 1998; 19:321–328
6. Grimes DA, Lang AE, Bergeron CB: Dementia as the most common presentation of cortical-basal ganglionic degeneration. Neurology 1999; 53:1969–1974
7. Rebeiz JJ, Kolodny EH, Richardson EP Jr: Corticodentatonigral degeneration with neuronal achromasia. Arch Neurol 1968; 18:20–33
8. Boeve BF, Lang A, Litvan I: Corticobasal degeneration and its relationship to progressive supranuclear palsy and frontotemporal dementia. Ann Neurol 2003; 54 (suppl 5):S15–S19
9. Volicer L, McKee A, Hewitt S: Dementia. Neurol Clin 2001; 19:867–885
10. DePold Hohler A, Ransom BR, Chun MR, et al: The youngest reported case of corticobasal ganglia degeneration. Parkinsonism Relat Disord 2003; 10:47–50
11. Litvan I, Agid Y, Goetz C, et al: Accuracy of the clinical diagnosis of corticobasal degeneration: a clinicopathologic study. Neurology 1997; 48:119–125
12. Cummings JL, Litvan I: Neuropsychiatric aspects of corticobasal degeneration. Adv Neurol 2000; 82:147–152
13. Litvan I, Cummings JL, Mega M: Neuropsychiatric features of corticobasal degeneration. J Neurol Neurosurg Psychiatry 1998; 65:717–721
14. Kertesz A, Martinez-Lage P, Davidson W, et al: The corticobasal degeneration syndrome overlaps progressive aphasia and frontotemporal dementia. Neurology 2000; 55:1368–1375
15. Graham NL, Bak TH, Hodges JR: Corticobasal degeneration as a cognitive disorder. Mov Disord 2003; 18:1224–1232
16. Hanna P, Doody R: Alien limb sign. Adv Neurol 2000; 82:135–145
17. Mendez MF: Corticobasal ganglionic degeneration with Balint's syndrome. J Neuropsychiatry Clin Neurosci 2000; 12:273–275
18. Monza D, Ciano C, Scaioli V, et al: Neurophysiological features in relation to clinical signs in clinically diagnosed corticobasal degeneration. Neurol Sci 2003; 24:16–23
19. Savoiardo M, Grisoli M, Girotti F: Magnetic resonance imaging in CBD, related atypical parkinsonian disorders, and dementias. Adv Neurol 2000; 82:197–208

20. Ikeda K, Iwasaki Y, Ichikawa Y: Cognitive and MRI aspects of corticobasal degeneration and progressive supranuclear palsy (letter). Neurology 2000; 54:1878
21. Groschel K, Hauser TK, Luft A, et al: Magnetic resonance imaging-based volumetry differentiates progressive supranuclear palsy from corticobasal degeneration. Neuroimage 2004; 21:714–724
22. Moretti R, Ukmar M, Torre P, et al: Cortico-basal ganglionic degeneration: a clinical, functional and cognitive evaluation (1-year follow-up). J Neurol Sci 2000; 182:29–35
23. Ukmar M, Moretti R, Torre P, et al: Corticobasal degeneration: structural and functional MRI and single-photon emission computed tomography. Neuroradiology 2003; 45:708–712
24. Yamauchi H, Fukuyama H, Nagahama Y, et al: Atrophy of the corpus callosum, cortical hypometabolism, and cognitive impairment in corticobasal degeneration. Arch Neurol 1998; 55:609–614
25. Wolters A, Classen J, Kunesch E, et al: Measurements of transcallosally mediated cortical inhibition for differentiating parkinsonian syndromes. Mov Disord 2004; 19:518–528
26. Trompetto C, Buccolieri A, Marchese R, et al: Impairment of transcallosal inhibition in patients with corticobasal degeneration. Clin Neurophysiol 2003; 114:2181–2187
27. Hosaka K, Ishii K, Sakamoto S, et al: Voxel-based comparison of regional cerebral metabolism between PSP and corticobasal degeneration. J Neurol Sci 2002; 199:67–71
28. Ishii K: Clinical application of PET for diagnosis of dementia. Ann Nucl Med 2002; 16:515–525
29. Taniwaki T, Yamada T, Yoshida T, et al: Heterogeneity of glucose metabolism in corticobasal degeneration. J Neurol Sci 1998; 161:70–76
30. Hirono N, Ishii K, Sasaki M, et al: Features of regional cerebral glucose metabolism abnormality in corticobasal degeneration. Dement Geriatr Cogn Disord 2000; 11:139–146
31. Lutte I, Laterre C, Bodart JM, et al: Contribution of PET studies in diagnosis of corticobasal degeneration. Eur Neurol 2000; 44:12–21
32. Garraux G, Salmon E, Peigneux P, et al: Voxel-based distribution of metabolic impairment in corticobasal degeneration. Mov Disord 2000; 15:894–904
33. Laureys S, Salmon E, Garraux G, et al: Fluorodopa uptake and glucose metabolism in early stages of corticobasal degeneration. J Neurol 1999; 246:1151–1158
34. Nagasawa H, Tanji H, Nomura H, et al: PET study of cerebral glucose metabolism and fluorodopa uptake in patients with corticobasal ganglia degeneration. J Neurol Sci 1996; 139:210–217
35. Frisoni GB, Pizzolato G, Zanetti O, et al: Corticobasal degeneration: neuropsychological assessment and dopamine D2 receptor SPECT analysis. Eur Neurol 1995; 35:50–54
36. Hossain AK, Murata Y, Zhang L, et al: Brain perfusion SPECT in patients with corticobasal degeneration: analysis using statistical parametric mapping. Mov Disord 2003; 18:697–703
37. Zhang L, Murata Y, Ishida R, et al: Differentiating between progressive supranuclear palsy and corticobasal degeneration by brain perfusion SPET. Nucl Med Commun 2001; 22:767–772
38. Okuda B, Tachibana H, Kawabata K, et al: Comparison of brain perfusion in corticobasal degeneration and Alzheimer's disease. Dement Geriatr Cogn Disord 2001; 12:226–231
39. Okuda B, Tachibana H, Kawabata K, et al: Cerebral blood flow in corticobasal degeneration and progressive supranuclear palsy. Alzheimer Dis Assoc Disord 2000; 14:46–52
40. Okuda B, Tachibana H, Kawabata K, et al: Cerebral blood flow correlates of higher brain dysfunctions in corticobasal degeneration. J Geriatr Psychiatry Neurol 1999; 12:189–193
41. Pirker W, Asenbaum S, Bencsits G, et al: [^{123}I]β-CIT SPECT in multiple system atrophy, progressive supranuclear palsy, and corticobasal degeneration. Mov Disord 2000; 15:1158–1167
42. Lai SC, Weng YH, Yen TC, et al: Imaging early stage corticobasal degeneration with [^{99m}Tc]TRODAT-1 SPET. Nucl Med Commun 2004; 25:339–345
43. Tedeschi G, Litvan I, Bonavita S, et al: Proton magnetic resonance spectroscopic imaging in progressive supranuclear palsy, Parkinson's disease and corticobasal degeneration. Brain 1997; 120:1541–1552
44. Abe K, Terakawa H, Takanashi M, et al: Proton magnetic resonance spectroscopy of patients with parkinsonism. Brain Res Bull 2000; 52:589–595
45. Kizu O, Yamada K, Nishimura T: Proton chemical shift imaging in Pick complex. Am J Neuroradiol 2002; 23:1387–1392
46. Coulier IM, de Vries JJ, Leenders KL: Is FDG-PET a useful tool in clinical practice for diagnosing corticobasal ganglia degeneration? Mov Disord 2003; 18:1175–1178

Recent Publications of Interest

Belfor N, Amici S, Boxer AL, et al: Clinical and neuropsychological features of corticobasal degeneration. Mech Ageing Dev 2006; 127:203–207
Reviews the history, clinical, cognitive, imaging, and neuropathological features of corticobasal degeneration, and presents the neuropsychological profile compared to Alzheimer's disease.

Eckert T, Barnes A, Dhawan V, et al: FDG PET in the differential diagnosis of parkinsonian disorders. Neuroimage 2005; 26:912–921
Compared regional cerebral metabolism, measured using positron emission tomography, in several groups of patients with parkinsonian symptoms in order to identify defining characteristics for each to aid in differential diagnosis. The defining feature for corticobasal degeneration was asymmetrical activation, with relative hypometabolism in cortex and basal ganglia contralateral to the most affected side.

Mahapatra RK, Edwards MJ, Schott JM, et al: Corticobasal degeneration. Lancet Neurol 2004; 3:736–743
Reviews the epidemiology, clinical presentation, differential diagnosis, neuropathology, and symptom-directed treatment for corticobasal degeneration.

Wakabayashi K, Takahashi H: Pathological heterogeneity in progressive supranuclear palsy and corticobasal degeneration. Neuropathology 2004; 24:79–86
Presents an overview of the neuropathological diagnostic criteria for progressive supranuclear palsy and corticobasal degeneration, as well as a discussion of the pathological heterogeneity that can present diagnostic challenges.

Reprinted from Seritan AL, Mendez MF, Silverman DHS, et al: "Functional Imaging as a Window to Dementia: Corticobasal Degeneration." *Journal of Neuropsychiatry and Clinical Neurosciences* 16: 393–399, 2004. Used with permission.

Chapter 15

METACHROMATIC LEUKODYSTROPHY

A Model for the Study of Psychosis

DEBORAH N. BLACK, M.D.
KATHERINE H. TABER, PH.D.
ROBIN A. HURLEY, M.D.

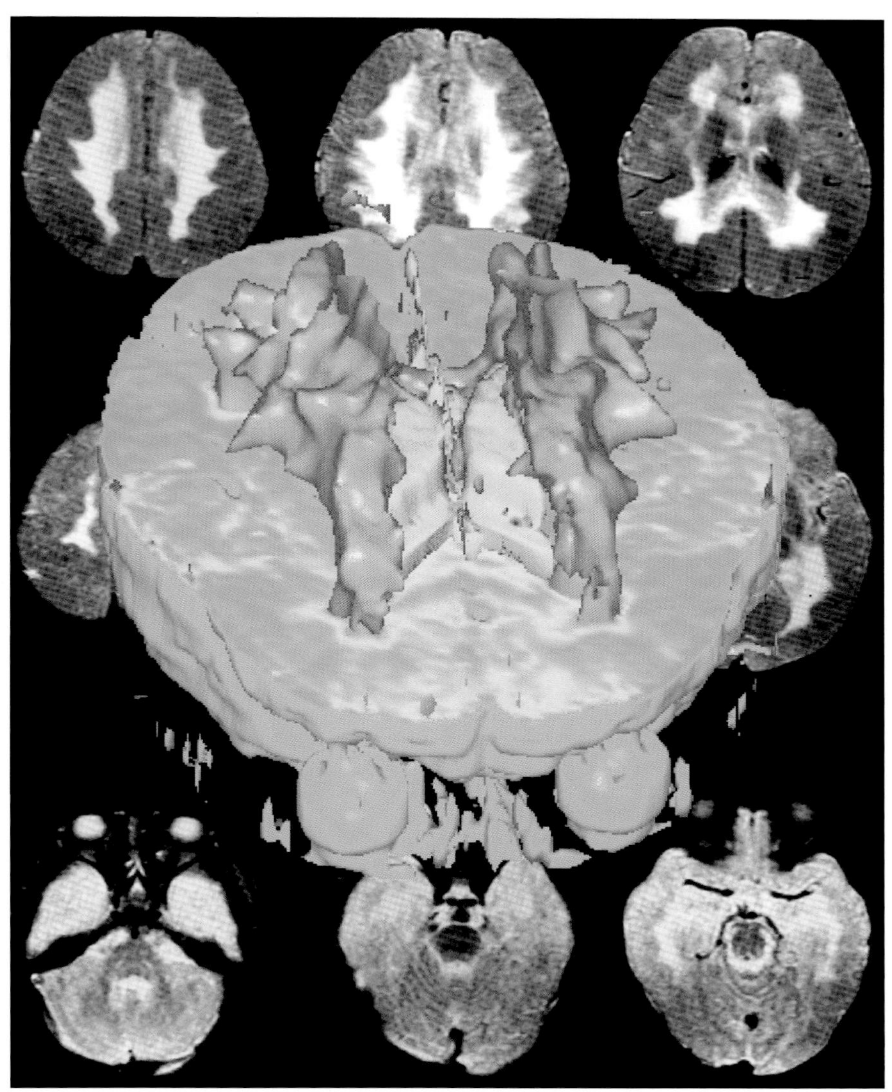

A three-dimensional reconstruction of the white matter lesions (*orange*) and ventricles (*yellow*) of a young child with metachromatic leukodystrophy. It is surrounded by the two-dimensional axial magnetic resonance images from which it was created. Reprinted with permission from Minamikawa-Tachino et al.[1]

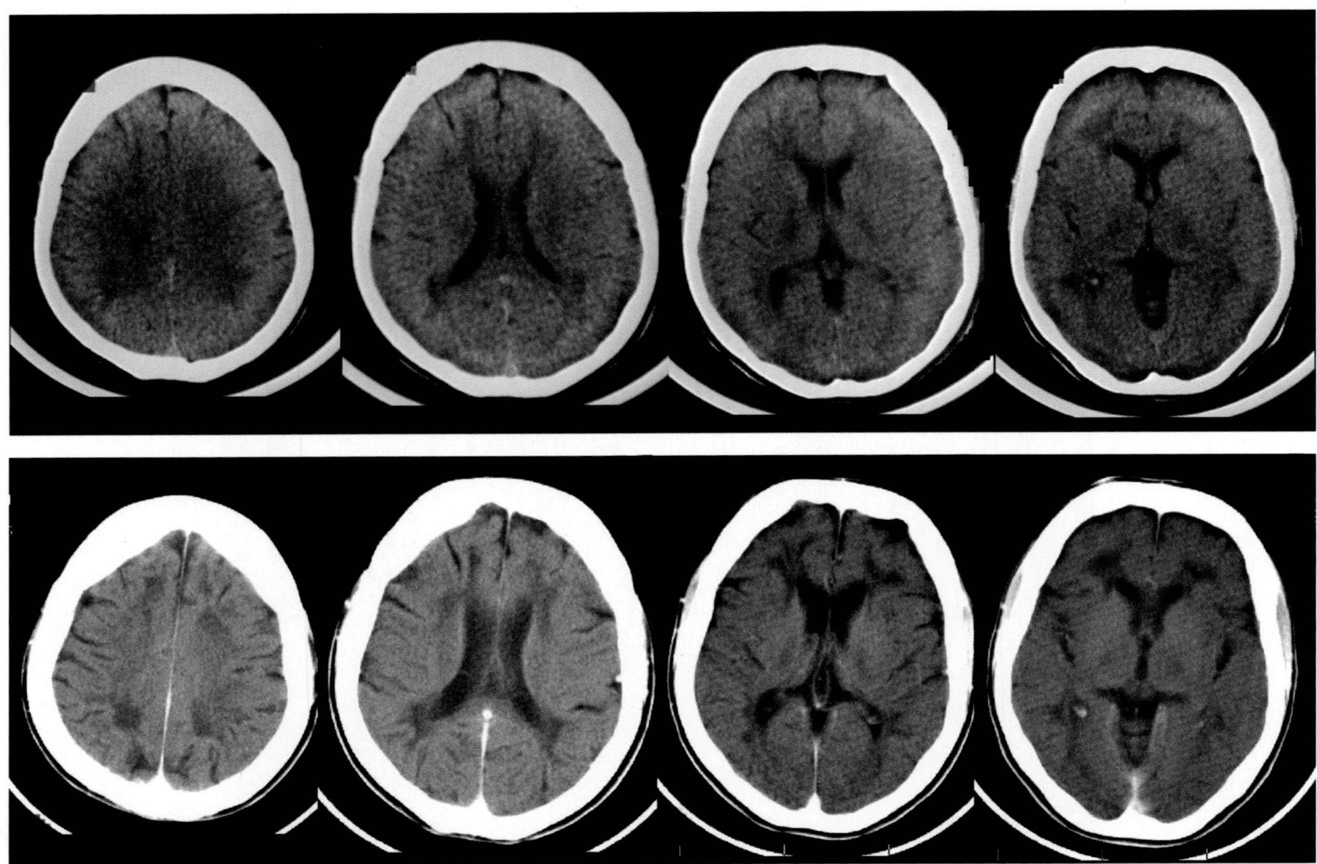

FIGURE 15–1. Serial CT in a young adult female patient with adult-onset MLD. Axial CT images (top) of a female with auditory hallucinations, agitation, and grandiose and paranoid delusions. Cognitive testing showed IQ 78, attentional errors, psychomotor slowing, impaired verbal and nonverbal memory, and concreteness. Behavioral changes began at age 17 with deterioration of school performance, promiscuity, and polysubstance abuse. Note the enlarged ventricles and white matter attenuation. Follow-up CT (bottom) 9 years later showed progression of white matter attenuation and increased ventricular size, consistent with cerebral atrophy. Concurrently she exhibited urinary and fecal incontinence, global deficiencies in self-care, marked apathy, and was unable to name the month or recite the alphabet. Pseudobulbar affect, imitation behavior, and primitive and brisk tendon reflexes without other neurological abnormalities were present. Arylsulfatase A was absent in leukocytes. An older brother was similarly but more severely affected.

Metachromatic leukodystrophy (MLD) is a demyelinating genetic disorder in which neuropsychiatric abnormalities, including psychotic features similar to those present in schizophrenia, are prominent symptoms. Although rare, it is a valuable model for the study of psychosis.[2] MLD occurs worldwide with an estimated frequency of 1 in 40,000, although several clusters of much higher frequency have been identified.[3] MLD is caused by an autosomal recessive mutation on chromosome 22q, resulting in the near-complete absence of the lysosomal enzyme arylsulfatase A (ARS-A). More than 57 mutations of the ARS-A gene have been identified, including 31 amino acid substitutions, 1 nonsense mutation, 3 deletions, 3 splice donor site mutations, and 1 combined missense-splice donor site mutation.[3,4] There is also an ARS-A pseudodeficiency, with a frequency of around 16% in the general population.[5] Patients with this pseudodeficiency, who appear clinically healthy, are thought to be compound heterozygotes for the deficient allele and another allele coding for low enzyme activity. MLD can be mimicked by genetically unrelated deficiency of cerebroside sulfatase activator and multiple sulfatase deficiency.

Metachromatic material (cerebroside sulfate) accumulates in brain oligodendrocytes and microglia, peripheral nerve Schwann cells, and kidneys, and it is excreted in urine. The accumulation of this material leads to abnormal myelin formation and myelin degeneration by unknown pathophysiological mechanisms. Diagnosis of MLD may be suspected when metachromatic granules are found in conjunctival or sural nerve biopsy.[6] Definitive di-

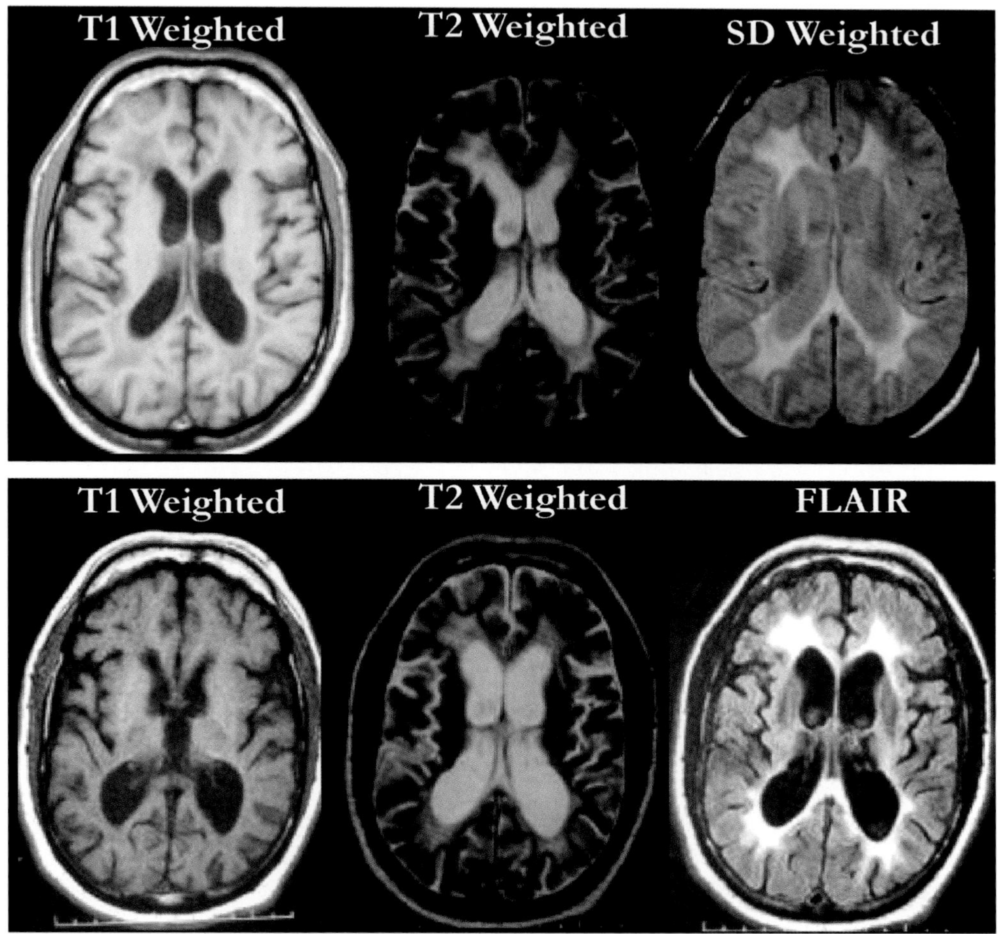

FIGURE 15–2. Serial MRI in a middle-aged male patient with adult-onset MLD. Axial magnetic resonance (MR) images (top) of a male who developed difficulty with walking and coordination. After a full neurological work-up and brain biopsy, the patient was determined to have adult-onset MLD. Note the ventricular enlargement and hyperintense signal around the ventricles on T_2 and spin density (SD) images, indicating white matter disease. Two years later, the patient developed psychiatric symptoms, including disinhibition, aggression, and depression. Follow-up MR images 4 years after onset (bottom) showed greatly enlarged ventricles and significant atrophy, consistent with the worsening of the patient's symptoms, including gait instability and bowel/bladder incontinence.

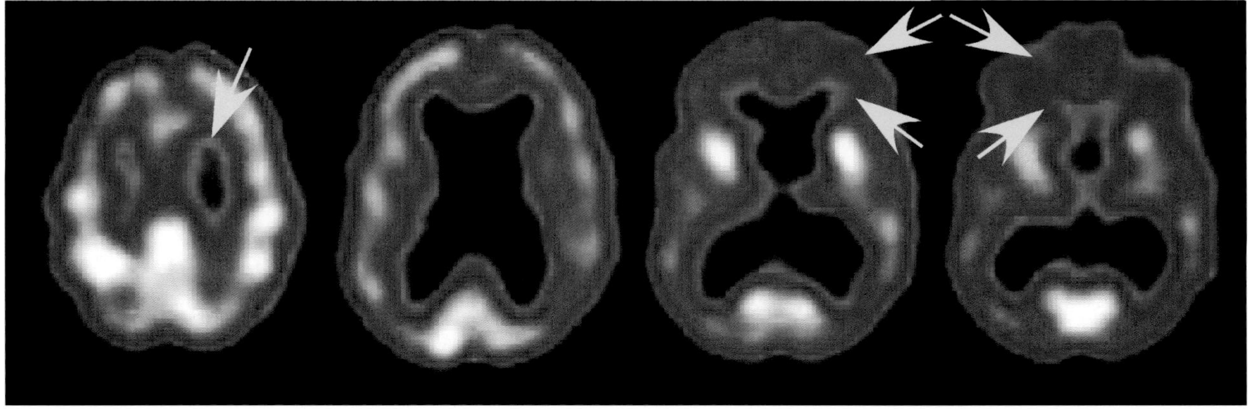

FIGURE 15–3. Companion single-photon emission computed tomography (SPECT) images. SPECT acquired at the same time as the second set of magnetic resonance images (Figure 15–2, bottom) showed ventricular enlargement, significant atrophy, and decreased perfusion, especially in frontal lobe gray and white matter (arrows).

agnosis relies on the confirmation of low ARS-A activity in leukocytes or cultured fibroblasts.[3] The clinical phenotype of MLD is divided into late infantile, juvenile, and adult-onset forms. The late infantile form, which is the most common, presents before age 2, with weakness, muscular hypotonia, and delayed motor and intellectual milestones. Death usually occurs before age 5 in a rigid, vegetative state. Juvenile MLD most commonly presents between 4 and 10 years of age. The distinction between juvenile and adult-onset MLD is arbitrarily set at age 16.

Both the juvenile and adult-onset forms are distinguished from late infantile MLD by slower progression, higher residual ARS-A activity, and a preponderance of neuropsychiatric abnormalities, including conduct disorder, nonverbal learning disability, alcohol or substance abuse, depression, and schizophrenia-like psychosis.[3,7,8] Baumann et al. described two distinct clinical patterns of adult MLD.[7] One presents with predominantly motor manifestations similar to those found in infantile cases. The other presents as a schizophrenia-like psychosis, with prominent negative signs (e.g., psychomotor slowing, apathy, apragmatism, poor judgment, and disorganized thinking). The cognitive profile resembles a subcortical dementia, including impaired verbal fluency, impaired memory retrieval, and executive dysfunction. Disinhibition, anosognosia, complex delusions, bizarre behavior, and auditory hallucinations may also occur.[7,9] Extrapyramidal symptoms, including choreoathetosis and dystonia, seizures, and peripheral neuropathy rarely occur. Some variability is probably related to different mutations within the ARS-A gene. For example, adult MLD patients with primarily psychiatric manifestations may carry mutations in regions of the ARS-A gene that are distinct from the common P426L mutation found in most patients with motor signs.[7] However, strict genotype-phenotype correlations do not apply in all cases, and genetic background probably modifies the clinical profile.[4] Whatever the age at onset, progression is the rule. Motor signs can be absent until decades into the illness despite the characteristic white matter appearance on neuroimaging.[10] The prominent behavioral disturbance and more subtle initial cognitive dysfunction combined with the lack of motor signs can make recognition of this degenerative dementia challenging. All cases eventually manifest dementia and spasticity.

It is unclear at this time whether the neuropsychiatric profile of adult MLD is a direct manifestation of low ARS-A activity or whether neuropsychiatric abnormalities, particularly psychosis, reflect disruption of brain white matter tracts. In favor of the low-ARS-A-activity-neuropsychiatric-phenotype model is the observation of increased psychopathology in some first-degree relatives of MLD patients. These individuals are presumably heterozygote carriers of one defective allele of the ARS-A gene.[8] Subtle deficits in visuospatial perception, construction, stereognosis, and visual search tasks have been found in MLD heterozygotes.[11]

Structural Imaging

Computed tomography (CT) findings in MLD consist of confluent attenuation of signal from hemispheric white matter (Figure 15–1). This is particularly marked in frontal and parietal regions. Later signs include progressive cortical and subcortical atrophy and ventricular dilatation ex vacuo.[9,12] White matter hypodensities on CT probably reflect myelin loss rather than pathological accumulation of cerebroside.[12]

Magnetic resonance imaging (MRI) is more sensitive than CT for the detection of white matter lesions of the brain (Figure 15–2).[13] MRI is particularly useful for the visualization of early lesions and involvement of posterior fossa structures (brainstem and cerebellum), and for evaluating the severity and extent of the disease.[14] On T_1 (inversion recovery)-weighted sequences, brain white matter has high signal, which reflects the presence of free water in the 150 nm spaces between the myelin lamellae. In contrast, brain white matter has low signal and cerebrospinal fluid (CSF) is hyperintense on T_2-weighted sequences, which are more useful than T_1 sequences for the detection of lesions of myelin.[13] Fluid attenuated inversion recovery (FLAIR) sequences produce T_2-weighted images with the additional advantage of suppressing the CSF signal, facilitating the distinction between white matter lesions and enlarged Virchow-Robin spaces and lacunes.[13]

Like other leukodystrophies, MLD is distinguished from the asymmetrical white matter changes of normal aging, small-vessel disease, and multiple sclerosis by relatively symmetrical and confluent involvement of the hemispheric white matter. Most cases show lack of enhancement after contrast agent administration, although Kim et al. reported linear enhancement of radial bands of intact perivascular myelin alternating with affected myelin in a tigroid or spotty pattern in 6 affected children, a pattern similar to Pelizaeus-Merzbacher leukodystrophy.[15] Progressive demyelination is believed to spread anteriorly to posteriorly, although exceptions to this pattern may occur.[15] Subcortical U-fibers are initially spared.[15] MLD has the added distinction of early and extensive involvement of the corpus callosum, internal capsules, corticospinal tracts in the brainstem, and deep cerebellar white matter.[13,15] Abnormal low signal in the thalami on T_2-weighted images has also been reported.[14,15] Despite these features, T_2-weighted MRI alone cannot definitively distinguish MLD from other dysmyelinating leukodystrophies, such as adrenoleukodystrophy and Krabbe's (globoid cell) leukodystrophy.[14]

Diffusion-weighted MRI (DWI), which is sensitive to the mobility of water in tissue, may be more specific than standard T_2-weighted MRI in distinguishing MLD from other leukodystrophies, although there are few studies at present.[16,17] The apparent diffusion constant (ADC) was reduced in the deep white matter (indicating more restricted diffusion) of an infant with MLD on images acquired at 10 and 16 months of age. Restriction of diffusion in the diseased white matter was similar to the changes seen in cytotoxic edema.[17] Reduced ADC within the corpus callosum and inner portions of the centrum semiovale was also found in a 4½-year-old child with MLD.[16] The authors suggest that the accumulation of lysosomal membrane–bound sulfatides may restrict the movement of water in affected tissue.[16] In addition, directionality of diffusion, which is normally high in white matter, was also very low. The authors suggest that this may result from the extremely restricted diffusion in the affected white matter. These results are in contrast to most other leukodystrophies examined in this study, in which the ADC was increased, indicating less restricted diffusion.

In late-onset MLD, where the clinical presentation may resemble a primary psychiatric disorder, MRI is particularly useful in indicating the presence of white matter disease; indeed, pathological involvement of white matter may be seen on MRI before the onset of typical clinical signs.[12] MRI may, therefore, be a useful adjunct to biochemical screening for early disease detection in affected families.[14] Serial MRI may be a useful adjunct to clinical neurobehavioral evaluation to document decrease or stabilization of white matter pathology following therapeutic bone marrow transplantation.[18]

Functional Imaging

Salmon et al. obtained positron emission tomography (PET) in a woman with enzymatically confirmed MLD who presented with cognitive changes in her mid-30s.[9] In contrast to the subcortical involvement of white matter on CT and MRI, hypometabolism was observed bilaterally in the thalamus, medial frontal cortex, frontal poles, and occipital cortex. This pattern differed from the characteristic dorsolateral prefrontal, parietal, and posterior temporal association cortical hypometabolism in Alzheimer's dementia (AD). Tamagaki et al. reported a similar lack of correlation between T_2-weighted MRI subcortical abnormalities and cortical hypoperfusion on single-photon emission computed tomography (SPECT) in a patient with adult-onset MLD who presented behavioral abnormalities, euphoria, personality changes, and dementia.[19] Widespread functionally interconnected cortical regions may be disconnected by subcortical lesions. The clinical repercussions may resemble a primary cortical lesion (diaschisis) (Figure 15–3).

A Model of Psychosis

Late-onset MLD has been proposed as a naturally occurring model of schizophrenia.[2,20] The psychotic and cognitive features of late-onset MLD are extremely similar to those of schizophrenia. Both disorders are characterized by widespread anatomic dysconnectivity and secondary functional disruption. The prominent executive dysfunction in both MLD and schizophrenia reflects extensive disruption of frontal-subcortical circuits, which subserve mood, motivation, behavioral regulation, planning, and judgment.[21] Although abundant evidence suggests that schizophrenia is predominantly a disease of gray matter and MLD is a disease of white matter, there is evidence of neuronal dysfunction in MLD and white matter abnormalities in schizophrenia.[22–24] Decreased fractional anisotropy in the inferior frontal white matter is inversely correlated with negative symptoms in schizophrenia.[25] Furthermore, the anatomical distinction between cortical and subcortical disease is not corroborated by either clinical observation or functional imaging. A functional disturbance of neuronal metabolism and activity at a remote site after injury to an anatomically connected area of brain (diaschisis) is frequently found, and it may be the explanation for the SPECT observation of thalamic and widespread cortical hypoperfusion in the adult case of MLD, above.[9,19]

Some patients with refractory schizophrenia have been shown to have ARS-A pseudodeficiency or intermediate ARS-A levels between normal and deficient.[8] This supports the suggestion that accumulation of cerebroside sulfate is toxic to the brain. However, these observations have not been consistently replicated, in part because of differing assay techniques, widely variable normal ARS-A levels, and poorly controlled case definition. Additionally, it has not been definitively established that ARS-A deficiency or pseudodeficiency is higher in the psychiatric population than in the general population.[5,8,26,27] One interpretation of these discrepant results, based on in vitro studies, is that low-enzyme activity individuals may be at greater risk of neuropsychiatric disability if they are exposed to environmental or endogenous stressors such as ethanol consumption.[8,11] An additional interpretation of these discrepant findings is that there may be a subgroup of patients with schizophrenia who have low ARS-A levels. These could be obscured by mean group comparisons.[28]

Evidence for the importance of white matter pathology in both schizophrenia and MLD is compelling. It has been proposed that schizophrenia is characterized by a developmentally mediated abnormal connectivity ("dysconnectivity") between the prefrontal and mesiotemporal cortex.[29,30] In this model, subtle disorganization of cortical cytoarchitecture leads to disruption of neuronal circuits in widely distributed, functionally interrelated brain regions.[31] Loss of the normally dense and reciprocal projections between the prefrontal and limbic cortex is supported by anatomical studies showing reversal of the normal positive correlation between the volumes of left prefrontal cortex, superior temporal cortex, and hippocampus in patients with schizophrenia.[32] Functional imaging studies suggest that hypoactivation of prefrontal cortex is associated with dysregulation of mesiotemporal and ventral striatal regions, overactivity of limbic dopaminergic systems, and the "positive" manifestations of psychosis, namely, hallucinations and delusions.[33,34] Secondary disruption of white matter tracts is suggested by the finding of reduced volume of the mid–corpus callosum, which conveys axonal projections between the temporal lobes.[35] Some diffusion tensor imaging studies in schizophrenic patients show lower diffusion anisotropy in the prefrontal white matter and in the splenium of the corpus callosum relative to healthy controls (but compare references 36–39). Disruption of white matter may be secondary to cortical neuronal dysfunction, or a primary deficit in myelin gene expression in oligodendroglia.[13,40,41]

Conclusion

There are several parallels between MLD and schizophrenia that support the value of MLD as a model for psychosis. To date, it is not clear whether MLD resembles schizophrenia because of widespread cortical and subcortical disconnection in both diseases or whether specific brain sites must be involved to cause the clinical phenotype of schizophrenia, independent of pathology. What is needed are comparisons of the areas of anatomical overlap between MLD and schizophrenia to define the necessary common ground for clinical disease. Suzuki et al., using three-dimensional MRI in a group of patients with schizophrenia, reported significant white matter decrease in the anterior limbs of the internal capsules and superior occipitofrontal fasciculus.[42] In contrast, Kim et al. described white matter changes in the posterior limb of the internal capsule in a group of seven children with infantile MLD.[15] The anterior limbs were spared in all cases. The anterior limb of the internal capsule conveys reciprocal connections between the dorsomedian thalamus and the prefrontal cortex, while the posterior limb of the internal capsule conveys mostly corticospinal and corticobulbar motor fibers. The schizophreniform psychosis in adult MLD may reflect involvement of the thalamus in this condition, with secondary repercussions in the prefrontal cortex.[9] Further careful anatomical and functional neuroimaging studies will be useful in defining the anatomical substrate for diverse neuropsychiatric disorders with overlapping clinical manifestations.

References

1. Minamikawa-Tachino R, Maeda Y, et al: Three-dimensional brain visualization for metachromatic leukodystrophy. Brain Dev 1996; 18:394–399
2. Hyde TM, Ziegler JC, Weinberger DR: Psychiatric disturbances in metachromatic leukodystrophy. Insights into the neurobiology of psychosis. Arch Neurol 1992; 49:401–406
3. McKusick VA: Metachromatic leukodystrophy. Online Mendelian Inheritance in Man, 2003
4. Berger J, Loschl B, et al: Occurrence, distribution, and phenotype of arylsulfatase A mutations in patients with metachromatic leukodystrophy. Am J Med Genet 1997; 69:335–340
5. Propping P, Friedl W, et al: The influence of low arylsulfatase A activity on neuropsychiatric morbidity—a large-scale screening in patients. Hum Genet 1986; 74:244–248
6. Blackwood W, Corsellis JAN: Greenfield's Neuropathology. London, Arnold, 1976
7. Baumann N, Turpin JC, et al: Motor and psycho-cognitive clinical types in adult metachromatic leukodystrophy: genotype/phenotype relationships? J Physiol Paris 2002; 96:301–306
8. Fluharty AL: The relationship of the metachromatic leukodystrophies to neuropsychiatric disorders. Molecular and Chemical Neuropathology 1990; 13:81–94
9. Salmon E, Van der Linden M, et al: Early thalamic and cortical hypometabolism in adult-onset dementia due to metachromatic leukodystrophy. Acta Neurologica Belgica 1999; 99:185–188
10. Finelli PF: Metachromatic leukodystrophy manifesting as a schizophrenic disorder—computed tomographic correlation. Annals of Neurology 1985; 18:94–95
11. Kohn H, Manowitz P, et al: Neuropsychological deficits in obligatory heterozygotes for metachromatic leukodystrophy. Human Genetics 1988; 79:8–12
12. Reider-Grosswasser I, Bornstein N: CT and MRI in late-onset metachromatic leukodystrophy. Acta Neurol Scand 1987; 75:64–69
13. Barkhof F, Scheltens P: Imaging of white matter lesions. Cerebrovascular Diseases 2002; 13:21–30
14. Demaerel P, Faubert C, et al: MR findings in leukodystrophy. Neuroradiology 1991; 33:368–371
15. Kim TS, Kim IO, et al: MR of childhood metachromatic leukodystrophy. Am J Neuroradiol 1997; 18:733–738
16. Engelbrecht V, Scherer A, et al: Diffusion-weighted MR imaging in the brain in children: findings in the normal brain and in the brain with white matter diseases. Radiology 2002; 222:410–418

17. Sener RN: Metachromatic leukodystrophy: diffusion MR imaging findings. Am J Neuroradiol 2002; 23:1424–1426
18. Stillman AE, Krivit W, et al: Serial MR after bone-marrow transplantation in 2 patients with metachromatic leukodystrophy. Am J Neuroradiol 1994; 15:1929–1932
19. Tamagaki C, Murata A, et al: Two siblings with adult-type metachromatic leukodystrophy: correlation between clinical symptoms and neuroimaging [in Japanese]. Seishin Shinkeigaku Zasshi 2000; 102:399–409
20. Holden C: Neuroscience: deconstructing schizophrenia. Science 2003; 299:333–335
21. Lim KO, Helpern JA: Neuropsychiatric applications of DTI—a review. NMR Biomed 2002; 15:587–593
22. Mega MS, Cummings JL: Frontal-subcortical circuits and neuropsychiatric disorders. J Neuropsychiatry Clin Neurosci 1994; 6:358–370
23. Alves D, Pires MM, et al: 4 Cases of late onset metachromatic leukodystrophy in a family—clinical, biochemical and neuropathological studies. J Neurol Neurosurg Psychiatry 1986; 49:1417–1422
24. Goebel HH, Argyrakis A, et al: Adult metachromatic leukodystrophy, 4: ultrastructural studies on the central and peripheral nervous-system. Eur Neurol 1980; 19:294–307
25. Wolkin A, Choi SJ, et al: Inferior frontal white matter anisotropy and negative symptoms of schizophrenia: a diffusion tensor imaging study. Am J Psychiatry 2003; 160:572–574
26. Lejoyeux M, Dubois G, et al: Arylsulfatase A activity among psychotic patients. Psychiatry Res 1989; 30:107–108
27. Shah SN: Arylsulfatase A (ASA) defect and psychiatric illness—a review. Mol ChemNeuropathol 1990; 12:121–129
28. Heavey AM, Philpot MP, et al: Leukocyte arylsulfatase-A activity and subtypes of chronic schizophrenia. Acta Psychiatr Scand 1990; 82:55–59
29. Meyer-Lindenberg A, Poline JB, et al: Evidence for abnormal cortical functional connectivity during working memory in schizophrenia. Am J Psychiatry 2001; 158:1809–1817
30. Bullmore ET, Frangou S, Murray RM: The dysplastic net hypothesis: an integration of developmental and dysconnectivity theories of schizophrenia. Schizophr Res 1997; 28:143–156
31. Weinberger DR, Lipska BK: Cortical maldevelopment, antipsychotic drugs, and schizophrenia—a search for common ground. Schizophr Res 1995; 16:87–110
32. Woodruff PW, Wright IC, et al: Structural brain abnormalities in male schizophrenics reflect fronto-temporal dissociation. Psychol Med 1997; 27:1257–1266
33. Epstein J, Stern E, Silbersweig D: Mesolimbic activity associated with psychosis in schizophrenia—symptom-specific PET studies. Advancing From the Ventral Striatum to the Extended Amygdala 1999; 877:562–574
34. Silbersweig DA, Stern E, et al: A functional neuroanatomy of hallucinations in schizophrenia. Nature 1995; 378:176–179
35. Woodruff PW, Pearlson GD, et al: A computerized magnetic resonance imaging study of corpus callosum morphology in schizophrenia. Psychol Med 1993; 23:45–56
36. Foong J, Maier M, et al: Neuropathological abnormalities of the corpus callosum in schizophrenia: a diffusion tensor imaging study. J Neurol Neurosurg Psychiatry 2000; 68:242–244
37. Buchsbaum MS, Tang CY, et al: MRI white matter diffusion anisotropy and PET metabolic rate in schizophrenia. Neuroreport 1998; 9:425–430
38. Agartz I, Andersson JLR, Skare S: Abnormal brain white matter in schizophrenia: a diffusion tensor imaging study. Neuroreport 2001; 12:2251–2254
39. Foong J, Symms MR, et al: Investigating regional white matter in schizophrenia using diffusion tensor imaging. Neuroreport 2002; 13:333–336
40. Steel RM, Bastin ME, et al: Diffusion tensor imaging (DTI) and proton magnetic resonance spectroscopy (1H MRS) in schizophrenic subjects and normal controls. Psychiatry Res 2001; 106:161–170
41. Holden C: Neuroscience. White matter's the matter. Science 2003; 299:334
42. Suzuki M, Nohara S, et al: Regional changes in brain gray and white matter in patients with schizophrenia demonstrated with voxel-based analysis of MRI. Schizophr Res 2002; 55:41–54

Recent Publications of Interest

Walterfang M, Wood SJ, Velakoulis D, et al: Diseases of white matter and schizophrenia-like psychosis. Aust N Z J Psychiatry 2005; 39:746–756

Analyzed the neurological and psychiatric literature on a broad range of white matter diseases (developmental, neoplastic, infective, immunological) in order to identify those that can present as a schizophrenia-like psychosis. They discuss the nature, location, and timing of white matter pathology as key factors in the development of psychosis and the implications for schizophrenia.

van der Voorn JP, Pouwels PJ, Kamphorst W, et al: Histopathologic correlates of radial stripes on MR images in lysosomal storage disorders. Am J Neuroradiol 2005; 26:442–446

Performed a histopathological study of the radially oriented hypointense stripes observed in the white matter on magnetic resonance imaging in some lysosomal storage diseases. They found that in metachromatic leukodystrophy these stripes correlate with perivascular regions containing spared myelin, macrophages, and lipid-containing glial cells.

Kumperscak HG, Paschke E, Gradisnik P, et al: Adult metachromatic leukodystrophy: disorganized schizophrenia-like symptoms and postpartum depression in 2 sisters. J Psychiatry Neurosci 2005; 30:33–36

Reports a case in which schizophrenia-like symptoms were the initial manifestation of metachromatic leukodystrophy in an 18-year-old female.

Patay Z: Diffusion-weighted MR imaging in leukodystrophies. Eur Radiol 2005;15:2284–2303

Provides an overview of the application of diffusion-weighted magnetic resonance imaging to lysosomal storage diseases, including metachromatic leukodystrophy.

Matzner U, Herbst E, Hedayati KK, et al: Enzyme replacement improves nervous system pathology and function in a mouse model for metachromatic leukodystrophy. Hum Mol Genet 2005; 14:1139–1152
Assessed the therapeutic potential of enzyme replacement therapy in a mouse model of metachromatic leukodystrophy. A series of four weekly injections were effective in reducing excess sulfatide storage in brain and spinal cord, suggesting that this approach may be worth pursuing as a therapeutic option.

Reprinted from Black DN, Taber KH, Hurley RA: "Metachromatic Leukodystrophy: A Model for the Study of Psychosis." *Journal of Neuropsychiatry and Clinical Neurosciences* 15:289–293, 2003. Used with permission.

Chapter 16

IDENTIFICATION OF HIV-ASSOCIATED PROGRESSIVE MULTIFOCAL LEUKOENCEPHALOPATHY

Magnetic Resonance Imaging and Spectroscopy

ROBIN A. HURLEY, M.D.
THOMAS ERNST, PH.D.
KAMEL KHALILI, PH.D.
LUIS DEL VALLE, M.D.
ISABELLA LAURA SIMONE, M.D.
KATHERINE H. TABER, PH.D.

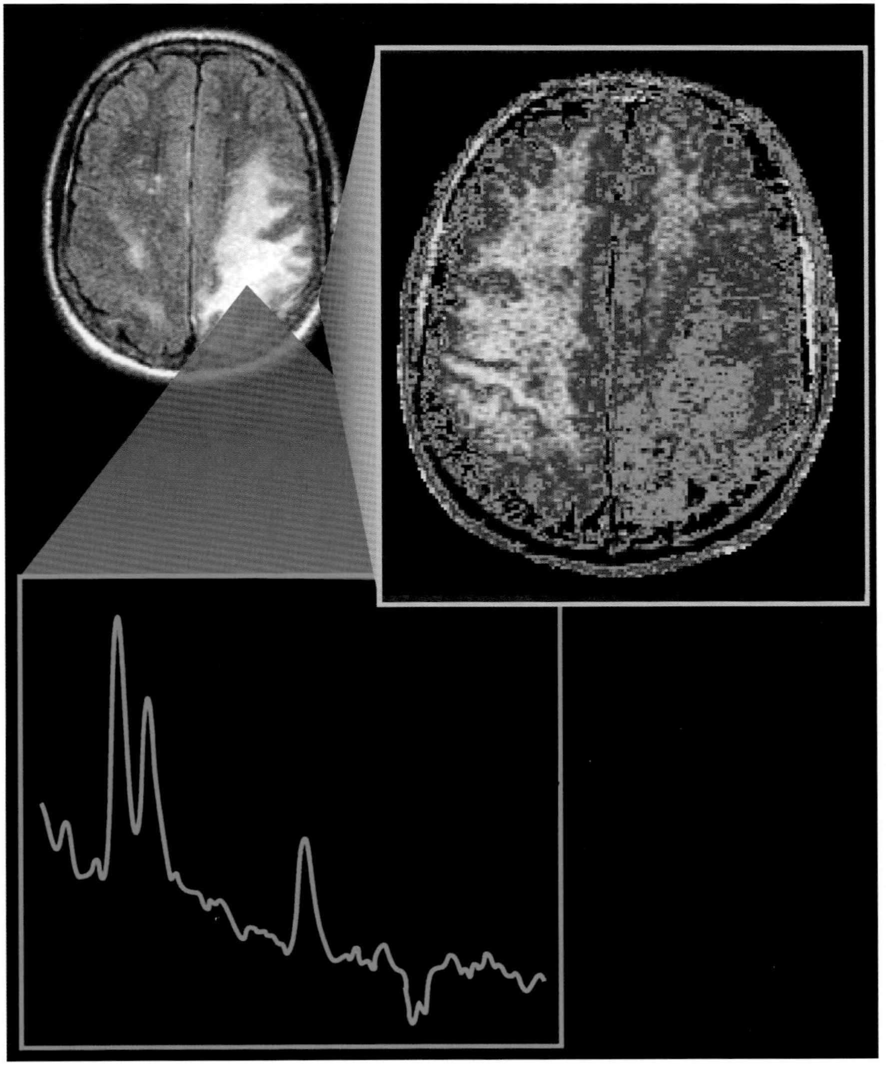

Companion axial fluid-attenuated inversion recovery (FLAIR) images (top left) and magnetization transfer ratio (MTR) images (top right) of progressive multifocal leukoencephalopathy (PML). A representative proton magnetic resonance spectrum (bottom left) is also shown.

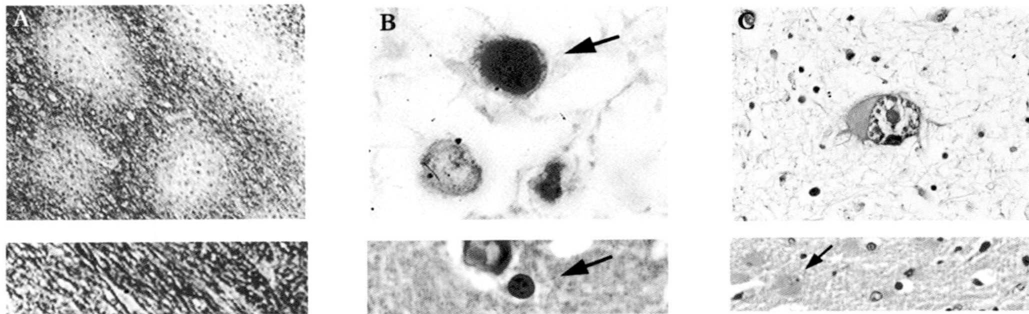

FIGURE 16–1. The histological characteristics of PML include destruction of myelin (A, myelin-stained section of subcortical white matter), loss of oligodendrocytes (B, enlarged oligodendrocytes harboring intranuclear eosinophilic inclusion bodies, at arrow), and bizarre reactive astrocytes (C, transformed bizarre reactive astrocyte). Companion normal images are shown beneath each panel for comparison.

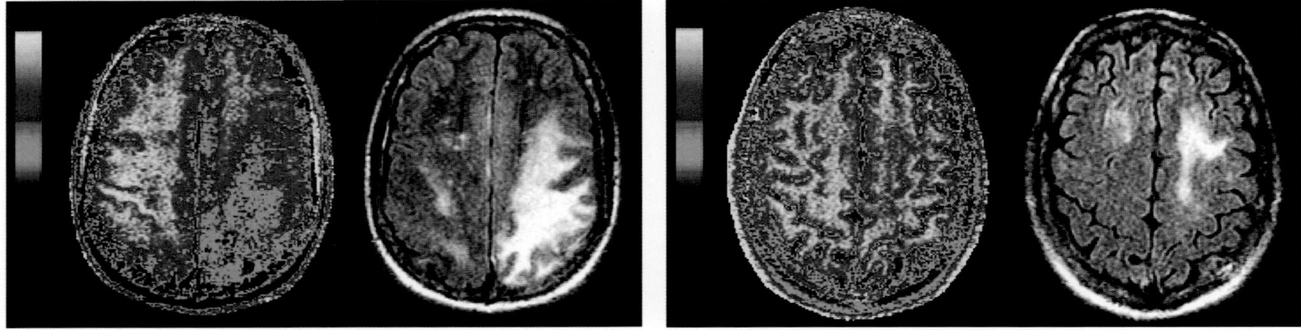

FIGURE 16–2. Companion magnetization transfer ratio (MTR, color) and FLAIR (grayscale) magnetic resonance images of PML (left set) and HIV–white matter lesions (right set). Although the areas of abnormality in the white matter look quite similar on the FLAIR images, they are clearly different on the MTR images. The MTR of the PML lesions is deeply decreased (*green* and *blue* areas in left set of images), consistent with the demyelinating nature of the disease. The lesions in HIV infection show very little decrease in MTR, as would be expected based on the less destructive nature of this pathology.

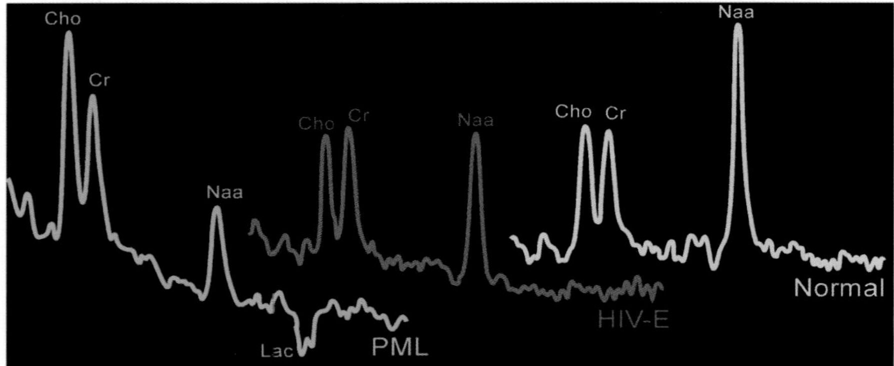

FIGURE 16–3. Illustrations of proton (^{1}H) magnetic resonance spectra acquired from normal brain (*white*), a white matter lesion in a patient with pure HIV infection (*red*), and a PML lesion (*green*). Spectra have been scaled so that creatine (Cr) peaks are similar heights. Note that the *N*-acetylaspartate (NAA) peak is decreased in both HIV and PML.

The human immunodeficiency virus (HIV) and resulting acquired immune deficiency syndrome (AIDS) is a leading cause of death worldwide. A recent estimate from the United Nations Programme on HIV/AIDS indicates that 40 million people worldwide have HIV/AIDS.[1] The advent of highly active antiretroviral therapy (HAART) has certainly increased survival. However, central nervous system (CNS) disorders remain a significant cause of morbidity and mortality in HIV/AIDS-infected patients. Current statistics indicate that 39%–70% of all AIDS patients develop neurological disorders, and these are the initial manifestations of AIDS in 7%–20%.[2] A large retrospective study of 450 AIDS autopsy cases (1984–1999) found that the brain continues to be second only to lung in pathology, with 28%–38% of cases having CNS findings.[3] Commonly occurring conditions include toxoplasma encephalitis, cryptococcal meningitis, primary CNS lymphoma, HIV-associated dementia, progressive multifocal leukoencephalopathy (PML), and other viral and opportunistic infections. Most authors agree that only some conditions have decreased with HAART. The incidence of PML has not changed over time, whereas some opportunistic infections such as toxoplasmosis and cytomegalovirus have had as much as a 50% decline.[3] Currently PML is estimated to occur in 1%–10% of AIDS patients, and in one study it occurred within 1 year of death in 91.7% of patients who were infected.[4,5]

A good brief overview of PML, with historical references, can be found in the review of Berger and Major.[4] This disorder is a multifocal demyelinating disease that is caused by a reactivation of the dormant JC virus (JCV), a DNA-containing polyomavirus. It was first described by a German neuropathologist, Hallervorden, in 1930. It was described as a syndrome in 1958 by Åstrom and Richardson and identified as a viral disease in 1965 by Zu-Rhein. The virus was isolated in 1971 by Padgett and Walker.[4,6] It was a rare disorder in immunocompromised patients until the AIDS epidemic, when its incidence greatly expanded. PML cases increased 400% in the decade between 1984 and 1994.[7] The rate varies considerably by country, being low in the United States (2%–5%) and higher in most European studies (4%–11%).[7] Additionally, PML was documented more often in intravenous drug users than non–drug users.[3] When PML develops in conjunction with HIV, it is particularly devastating, with survival times in the absence of treatment of only a few months.[8] Most adults (70%–90%) have IgG antibodies to JCV by middle age.[4,9] The initial infection has not been identified, but one proposal is that the acute infection may be in the tonsils.[4] JCV is also present in the kidneys.[10,11]

Because the disease is multifocal, symptoms will depend on the areas demyelinated; however, common complaints are present.[4] Weakness, disturbances of speech, cognitive abnormalities, headaches, gait disorders, seizures, sensory loss, and visual impairments (field loss, diplopia) are reported. Limb weakness was estimated in more than 50% of cases; cognitive and gait disorders in 25%–33%; seizures in 10%. HIV-associated dementia and other CNS disorders can certainly have similar presentations. It is therefore necessary to quickly identify this rapidly fatal disease in the least possibly invasive way. Recent improvements in cerebrospinal fluid (CSF) testing and newer imaging techniques are replacing the older biopsy method.

Pathology

Recent laboratory findings culminated in a proposed cycle for the development and progression of PML.[10,11] The virus has an icosahedral capsid covering a double-stranded DNA, which can be divided into three regions: early and late coding regions and a regulatory (noncoding) region. JCV DNA is present in the peripheral blood lymphocytes in more than 95% of PML cases. Activated B cells cross the blood–brain barrier. Immunohistochemical staining of tissue samples indicates that JCV is predominantly found in the oligodendrocytes, while HIV-1 is primarily found in the microglia, monocytes, and astrocytes.[10–12] Controversy remains as to whether or not glia can be a latent site for harborization. Once the virus is inside the CNS, replication begins in the glial cells. Recent theory, greatly simplified, is that the HIV-infected cells produce Tat, a transregulatory protein.[10,11] Tat is released from its host cell and taken up by the neighboring oligodendrocytes. Tat then induces the JCV promoter. Thus, JCV replication is increased. Host cells are lysed, and the cycle continues. Additionally, Tat induces the production of several cytotoxic proteins, including tumor necrosis factor, interleukin-1, and transforming growth factor β, that not only destroy neighboring cells but also stimulate further viral production.

Classic histological examination indicates extensive demyelinated plaques, oligodendrocytes with eosinophilic intranuclear JCV inclusions, and atypical hypertrophic astrocytes (Figure 16–1).[10,11] Less commonly, microglial nodules, perivascular lymphocytic cuffing, and cavity formation are found. Mossakowski and Zelman[7] autopsied 20 cases of PML. They found that PML was coexistent with other opportunistic AIDS-related brain diseases in 14 of the 20 cases. They divided the results into early, atypical, and late forms. The early form had multiple scattered foci, commonly near the corticosubcortical junctions or deep white matter. The oligodendrocytes were consistently abnormal, with the classic enlarged metachromatic nuclei. The astrocytes were mildly enlarged. The atypical form was more unifocal, with the classic findings in the glia. The late, severe group had much more demyelination, with bilateral, asymmetric lesions in the cerebrum and, less commonly, the brainstem and cerebellum. The glia were very abnormal, with JCV virions within the oligodendrocytes, hypertrophic astrocytes, cavitary lesions, and macrophage/lymphocytic invasion. The authors also noted that in their experience, PML destruction is more severe in AIDS than in other immunocompromising diseases, citing a synergy with the HIV virus itself.

Diagnostic Advances

Definitive diagnosis of PML can be made only by brain biopsy. However, this is invasive and can have associated with it occasional morbidity (hemorrhage or infection within 30 days), rare mortality, or lesion of brain circuitry. In a recent review of brain biopsies of 435 patients (47 local and 388 by literature review), Skolasky et al.[13] determined that biopsies have an 88% definitive diagnostic yield. However, morbidity and mortality were high and varied from site to site. Morbidity ranged from 3.3% to 30.8% (average 8.4%); mortality ranged from 0% to 5.3% (average 2.9%). In this survey, 25% of patients were diagnosed with PML. Currently, noninvasive techniques are increasing. Radiologic imaging and CSF analysis are emerging as potential tools to replace biopsy in many cases.

Magnetic Resonance Imaging

Both PML and HIV encephalopathy are associated with nonenhancing lesions in the cerebral white matter that show little or no mass effect and are hyperintense on T_2-weighted and fluid attenuated inversion recovery (FLAIR) magnetic resonance (MR) images.[8,14] However, PML can be differentiated from HIV encephalopathy because the PML lesions are commonly hypointense on T_1-weighted MR images, while in pure HIV infection, lesions are isointense. Serial imaging indicates the PML lesions become more hypointense as the disease progresses; markedly low signal intensity may indicate particularly aggressive infection.[8] In addition, PML lesions are focal and, if bilateral, they are asymmetric. They are located predominantly in the subcortical white matter just below the cortical ribbon, involve the arcuate (U) fibers (although brainstem and cerebellar lesions are also found), and present little or no atrophy.[15] In contrast, white matter lesions in HIV encephalopathy are diffuse and symmetric and do not involve the arcuate fibers. In addition, both cortical and subcortical (particularly caudate) atrophy are common.[8,12,14]

A new type of MR imaging, magnetization transfer (MT) imaging, appears to be much more sensitive than standard MR imaging to the demyelinating process that occurs in PML. MT imaging is based on the cross-relaxation between protons that are essentially immobile because they are bound to tissue ("solid-like" pool) and free protons ("liquid-like" pool), and thus it provides different information than is available from standard clinical MR images.[16–18] Most of the signal used to create any MR image comes from the free pool of protons. For MT imaging, specially designed saturation pulses are included in the imaging sequence to alter the magnetization of the bound protons. This in turn causes a decrease in the signal coming from the free protons and thus changes the signal intensity on the resulting MR image. Most commonly, this is expressed as the change in signal intensity relative to the normal MR image (magnetization transfer ratio, MTR, usually expressed as a percentage). The decrease in signal in the saturated image is large for complex tissues (gray matter, white matter) and small for areas that are mostly fluid (CSF, blood). The MTR is greater for white matter than for gray matter because of the high membrane content. MT imaging is sensitive to any process that disrupts the structural integrity of tissue, particularly the myelin sheath and axon.[19–21]

Two studies have shown that MT imaging can distinguish the demyelinating lesions of PML from both the diffuse lesions of HIV encephalopathy and nonspecific white matter lesions that may be present (Figure 16–2, left and right).[22,23] There were differences between the two studies in both methodology and patient selection. In one study, the pure HIV group all had cognitive deficits, while in the other, none did. Nevertheless, the MT imaging results were similar. Both found the average MTR for normal white matter to be 47%–48%. Both found the MTR of PML lesions to be profoundly decreased (average MTR 22%–26%). White matter lesions related purely to HIV, with or without accompanying cognitive deficits, had mildly reduced MTR (average MTR 38%–40%). These results indicate that MT imaging has the potential to distinguish the destructive demyelinating lesions of PML from the edematous lesions of HIV. Thus, it shows promise for differential diagnosis, prognosis, or monitoring of therapy by serial assessment.

Magnetic Resonance Spectroscopy

Proton (^{1}H) MR spectroscopy provides measures of several neurochemicals related to neuronal viability. Signal is present from *N*-acetylaspartate (NAA, located primarily in neurons, a marker for neuron and axon viability), choline (Cho, principally phosphatidyl choline, a membrane constituent), and creatine (Cr, used as an internal standard because its level is usually stable). An additional peak may be present from lactate (Lac, metabolite associated with inflammation or neuronal mitochondrial dysfunction and related to activated anaerobic glycolytic metabolism). If a short echo-time acquisition is used, it is possible to observe *myo*-inositol (MI, putative glial marker). The absolute amount of signal in each spectral peak is highly dependent on the acquisition parameters, so for comparison purposes the signals of interest (NAA, Cho) are commonly expressed relative to Cr. It is also possible to measure absolute metabolite concentrations, but the acquisition is more complex. The Cho/Cr peak reflects membrane metabolism and has been found to be elevated both during degradation (demyelination) and rapid synthesis. The NAA/Cr peak reflects neuronal and axonal density. Studies vary considerably in design and methodology, including differences in how spectra are acquired, what part of brain (lesion or normal appearing) was examined, and the types of spectral comparisons done. Nevertheless, the results are in reasonable agreement across studies.

In early HIV, when clinical symptoms are absent or mild, NAA/Cr is unchanged (92%–98% of normal value).[24–26] In late-stage HIV, when clinical symptoms are severe, NAA/Cr decreases (62%–84% of normal value).[24–28] Decreased NAA/Cr is found both in lesions and in normal-appearing brain.[24–30] These results are compatible with pathological findings that neuronal loss (which should result in a decrease in NAA/Cr) occurs in the late stage of HIV.[31] It is possible that in some cases decreased NAA/Cr indicates neuronal dysfunction rather than destruction. A return to normal levels was found concomitant with resolution of clinical symptoms following treatment with zidovudine in one study.[32] In contrast, Cho/Cr elevations were similar within studies in the presence and absence of symptoms and in the presence or absence of lesions on diagnostic images, although the size of the increase varied across studies.[24–26] This elevation may reflect an increase in membrane density due to glial changes and/or inflammatory cells.[24] These results suggest that the Cho peak of the spectrum may indicate the presence of subclinical HIV. MI and MI/Cr of normal-appearing white matter are also elevated in early HIV, but higher elevations are correlated with more severe clinical symptoms.[30] Thus increased MI may also indicate subclinical HIV, perhaps reflecting glial activation in response to inflammation.

Only a few studies have included patients with PML.[28,33,34] Both groups reporting on PML patients have found substantial decreases in NAA, whether measured in relation to Cr, to the contralateral NAA value, or by absolute quantification. This decrease is consistent with the destructive nature of the PML infection. Both groups have also found Cho to be elevated, perhaps reflecting myelin destruction. Lac was present in 75% of spectra, also consistent with the severe nature of PML.[28,34] Both increases and decreases in MI were found in the one study that measured it.[33] Interestingly, the study that used absolute quantification found that Cr was decreased.[34] If this is a general finding, it will require reevaluation of studies in which ratios were used.

Only one study has directly compared spectral changes in pure HIV with those in PML (Figure 16–3).[28] The results suggest that this technique may be helpful in differentiating PML from other entities. PML lesions had a more profound decrease in NAA than those associated with HIV encephalopathy, whereas lesions in HIV encephalopathy had a more consistent increase in Cho. In addition, PML lesions had an increased Lac peak.

CSF Analysis

JCV can be detected by polymerase chain reaction (PCR) testing of the CSF.[35] A recent review summarized the sensitivity as 90%–100%, with a specificity of 92%–100%.[9] However, other reports indicate that sensitivity may be lower in some circumstances.[8,23,28] PCR testing for JCV has potential as a prognostic tool because lower survival correlates with higher levels of JCV in the CSF.[9,36,37] Patients with a JCV load <4.7 log (log copies per mL of CSF) survived much longer than those with log >4.7 at time of diagnosis.[36,37] In one report, JCV load did not correlate with lesion load as measured from T_2-weighted MR images.[37] In this study of 12 patients, the volume of lesions did not correlate with JCV load even when CD4 count, treatment with HAART, plasma HIV load, age, and location of lesions were controlled for. Three of the 12 patients had more than one viral load measured. Two of the three had longitudinal correlation of viral load with lesion volume, and the third was inverse. The authors recommend further longitudinal examinations in larger patient groups for any correlations with lesion volume to be found. It might also be interesting to quantify lesion load by using MT imaging.

Conclusion

As newer imaging techniques and CSF testing become the mainstay of PML identification, it will be important for treatment to improve also. In some cases, HAART alone has been effective treatment for PML. However, Miralles et al.[38] report that approximately one-third of patients die despite treatment and improved CD4 cell counts (>200 cells/mm^3). Additionally, PML can develop following initiation of HAART, with a paradoxical worsening of inflammatory changes that are not typical for untreated PML.[39,40] It has been suggested that improved immune system function may be important in activating latent infection.[39] In these cases, at least, adjunct therapy is required. Cidofovir, an antiviral agent, has shown some promise in this regard.[39,41] Serial assessment with some combination of MT imaging, MR spectroscopy, and CSF testing may provide a more rapid and reliable tailoring of individual therapy, thus affecting management and prognosis. It is very likely, too, that MT imaging and MR spectroscopy will provide similarly important insights into other demyelinating conditions.

References

1. Stover J, Walker N, Garnett GP, et al: Can we reverse the HIV/ AIDS pandemic with an expanded response? Lancet 2002; 360:73–77
2. Maschke M, Kastrup O, Esser S, et al: Incidence and prevalence of neurological disorders associated with HIV since the introduction of highly active antiretroviral therapy (HAART). J Neurol Neurosurg Psychiatry 2000; 69:376–380
3. Jellinger KA, Setinek U, Drlicek M, et al: Neuropathology and general autopsy findings in AIDS during the last 15 years. Acta Neuropathol (Berl) 2000; 100:213–220
4. Berger JR, Major EO: Progressive multifocal leukoencephalopathy. Semin Neurol 1999; 19:193–200
5. Welch K, Morse A, Adult Spectrum of Disease Project in New Orleans: The clinical profile of end-stage AIDS in the era of highly active antiretroviral therapy. AIDS Patient Care STDs 2002; 16:75–81
6. Henson JW, Louis DN: Edward Peirson Richardson Jr (1918–1998) and the discovery of PML. J Neurovirol 1999; 5:325–326
7. Mossakowski MJ, Zelman IB: Pathomorphological variations of the AIDS-associated progressive multifocal leukoencephalopathy. Folia Neuropathol 2000; 38:91–100
8. Post MJ, Yiannoutsos C, Simpson D, et al: Progressive multifocal leukoencephalopathy in AIDS: are there any MR findings useful to patient management and predictive of patient survival? AJNR Am J Neuroradiol 1999; 20:1896–1906
9. Mamidi A, DeSimone JA, Pomerantz RJ: Central nervous system infections in individuals with HIV-1 infection. J Neurovirol 2002; 8:158–167
10. Sweet TM, Del Valle L, Khalili K: Molecular biology and immunoregulation of human neurotropic JC virus in CNS. J Cell Physiol 2002; 191:249–256
11. Del Valle L, Croul S, Morgello S, et al: Detection of HIV-1 Tat and JVC capsid protein, VP1, in AIDS brain with progressive multifocal leukoencephalopathy. J Neurovirol 2000; 6:221–228
12. Paul R, Cohen R, Navia B, et al: Relationships between cognition and structural neuroimaging findings in adults with human immunodeficiency virus type-1. Neurosci Biobehav Rev 2002; 26:353–359
13. Skolasky RL, Dal Pan GJ, Olivi A, et al: HIV-associated primary CNS lymorbidity and utility of brain biopsy. J Neurol Sci 1999; 163:32–38
14. Sarrazin JL, Soulie D, Derosier C, et al: [MRI aspects of progressive multifocal leukoencephalopathy] (French). J Neuroradiol 1995; 22:172–179
15. Kastrup O, Maschke M, Diener HC, et al: Progressive multifocal leukoencephalopathy limited to the brain stem. Neuroradiology 2002; 44:227–229
16. Dousset V, Armand JP, Huot P, et al: Magnetization transfer imaging in AIDS-related brain diseases. Neuroimaging Clin N Am 1997; 7:447–460
17. Van Buchem MA, Tofts PS: Magnetization transfer imaging. Neuroimaging Clin N Am 2000; 10:771–788
18. Filippi M, Grossman RI: MRI techniques to monitor MS evolution: the present and the future. Neurology 2002; 58:1147–1153
19. Dousset V, Grossman RI, et al: Experimental allergic encephalomyelitis and multiple sclerosis: lesion characterization with magnetization transfer imaging. Radiology 1992; 182:483–491
20. Lexa FJ, Grossman RI, Rosenquist AC: MR of wallerian degeneration in the feline visual system: characterization by magnetization transfer rate with histopathologic correlation. Am J Neuroradiol 1994; 15:201–212
21. Dousset V, Brochet B, Vital A, et al: Lysolecithin-induced demyelination in primates: preliminary in vivo study with MR and magnetization transfer. AJNR Am J Neuroradiol 1995; 16:225–231
22. Dousset V, Armand JP, Lacoste D, et al: Magnetization transfer study of HIV encephalitis and progressive multifocal leukoencephalopathy. AJNR Am J Neuroradiol 1997; 18:895–901
23. Ernst T, Chang L, Witt M, et al: Progressive multifocal leukoencephalopathy and human immunodeficiency virus–associated white matter lesions in AIDS: magnetization transfer MR imaging. Radiology 1999; 210:539–543
24. Menon DK, Ainsworth JG, Cox IJ, et al: Proton MR spectroscopy of the brain in AIDS dementia complex. J Comput Assist Tomogr 1992; 16:538–542
25. Chong WK, Sweeney B, Wilkinson ID, et al: Proton spectroscopy of the brain in HIV infection: correlation with clinical, immunologic, and MR imaging findings. Radiology 1993; 188:119–124
26. Tracey I, Carr CA, Guimaraes AR, et al: Brain choline-containing compounds are elevated in HIV-positive patients before the onset of AIDS dementia complex: a proton magnetic resonance spectroscopic study. Neurology 1996; 46:783–788
27. Jarvik JG, Lenkinski RE, Grossman RI, et al: Proton MR spectroscopy of HIV-infected patients: characterization of abnormalities with imaging and clinical correlation. Radiology 1993; 186:739–744
28. Simone IL, Federico F, Tortorella C, et al: Localised ^{1}H-MR spectroscopy for metabolic characterisation of diffuse and focal brain lesions in patients infected with HIV. J Neurol Neurosurg Psychiatry 1998; 64:516–523
29. Menon DK, Baudouin CJ, Tomlinson D, et al: Proton MR spectroscopy and imaging of the brain in AIDS: evidence of neuronal loss in regions that appear normal with imaging. J Comput Assist Tomogr 1990; 14:882–885
30. Chang L, Ernst T, Leonido-Yee M, et al: Cerebral metabolite abnormalities correlate with clinical severity of HIV-1 cognitive motor complex. Neurology 1999; 52:100–108

31. Everall IP, Luthert PJ, Lantos PL: Neuronal loss in the frontal cortex in HIV infection. Lancet 1991; 337:1119–1121
32. Vion-Dury J, Nicoli F, Salvan AM, et al: Reversal of brain metabolic alterations with zidovudine detected by proton localised magnetic resonance spectroscopy. Lancet 1995; 345:60–61
33. Chang L, Miller BL, McBride D, et al: Brain lesions in patients with AIDS: H-1 MR spectroscopy. Radiology 1995; 197:525–531
34. Chang L, Ernst T, Tornatore C, et al: Metabolite abnormalities in progressive multifocal leukoencephalopathy by proton magnetic resonance spectroscopy. Neurology 1997; 48:836–845
35. Giri JA, Gregoresky J, Silguero P, et al: Polyoma virus JC DNA detection by polymerase chain reaction in CSF of HIV infected patients with suspected progressive multifocal leukoencephalopathy. Am Clin Lab 2001; 20:33–35
36. De Luca A, Giancola ML, Ammassari A, et al: The effect of potent antiretroviral therapy and JC virus load in cerebrospinal fluid on clinical outcome of patients with AIDS-associated progressive multifocal leukoencephalopathy. J Infect Dis 2000; 182:1077–1083
37. Garcia de Viedma D, Diaz Infantes M, Miralles P, et al: JC virus load in progressive multifocal leukoencephalopathy: analysis of the correlation between the viral burden in cerebrospinal fluid, patient survival, and the volume of neurological lesions. Clin Infect Dis 2002; 34:1568–1575
38. Miralles P, Berenguer J, Lacruz C, et al: Inflammatory reactions in progressive multifocal leukoencephalopathy after highly active antiretroviral therapy. AIDS 2001; 15:1900–1902
39. Razonable RR, Aksamit AJ, Wright AJ, et al: Cidofovir treatment of progressive multifocal leukoencephalopathy in a patient receiving highly active antiretroviral therapy. Mayo Clin Proc 2001; 76:1171–1175
40. Clifford DB, Yiannoutsos C, Glicksman M, et al: HAART improves prognosis in HIV-associated progressive multifocal leukoencephalopathy. Neurology 1999; 52:623–625
41. Segarra-Newnham M, Vodolo KM: Use of cidofovir in progressive multifocal leukoencephalopathy. Ann Pharmacother 2001; 35:741–744

Recent Publications of Interest

Berger JR, Houff S: Progressive multifocal leukoencephalopathy: lessons from AIDS and natalizumab. Neurol Res 2006; 28:299–305

Summarizes the recent evidence that administration of natalizumab (a monoclonal antibody that blocks inflammatory cell entry into the brain) increases the risk of developing progressive multifocal leukoencephalopathy and discusses the possible mechanisms of action.

Roberts MT: AIDS-associated progressive multifocal leukoencephalopathy: current management strategies. CNS Drugs 2005; 19:671–682

Provides an overview of the clinical course and clinical management of progressive multifocal leukoencephalopathy.

Huisman TA, Boltshauser E, Martin E, et al: Diffusion tensor imaging in progressive multifocal leukoencephalopathy: early predictor for demyelination? AJNR Am J Neuroradiol 2005; 26:2153–2156

Presents a case in which diffusion tensor magnetic resonance imaging was able to visualize white matter pathology prior to conventional magnetic resonance imaging, suggesting that this imaging approach could potentially be used to guide and monitor treatment.

Koralnik JJ: New insights into progressive multifocal leukoencephalopathy. Curr Opin Neurol 2004; 17:365–370

Reviews the epidemiology, clinical presentation, immunology, treatment, and pathology of progressive multifocal leukoencephalopathy.

Katz-Brull R, Lenkinski RE, Du Pasquier RA, et al: Elevation of myoinositol is associated with disease containment in progressive multifocal leukoencephalopathy. Neurology 2004; 63:897–900

Compares magnetic resonance imaging, magnetic resonance spectroscopy, and immunologic and virologic results between patients who survived progressive multifocal leukoencephalopathy and those who did not. In the acute stage, lesions in patients who would survive had a much higher ratio of myo-inositol (a presumed glial marker) to creatine than lesions in those who would not survive, suggesting that inflammation limits disease progression.

Reprinted from Hurley RA, Ernst T, Khalili K, et al: "Identification of HIV-Associated Progressive Multifocal Leukoencephalopathy: Magnetic Resonance Imaging and Spectroscopy." *Journal of Neuropsychiatry and Clinical Neurosciences* 15:1–6, 2003. Used with permission.

Chapter 17

THE EXPANDING ROLE OF IMAGING IN PRION DISEASE

KATHERINE H. TABER, PH.D.
PIETRO CORTELLI, M.D., PH.D.
WOLFGANG STAFFEN, M.D.
ROBIN A. HURLEY, M.D.

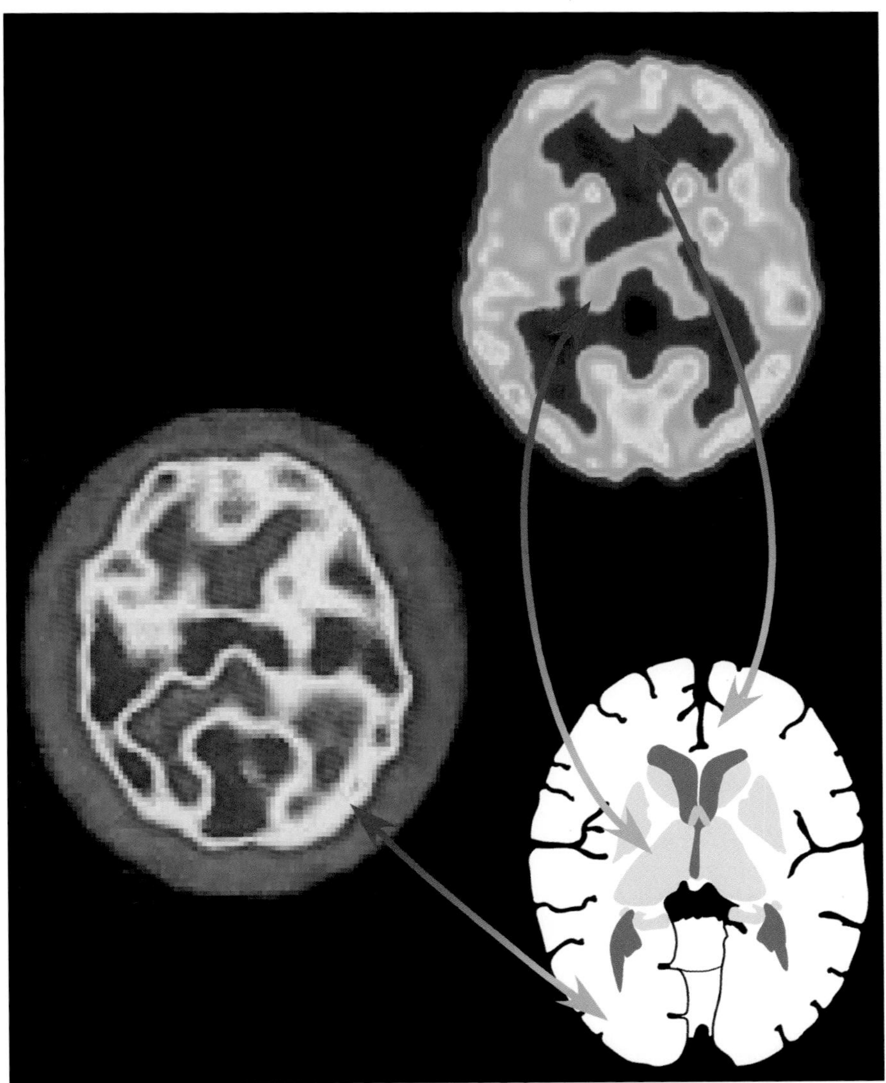

Axial SPECT (left) and PET (top right) images contrast regional changes in prion disease variants. While frontal cortex is abnormal in both images, the image on the left shows marked hypoperfusion in occipital cortex, while the one on the right shows hypometabolism in cingulate cortex and thalamus (indicated by arrows). The approximate axial section is illustrated (bottom right).

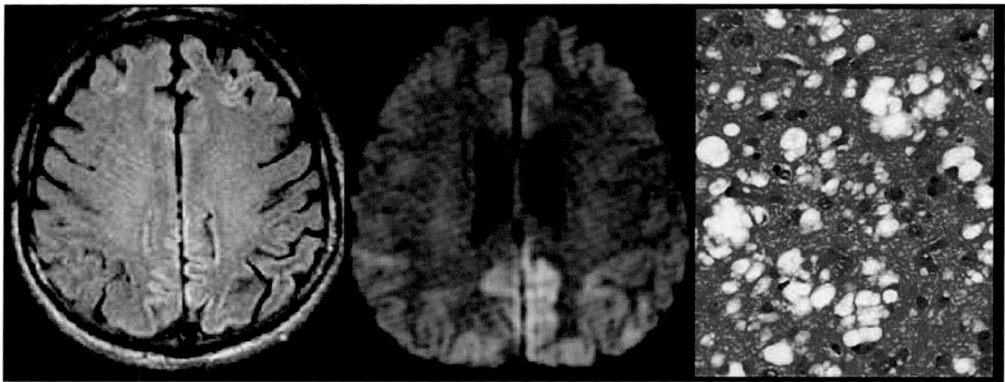

FIGURE 17–1. Increased signal is clearly present in the cortical ribbon on the FLAIR (left) and the diffusion-weighted (middle) magnetic resonance images, particularly in the posterior regions. Diagnosis of Creutzfeldt-Jakob disease was confirmed by presence of marked spongiform changes (right) in the brain at biopsy.[1]

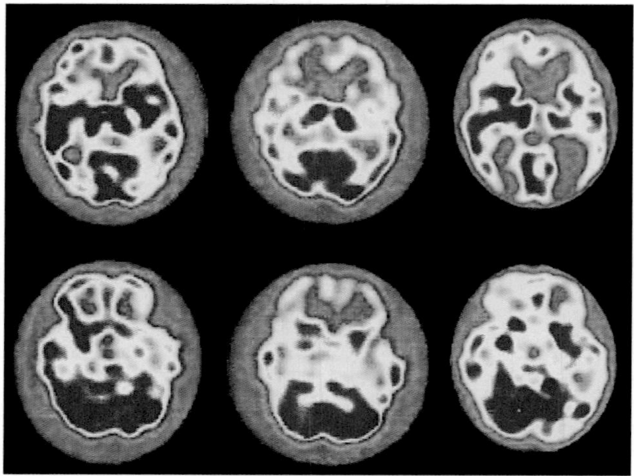

FIGURE 17–2. Images of regional cerebral blood flow (rCBF) were acquired monthly for 3 months by using technetium-99m hexamethylpropyleneamine oxime ([^{99m}Tc]HMPAO) SPECT in a patient with sCJD, Heidenhain subtype. One month after symptom onset (left) there was clearly decreased rCBF in the frontal and left temporal cortices. Decreases were more widespread one month later (middle). By one month before death (right) rCBF was diminished throughout the cerebral cortex, particularly in the temporo-occipital regions. Modified with permission from Staffen et al.[2]

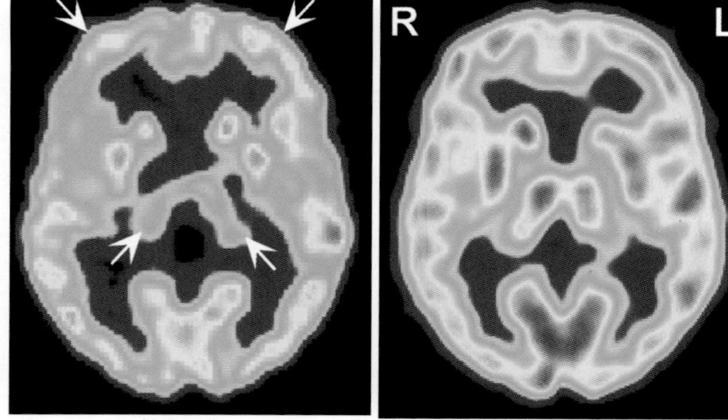

FIGURE 17–3. Regional cerebral glucose metabolism was imaged utilizing [^{18}F]-2-fluoro-2-deoxy-D-glucose (FDG) PET in a patient with fFI of 10 months' duration (left). Note the severe thalamic hypometabolism and milder secondary impairment in frontal and cingulate cortices (arrows). An image of a normal individual (right) is shown for comparison. Images courtesy of Dr. Perani, HSR Milan.

The transmissible spongiform encephalopathies (TSEs) are invariably fatal rare neurodegenerative diseases. The most accepted theory is that TSEs are caused by abnormal forms of a naturally occurring glycoprotein. These proteinaceous infectious agents (or prions) are altered forms (PrP^{TSE}) of the normal cellular prion protein (PrP^{C}).[3,4] Both isoforms have the same primary sequence, but their three-dimensional conformations are quite different (PrP^{C} has 3% β-sheets, whereas PrP^{TSE} has 43%), as are their biochemical and biophysical properties.[3,5] In particular, the PrP^{TSE} form is extremely resistant to inactivation by methods ranging from chemical (such as formalin) to heat (including autoclaving) to radiation (both ionizing and ultraviolet).[3] According to the prion shear theory, infection spreads as a result of PrP^{TSE}-induced unfolding and refolding of the normal PrP^{C} into the infectious form. Chaperone proteins may also play a role. There are a number of different PrP^{TSE} strains with distinctly different clinical and pathological phenotypes. This has been difficult to reconcile with the protein-only prion hypothesis, but may relate to differences in three-dimensional conformation.[3,5,6] The sporadic form of Creutzfeldt-Jakob disease (sCJD), for instance, has at least six major variations based on a combination of different forms of the protease-resistant core of PrP^{TSE} (type 1 and type 2) and the genotype at codon 129 of the PrP gene (homozygous or heterozygous for methionine or valine).[7,8] These strains vary along many dimensions, including average age at onset, disease duration, constellation of clinical symptoms, neuropathological characteristics, presence of electroencephalographic (EEG) abnormality, diagnostic imaging appearance, and cerebrospinal fluid (CSF) findings.[7,9]

The TSEs are caused by spontaneous conversion of PrP^{C} to PrP^{TSE} (sporadic form), by inherited germ-line mutation (genetic or familial form), and by inoculation (iatrogenic or dietary forms). Sporadic cases (unknown etiology) are the most common (>85%), followed by familial cases (12%–14%); iatrogenic cases are least common.[5] Many different mutations in the PrP gene (*PRNP*) have been identified. The predominant forms in humans are Creutzfeldt-Jakob disease (CJD), Gerstmann-Straüssler-Scheinker syndrome (GSS), fatal insomnia (FI), kuru, and new variant Creutzfeldt-Jakob disease (vCJD). Familial GSS is associated with codon 102, 105, 117, 198, and 217 mutations.[10] The familial form of CJD (fCJD) is associated with codon 53, 178, and 200 mutations. The familial form of FI (fFI) is also associated with mutation at codon 178. In addition, the genotype at codon 129 of the PrP gene (homozygous or heterozygous for methionine or valine) drastically affects disease course.[11] Individuals with the codon 178 mutation who are homozygous for valine express fCJD, while those who are heterozygous or homozygous for methionine express fFI.[10,12] Patients heterozygous at codon 129 have a slower disease progression (21±15 months) than those who are homozygous for methionine (12±4 months).[11,1314]

There is much debate in the medical literature about the existence of some variants of the disease, the true epidemiology, and transmissibility of the infectious agent from one species to another.[15–17] Scrapie has been recognized in sheep from the 1700s onward.[18] A few cases of what would now be considered human TSE were reported in the 1920s and 1930s. The discovery in the 1950s of kuru, with its clinical similarities to scrapie, resulted in a wider recognition of the human forms of TSE. The emergence of bovine spongiform encephalopathy (BSE) in cattle in Great Britain in the 1980s heightened awareness of the TSEs and created concern about the potential for transmission to humans. The identification of vCJD in humans has spurred a resurgence of both concern and research. A PubMed search of TSEs in humans produced 3,636 articles in English; 464 of these were written since January 2001. Currently, many nations have "surveillance units" to follow any suspected cases and to monitor for potential outbreaks.

The worldwide incidence of these rare diseases is estimated as one case per million population. Iatrogenic cases have been described in patients receiving cadaver pituitary growth hormone extracts (cadaver extracts are now illegal in most countries, replaced by synthetic growth hormone), insertion of EEG depth electrodes, and corneal and dura mater transplants from persons later found to have infection.[19] Sporadic cases generally occur in the elderly (sixth to seventh decade); the transplant and new variant cases occur in younger adults. Incubation time can be years, with death rapidly occurring once symptoms begin (generally within 9 months of symptom onset).[9,20]

Although prion diseases are rare, the differential diagnosis includes common conditions such as Alzheimer's disease and vascular dementia. They serve as examples of the importance of newer imaging techniques and diagnostic testing in clinical neuropsychiatry. Additionally, the public health implications of a missed identification of a patient with prion disease are troublesome.

Clinical Features

As noted earlier, prion diseases are fatal encephalopathies. The clinical features vary according to the individual diagnosis, and many patients exhibit variations of a central theme according to the form of protein mutation. However, common clinical characteristics exist. An excellent clinical review can be found in the monograph series by Knight and Collins.[21] The following brief overview of this summary can be helpful as an initial framework for study or patient screening in suspected cases.

A diagnostic progression has been developed for CJD in which the diagnosis is definite (confirmed by biopsy or autopsy), probable, or possible. The probables are approximately 95% certain for sporadic CJD, with clinical and EEG or CSF markers. The possibles have less specific clinical and diagnostic findings. The hallmark features of sCJD include a rapidly progressive dementia with visual/cerebellar features (including ataxia), myoclonus, pyramidal/extrapyramidal features, and progression to akinetic mutism. Other vague markers include initial depression, insomnia, or headaches. The variant form has a slower progression and is reported to have unexplained pain and more psychiatric findings (including delusions, hallucinations, agitation, anxiety, and depression), with less akinetic mutism. Positive EEG and CSF findings are less likely.[21]

GSS symptoms include a pancerebellar dysfunction with dementia, akinetic mutism, and occasionally aggression or emotional lability. Classic EEG findings are present in some cases. FI has a progressive loss of the normal sleep–wake cycle with eventual inability to attain normal sleep. The patients have hallucinations, parasomnias, and severe sympathetic overactivity (including salivation, rhinorrhea, hyperthermia, tachycardia, and hypertension). Hormonal abnormalities include increased serum cortisol and decreased melatonin or thyrotropin. Abnormal cycles of other hormones, including prolactin and the gonadal hormones, occur. Eventual cerebellar dysfunction, myoclonus, altered respirations, dementia, coma, and death ensue. Polysomnographic testing demonstrates lack of stage 2 and non-REM sleep and only brief REM sleep episodes (often associated with oneiric behavior). Classic EEG and CSF findings are not present. Kuru has a prominent pancerebellar dysfunction with initial ataxia and eventual loss of all voluntary muscle control, gross tremors, movements similar to shivering, euphoria, and late-onset cognitive decline and emotional lability.[21]

Diagnostic Testing

To date, limited medical testing is available to support a proposed diagnosis of TSE.[7] Periodic sharp and slow wave complexes (PSWCs) are frequently found on EEGs but may not be present in the early or late stages of the disease. They are not pathognomonic, as they have been reported in many conditions, including Alzheimer's disease. Serial EEGs are recommended in order to have the best chance for demonstration of PSWCs. Test sensitivity is 30%–100%, and eventual identification of the complexes occurs in approximately two-thirds of sCJD cases. Variant CJD and FI patients do not generally have PSWCs.[21,22]

Routine CSF studies are normal in prion diseases. The TSEs are unusual in that the immune system is not activated by the infection.[3] Two CSF neuronal proteins (neuron-specific enolase [NSE] and S-100) have been found commonly in patients with prion diseases. However, recent comparisons to another marker, 14–3–3, have established it as being more reliable. 14–3–3 has a sensitivity of 89%–93% and a specificity of 93%–100% for sCJD.[22,23] Several conditions may give false positives, including herpes encephalitis, multiple sclerosis, and cerebral infarction, but they can be eliminated by other diagnostic tests. Although 14–3–3 results are helpful, particularly in cases that do not show all of the classic clinical symptoms, definitive confirmation of the diagnosis requires neuropathological demonstration of the characteristic spongiform changes (Figure 17–1).

Computed tomography (CT) is used as a screening tool to rule out other illnesses with similar initial presentations. Magnetic resonance (MR) imaging is becoming increasingly useful in the diagnosis of TSEs. A recent large study assessed the presence of high signal intensity within the basal ganglia on T_2-weighted MR imaging in patients with sCJD and those with non-CJD-related dementia.[24] This appearance was found in 67% (109/162) of patients with sCJD but only 7% (4/58) of patients with dementia due to another cause. A similar frequency was found in a previous review of case reports of sCJD with extrapyramidal signs, while an earlier study found increased signal intensity within the basal ganglia in 79% (23/29) of CJD patients.[25,26] Thus the presence of high signal intensity within the basal ganglia has reasonable sensitivity and high specificity for diagnosis of sCJD. High signal intensity may also be found in the thalamus (particularly in vCJD) and within the cortical ribbon (Figure 17–1). Several studies indicate that a variation on T_2-weighted MR in which the high signal intensity from CSF is removed (fluid attenuated inversion recovery [FLAIR]) is even more sensitive to these changes (Figure 17–1).[27] Neuropathological studies indicate that this appearance is associated with gliosis more than spongiform changes.[24,26] Thus T_2-weighted and FLAIR MR imaging would be expected to be most sensitive to TSEs in the later stages of disease progression.

A new type of MR imaging, diffusion-weighted (DW) MR imaging, may provide a way to image changes much earlier in disease progression. Several studies have shown that high signal intensity areas (indicating restricted diffusion) are present on DW MR images prior to the appearance of abnormality on other MR imaging methods (Figure 17–1).[28–31] In one study they were present even before the appearance of PSWCs in the EEG or increased protein 14–3–3 in the CSF.[32] Neuropathological studies indicate that this appearance is associated with the microvesicular spongiform changes that occur earlier in disease progression.[31,32] DW MR images are also affected by T_2 weighting, so areas with both restricted diffusion and prolonged T_2 will be even brighter.[28] This may be an additional reason why DW MR images are more sensitive early in disease progression. Sequential imaging in one case demonstrated that very late in disease progression this distinctive appearance on DW MR images can disappear.[30] No histopathology was presented, but the authors suggest that this may be due to the development of gliosis. Thus, DW MR imaging shows promise both for the early diagnosis of TSEs and for monitoring of disease progression.

Functional brain imaging (positron emission tomography [PET], single-photon emission computed tomography [SPECT]) also appears to be quite sensitive to the changes that occur early in the TSEs. Several studies have shown functional decreases (in blood flow or metabolic rate) prior to development of clear abnormalities on structural imaging, EEG, and/or level of 14–3–3 in CSF.[2,33–38] The pattern of abnormalities may be relatively specific to the TSE clinical variant. In sCJD hypoperfusion/hypometabolism primarily in frontal and temporoparietal cortices early in the disease progresses to global decreases by later stages.[33,36,39] Benzodiazepine receptor binding (as measured with ^{123}I-iomazenil SPECT) is also severely decreased, suggesting widespread neuronal degeneration.[39] In iatrogenic CJD (iCJD) cerebellar clinical signs are common.[19] Cerebellar hypoperfusion has been shown early in disease progression.[36] In sCJD-Heidenhain variant, which is characterized by visual disturbances (including isolated homonymous hemianopsia), hypometabolism/hypoperfusion is found in occipital cortex (Figure 17–2).[2,37,38] In fFI the most common early metabolic changes are in thalamus (particularly anterior) and cingulate cortex (Figure 17–3).[11] Neuropathological studies strongly link the autonomic dysfunction and disruption of the sleep–waking cycle that characterize this disease with anterior thalamic degeneration. The authors of this study comment: "The presence of significant hypometabolism in the thalamus and cingulate cortex in all fFI patients, regardless of symptom duration and the codon 129 genotype, indicates that the disease arises relatively early in these structures and subsequently spreads to other areas of the brain." If this holds true for all the TSE variants, as seems likely, functional imaging may provide a basis for early differential diagnosis.

MR spectroscopy provides another way of assessing cerebral function, by measuring the levels of certain brain metabolites. Most of the few TSE cases examined with this technique were in a fairly advanced state of the disease, with widespread neuronal loss that was reflected by decreases in measured *N*-acetylaspartate (NAA, a neuronal marker).[40–42] Two cases have been reported in which NAA was decreased in brain regions that still appeared normal by other techniques.[41,43] In a case of CJD the cortical neuronal number (assessed from a brain biopsy) was normal, but NAA was decreased by 27%.[41] Similarly, NAA was decreased in all areas surveyed (frontal cortex, putamen, cerebellum) in a case of GSS at a time when cerebral blood flow in these areas was normal (as measured by SPECT).[43] Thus MR spectroscopy shows some promise for earlier diagnosis of TSEs and may also help to differentiate TSE from other dementing illnesses.

Conclusion

Diagnosis of the transmissible spongiform encephalopathies is challenging because there is a wide range of potential presentations, many of which do not fulfill the most widely used criteria, and there is no definitive imaging or laboratory finding. Thus it is likely that TSEs are underreported. Both diffusion-weighted magnetic resonance and functional imaging show promise for early differential diagnosis. They may also be useful in improving targeting of brain biopsy sites. Other tests also show some promise, such as tonsillar biopsy for new variant Creutzfeldt-Jakob disease and peripheral blood immunoassays for PrP^{TSE}.[22] Additionally, one in vitro study suggests that chlorpromazine and quinacrine (an antimalarial agent) reduce the conversion of PrP^{C} to PrP^{TSE} and may enhance clearance of the abnormal form, perhaps in part by blocking transport across the plasma membrane.[44,45] Initial trials in two patients resulted in symptom reduction in one.[45,46]

References

1. Case courtesy of Drs. Fatima Janjua and Dennis Mosier, Baylor College of Medicine: www.bcm.tmc.edu/neurol/challeng/pat52 /menu.html
2. Staffen W, Trinka E, Iglseder B, et al: Clinical and diagnostic findings in a patient with Creutzfeldt-Jakob disease (type Heidenhain). J Neuroimaging 1997; 7:50–54
3. Prusiner SB: An introduction to prion biology and diseases, in Prion Biology and Diseases Edited by Prusiner SB. Cold Spring Harbor, NY, Cold Spring Harbor Laboratory Press, 1999, pp 1–66
4. Riesner D: The prion theory: background and basic information, in Prions: A Challenge for Science, Medicine and Public Health System. Edited by Rabenau HF, Cinatl J, Doerr HW. Basel, Karger, 2001, pp 7–20
5. Cappai R, Jobling MF, Barrow CJ, et al: Structural biology of prions, in Prions: A Challenge for Science, Medicine and Public Health System. Edited by Rabenau HF, Cinatl J, Doerr HW. Basel, Karger, 2001, pp 32–47
6. Hill AF, Collinge J: Strain variations and species barriers, in Prions: A Challenge for Science, Medicine and Public Health System. Edited by Rabenau HF, Cinatl J, Doerr HW. Basel, Karger, 2001, pp 48–57
7. Zerr I, Schulz-Schaeffer WJ, Giese A, et al: Current clinical diagnosis in Creutzfeldt-Jakob disease: identification of uncommon variants. Ann Neurol 2000; 48:323–329
8. Parchi P, Capellari S, Gambetti P: Intracerebral distribution of the abnormal isoform of the prion protein in sporadic Creutzfeldt-Jakob disease and fatal insomnia. Microscopy Research and Technique 2000; 50:16–25
9. Kordek R: The diagnosis of human prion diseases. Folia Neuropathol 2000; 38:151–160
10. Monari L, Chen SG, Brown P, et al: Fatal familial insomnia and familial Creutzfeldt-Jakob disease: different prion proteins determined by a DNA polymorphism. Proc Natl Acad Sci USA 1994; 91:2839–2842
11. Cortelli P, Perani D, Parchi P, et al: Cerebral metabolism in fatal familial insomnia: relation to duration, neuropathology, and distribution of protease-resistant prion protein. Neurology 1997; 49:126–133
12. Parchi P, Petersen RB, Chen SG, et al: Molecular pathology of fatal familial insomnia. Brain Pathol 1998; 8:539–548

13. Montagna P, Cortelli P, Avoni P, et al: Clinical features of fatal familial insomnia: phenotypic variability in relation to a polymorphism at codon 129 of the prion protein gene. Brain Pathol 1998; 8:515–520
14. Cortelli P, Gambetti P, Montagna P, et al: Fatal familial insomnia: clinical features and molecular genetics. J Sleep Res 1999; 8:23–29
15. van Duijn CM, Delasnerie-Lauprêtre N, Masullo C, et al: Case-control study of risk factors of Creutzfeldt-Jakob disease in Europe during 1993–95. Lancet 1998; 351:1081–1085
16. Coulthart MB, Cashman NR: Variant Creutzfeldt-Jakob disease: a summary of current scientific knowledge in relation to public health. CMAJ Can Med Assoc J 2001; 165:51–58
17. Venters GA: New variant Creutzfeldt-Jakob disease: the epidemic that never was. BMJ 2001; 323:858–861
18. Brown P, Bradley R: 1755 and all that: a historical primer of transmissible spongiform encephalopathy. BMJ 1998; 317:1688–1692
19. Brown P, Preece M, Brandel JP, et al: Iatrogenic Creutzfeldt-Jakob disease at the millennium. Neurology 2000; 55:1075–1081
20. Zerr I, Poser S: Epidemiology and risk factors of transmissible spongiform encephalopathies in man, in Prions: A Challenge for Science, Medicine and Public Health System. Edited by Rabenau HF, Cinatl J, Doerr HW. Basel, Karger, 2001, pp 93–104
21. Knight R, Collins S: Human prion diseases: cause, clinical and diagnostic aspects, in Prions: A Challenge for Science, Medicine and Public Health System. Edited by Rabenau HF, Cinatl J, Doerr HW. Basel, Karger, 2001, pp 68–92
22. Collins S, Boyd A, Fletcher A, et al: Recent advances in the premortem diagnosis of Creutzfeldt-Jakob disease. J Clin Neurosci 2000; 7:195–202
23. Poser S, Mollenhauer B, Kraub A, et al: How to improve the clinical diagnosis of Creutzfeldt-Jakob disease. Brain 1999; 122: 2345–2351
24. Schröter A, Zerr I, Henkel K, et al: Magnetic resonance imaging in the clinical diagnosis of Creutzfeldt-Jakob disease. Arch Neurol 2000; 57:1751–1757
25. Finkenstaedt M, Szudra A, Zerr I, et al: MR imaging of Creutzfeldt-Jakob disease. Radiology 1996; 199:793–798
26. Urbach H, Klisch J, Wolf HK, et al: MRI in sporadic Creutzfeldt-Jakob disease: correlation with clinical and neuropathological data. Neuroradiology 1998; 40:65–70
27. de Priester JA, Jansen GH, de Kruijk JR, et al: New MRI findings in Creutzfeldt-Jakob disease: high signal in the globus pallidus on T_1-weighted images. Neuroradiology 1999; 41:265–268
28. Bahn MM, Parchi P: Abnormal diffusion-weighted magnetic resonance images in Creutzfeldt-Jakob disease. Arch Neurol 1999; 56:577–583
29. Demaerel P, Heiner L, Robberecht W, et al: Diffusion-weighted MRI in sporadic Creutzfeldt-Jakob disease. Neurology 1999; 52:205–208
30. Matoba M, Tonami H, Miyaji H, et al: Creutzfeldt-Jakob disease: serial changes on diffusion-weighted MRI. J Comput Assist Tomogr 2001; 25:274–277
31. Mao-Draayer Y, Braff SP, Nagle KJ, et al: Emerging patterns of diffusion-weighted MR imaging in Creutzfeldt-Jakob disease: case report and review of the literature. AJNR Am J Neuroradiol 2002; 23:550–556
32. Mittal S, Farmer P, Kalina P, et al: Correlation of diffusion-weighted magnetic resonance imaging with neuropathology in Creutzfeldt-Jakob disease. Arch Neurol 2002; 59:128–134
33. Ogawa T, Inugami A, Fujita H, et al: Serial positron emission tomography with fludeoxyglucose F 18 in Creutzfeldt-Jakob disease. AJNR Am J Neuroradiol 1995; 16:978–981
34. de Silva R, Patterson J, Hadley D, et al: Single photon emission computed tomography in the identification of new variant Creutzfeldt-Jakob disease: case reports. BMJ 1998; 316:593–594
35. Miller DA, Vitti RA, Maslack MM: The role of 99m-Tc HMPAO SPECT in the diagnosis of Creutzfeldt-Jakob disease. AJNR Am J Neuroradiol 1998; 19:454–455
36. Matsuda M, Tabata K-I, Hattori T, et al: Brain SPECT with ^{123}I-IMP for the early diagnosis of Creutzfeldt-Jakob disease. J Neurol Sci 2001; 183:5–12
37. Jacobs DA, Lesser RL, Mourelatos Z, et al: The Heidenhain variant of Creutzfeldt-Jakob disease: clinical, pathologic, and neuroimaging findings. J Neuroophthalmol 2001; 21:99–102
38. Mathews D, Unwin DH: Quantitative cerebral blood flow imaging in a patient with the Heidenhain variant of Creutzfeldt-Jakob disease. Clin Nucl Med 2001; 26:770–773
39. Itoh Y, Amano T, Shimizu T, et al: Single-photon emission computed tomography image of benzodiazepine receptors in a patient with Creutzfeldt-Jakob disease. Intern Med 1998; 37:896–900
40. Bruhn H, Weber T, Thorwirth V, et al: In-vivo monitoring of neuronal loss in Creutzfeldt-Jakob disease by proton magnetic resonance spectroscopy. Lancet 1991; 337:1610–1611
41. Graham GD, Petroff OAC, Blamire AM, et al: Proton magnetic resonance spectroscopy in Creutzfeldt-Jakob disease. Neurology 1993; 43:2065–2068
42. Shyu W-C, Lee C-C, Hsu Y-D, et al: Panencephalitic Creutzfeldt-Jakob disease: unusual presentation of magnetic resonance imaging and proton magnetic resonance spectroscopy. J Neurol Sci 1996; 138:157–160
43. Konaka K, Kaido M, Okuda Y, et al: Proton magnetic resonance spectroscopy of a patient with Gerstmann-Straussler-Scheinker disease. Neuroradiology 2000; 42:662–665
44. Korth C, May BCH, Cohen F, et al: Acridine and phenothiazine derivatives as pharmacotherapeutics for prion disease. Proc Natl Acad Sci USA 2001; 98:9836–9841
45. Amaral L, Kristiansen JE: Phenothiazines: potential management of Creutzfeldt-Jacob disease and its variants. Int J Antimicrob Agents 2001; 18:411–417
46. Josefson D: Drugs for malaria and psychosis may offer hope to people with CJD. BMJ 2001; 323:416

Recent Publications of Interest

Trevitt CR, Collinge J: A systematic review of prion therapeutics in experimental models. Brain 2006; 129:2241–2265

Provides a comprehensive review of experimental approaches to therapeutics for prion diseases.

Caramelli M, Ru G, Acutis P, et al: Prion diseases: current understanding of epidemiology and pathogenesis. CNS Drugs 2006; 20:15–28

Reviews the epidemiology of prion diseases, with particular emphasis on vCJD, the pathogenesis of the transmissible spongiform encephalopathies, and potential therapeutic strategies.

Weissmann C, Aguzzi A: Approaches to therapy of prion diseases. Annu Rev Med 2005; 56:321–344

Provides a broad-based discussion of the transmissible spongiform encephalopathies, including description, diagnosis, genetics, incidence, pathogenic mechanisms, and possible approaches to prevention and therapy.

Ironside JW, Ritchie DL, Head MW: Phenotypic variability in human prion diseases. Neuropathol Appl Neurobiol 2005; 31:565–579

Reviews the factors that have been linked to particular disease subtypes, particularly polymorphism at codon 129 in the prion protein and multiple isoforms of the prion protein.

Legname G, Baskakov IV, Nguyen HO, et al: Synthetic mammalian prions. Science 2004; 305:673–676

Successfully induced neurologic dysfunction and neuropathological changes in mice consistent with prion disease utilizing a synthetic prion, providing strong evidence that prions are infectious proteins.

Reprinted from Taber KH, Cortelli P, Staffen W, et al: "The Expanding Role of Imaging in Prion Disease." *Journal of Neuropsychiatry and Clinical Neurosciences* 14:371–376, 2002. Used with permission.

Chapter 18

APPLICATIONS OF FUNCTIONAL IMAGING TO CARBON MONOXIDE POISONING

ROBIN A. HURLEY, M.D.
RAMONA O. HOPKINS, PH.D.
ERIN D. BIGLER, PH.D.
KATHERINE H. TABER, PH.D.

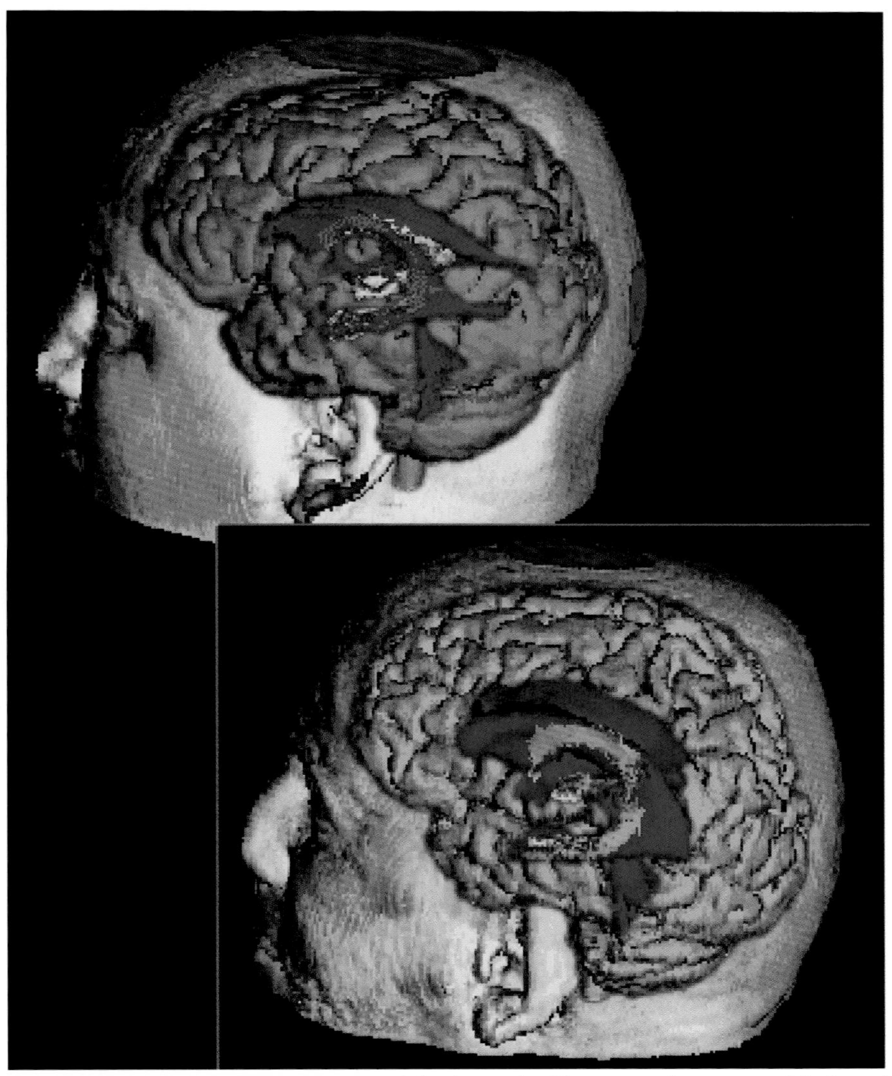

Three-dimensional surface rendering of the brain (*pink*), ventricular system (*blue*), and hippocampus (*yellow*) of a normal subject (top) and of a patient 1 year following carbon monoxide exposure (bottom). Note the ventricular enlargement and atrophy of the hippocampus in the patient.

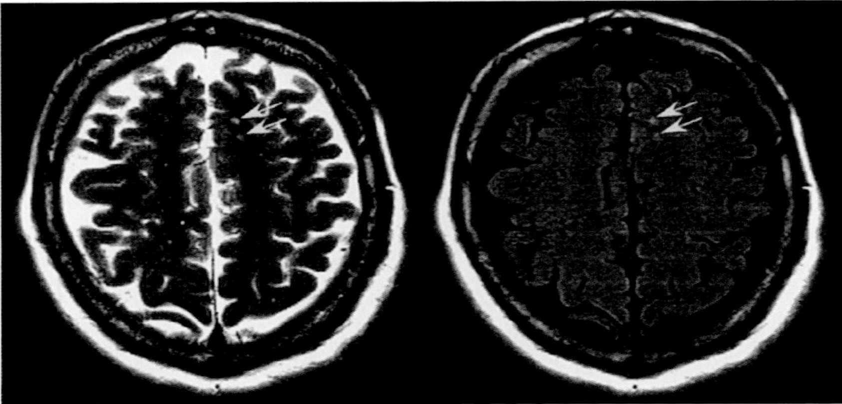

FIGURE 18–1. T_2-weighted (left) and FLAIR (right) axial magnetic resonance imaging scans obtained from a 47-year-old male 2 years after carbon monoxide poisoning. Although the patient has a normal IQ, there are still significant verbal and visual memory impairments. Note that the high-intensity lesions in the white matter (arrows) are much more easily identified on the FLAIR image.

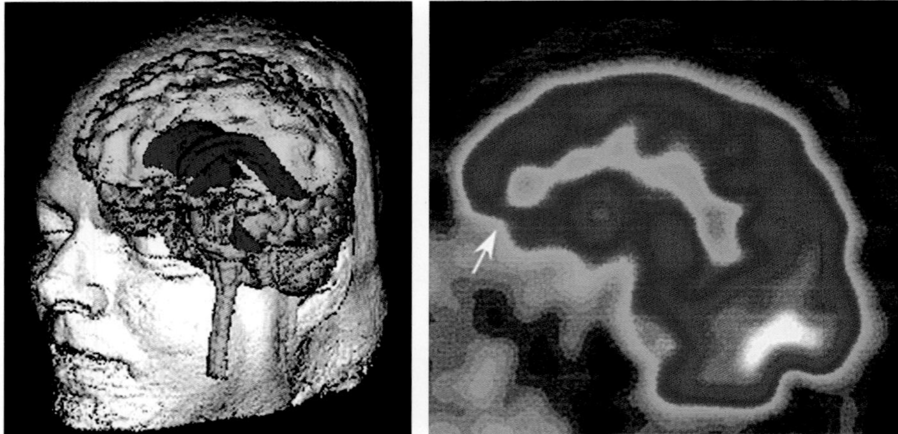

FIGURE 18–2. Three-dimensional surface rendering (left) of the same patient showing the brain (*pink*), ventricular system (*blue*), high-intensity lesions in the white matter (*red*), and the area of diminished perfusion on SPECT scanning (*yellow*). Sagittal SPECT scan (right) showing global cortical hypoperfusion (*blue*). Note the profound orbitofrontal hypoperfusion (*arrow*).

The functional anatomy of the brain, especially of the subcortical structures, is one of the least understood areas in medical science. Although there has been much debate over the years regarding the need for clinical imaging of patients with psychiatric symptoms, much of our understanding of functional anatomy is derived from study of patients whose brains have been damaged by injury or illness. This approach has been more fruitful in illuminating the functions of cortical areas rather than subcortical. The limited functional information regarding subcortical nuclei is due to the relatively small size of most subcortical nuclei and the density of adjacent tracts. Most injuries affect more than one subcortical structure. The exceptions to this are the disease and injury processes that target very specific brain areas.

Carbon monoxide (CO) poisoning, with its traditional symptom clusters and classic predilection for the basal ganglia and subcortical white matter, provides insight into the functional anatomy of this complex area. Patients who survive the initial CO poisoning provide a population in which imaging findings can be studied in relation to clinical symptoms. This is particularly valuable in view of the continuing controversy over the significance of small areas of abnormality on images, particularly areas of hyperintense signal on T_2-weighted magnetic resonance (MR) images (see Figure 18–1).

Carbon monoxide is a colorless, odorless gas produced as a by-product of combustion. Poisoning usually occurs

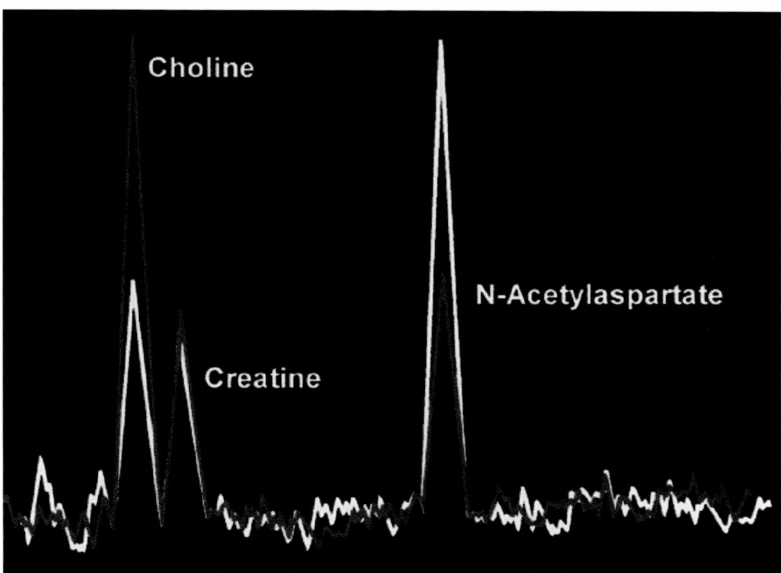

FIGURE 18–3. Simulated proton magnetic resonance spectrum (*red*) showing the changes that have been seen in the subcortical white matter following carbon monoxide poisoning. A simulated spectrum from white matter of a normal control subject (*white*) is provided to facilitate comparison. There is an increase in the choline and a decrease in the *N*-acetylaspartate peaks when compared with the control spectra.

from exposure to automobile engine exhaust, cigarette smoking, furnaces, or other unvented gas exhausts. Carbon monoxide is the major cause of poisoning deaths (accidental and deliberate) in the United States and Europe, with more cases occurring during the winter months.[1,2] Although estimates vary, in the United States 2,000–6,000 deaths and 40,000 emergency room visits occur each year from CO poisoning.[1]

As with most types of poisoning, outcome depends on the length and intensity of exposure. Commonly, initial symptoms include severe headache, nausea, weakness, confusion, arrhythmias, metabolic acidosis, coma, or death.[3,4] If the patient survives the initial insult, 2%–40% will develop a delayed or interval CO encephalopathy 2–40 days later. The most commonly reported sequelae include parkinsonism; dystonias or other motor impairments; cognitive or executive function deficits; akinetic mutism; mood disorders (including depression, anxiety, and emotional lability); memory deficits; and personality changes.[5–8]

Recovery varies; most patients achieve at least partial recovery within 6–12 months. However, studies examining neuropsychological functioning have been limited.[1,7,8] Recent studies using more detailed neuropsychological assessment indicate that subtle but significant decrements in cognitive performance may be common even years after recovery from the major symptoms.[1,7] Thus, while these individuals may appear normal and may have returned to independent living, some are functioning at a clearly diminished level. One study reported a significant correlation between neuropsychological impairments and abnormalities in cerebral perfusion, clinical MR, and/or brain volumetric measures (see images at opening to this chapter and Figure 18–2).[1] Prospective studies from the same group suggest that specific atrophic changes in white matter structures may correlate with some cognitive impairments at 6 months post–CO exposure.[9,10]

Clinicians generally have examined carboxyhemoglobin (COHb) levels for guidance on acute treatment and for prediction of long-term deficits. Recent work has shown that COHb levels do not correlate with clinical symptoms but can be helpful in guiding initial emergent care (i.e., the need for hyperbaric oxygen versus 100% oxygen at ambient pressure).[2,4]

For a fuller appreciation of the imaging findings in CO poisoning, a brief review of pathophysiology is helpful.[11] Carbon monoxide poisoning causes profound tissue hypoxia by both direct and indirect mechanisms. It competitively binds to hemoglobin, replacing oxygen, forming COHb. Although CO binds more slowly than oxygen, the binding is estimated to be more than 200 times stronger. As CO replaces oxygen on hemoglobin, less oxygen is available for transport to tissue. The bound CO also increases the stability of the oxyhemoglobin complex (shifts the oxygen dissociation curve to the left), allowing the hemoglobin to release less of the bound oxygen it carries to tissues. In addition, the stability of the COHb complex results in CO remaining bound to hemoglobin, reducing the amount of hemoglobin that is free to pick up carbon dioxide (CO_2) from tissue. As a result, the CO_2 concentration of the blood is lowered. The low blood CO_2 decreases the direct stimulation of the respiratory centers and thus lowers the respiratory rate. Although delivery of oxygen to tissue is low, the carotid sinus is not stimulated, since the oxygen partial pressure in the blood is normal. Carbon monoxide also combines with cytochromes and myoglobin. It inhibits cellular actions such as mitochondrial metabolism and promotes production of free radicals.[4] It may be the combination of these mechanisms that leads to the brain injury from CO poisoning.[12]

The brain and heart are particularly vulnerable to the destructive forces of this poison. The myocardium binds CO more strongly than skeletal muscle, leading to noticeable oxygen deprivation and symptoms of angina, arrhythmias, and markers of cellular death. If the patient survives the initial insult, demyelination of subcortical white matter and necrosis of the basal ganglia are common. In part, this may be because these areas have limited vascularity and a "watershed" blood supply. Cortical, hippocampal, and cerebellar insult occur with more extensive exposures.

For many years, MR and computed tomographic (CT) imaging have been performed in patients with CO poisoning. The findings generally have been reported in limited numbers or as single case reports, owing to the small number of poisoning cases that will come into a single emergency room or academic institution. Recently, the focus has shifted from simply reporting findings to examining their use as predictors of outcome, an important advance in understanding the functional role(s) of the basal ganglia. Imaging studies have been done both acutely and during later stages, when delayed parkinsonian and other symptoms are expected. The recent addition of methods more sensitive to brain function (i.e., imaging of cerebral blood flow and cerebral metabolism) may also provide valuable prognostic information.

Two recent studies present sufficient cases to assess the frequency of visualizing different types of brain injury during the first week after CO poisoning.[2,13] Although the imaging techniques used (MR, CT) provide quite different levels of anatomic detail, the results were rather similar. In both reports, slightly more than one-third of patients had normal imaging studies. The globus pallidus was the most frequently injured area (39%–63%), followed by the deep subcortical white matter (28%–32%). Cortical, mesial temporal lobe, and other subcortical lesions were occasionally seen.

Patients without imaging abnormalities had a favorable prognosis in both of these studies. In contrast, Lee and Marsden[14] did not find a better prognosis in patients with normal initial CT scans who were symptomatic in the first week. In general, the literature indicates that patients with more areas of injury have a poorer clinical course and are more likely to have significant neuropsychiatric abnormalities later. However, like the level of COHb in the blood and the initial duration of impaired consciousness, the results of imaging in the acute stage are not presently reliable predictors of outcome. This situation may change as MR techniques that are more sensitive to white matter damage come into clinical use. Murata et al.[15] reported a case in which standard clinical MR images (i.e., T_1- and T_2-weighted images) appeared normal at the same time that abnormalities were clearly present in the white matter on fluid-attenuated inversion recovery (FLAIR) images (see Figure 18–1). In the future, correlations between initial imaging abnormalities and outcome may improve.

Measures of cerebral blood flow, using positron emission tomography (PET), single-photon emission computed tomography (SPECT), or xenon-enhanced computed tomography (Xe-CT), may be more immediately useful in estimating prognosis during the acute stage. Several recent studies, using modern scanners that allow visualization of subcortical as well as cortical blood flow, have shown that regional cerebral blood flow abnormalities may be present in the absence of abnormality on CT or MR imaging.[16–18] In one study, cerebral blood flow abnormalities related to CO poisoning were present in two patients who had bad outcomes (death, long-term memory impairment), but not in one patient who recovered fully.[12] Two of these patients were studied the day of admission, the other patient 4 days after admission. Kao et al.,[17] who measured cerebral blood flow within a few hours of admission, also found that their two patients with normal cerebral blood flow had a good recovery. In contrast, Sesay et al.[16] did not find cerebral blood flow measurements taken 3–5 days after insult to be predictive of outcome.

One study indicates that there may be a good correlation between the areas that are hypoperfused during the acute stage and the neuropsychiatric symptoms that develop later.[17] Parkinsonian symptoms developed only in the patients with decreased perfusion of the basal ganglia. Cognitive deficits (confusion, disorientation, memory deficits) developed in patients with decreased cerebral blood flow in cortical areas.

As noted earlier, there can be delayed development of symptoms after a period of apparent recovery (the interval or delayed form). The most common locations of imaging abnormality may be different in this later stage. Some studies have found more lesions in the white matter (58%–64%) than in the globus pallidus (9%–26%), whereas others have found an equal incidence.[5,8,14]

MR and CT studies done when these delayed symptoms appear indicate that there is not a clear correlation between symptoms and imaging abnormalities. Pavese et al.[5] found that at 1 month post–CO poisoning, 50% of patients (11/22) had abnormalities on MR imaging, but only 27% were symptomatic. All patients with normal MR imaging were asymptomatic at 1 month, although one patient with a normal and one with an abnormal MR study became symptomatic later. Other authors have reported that many patients with delayed symptoms (30%–42%) have normal imaging examinations.[8,14]

As in the acute stage, measures of cerebral blood flow may be more sensitive to CO poisoning–related delayed changes than standard diagnostic imaging (Figure 18–2). A recent SPECT study found patchy hypoperfusion in all patients (13/13) examined after appearance of delayed symptoms.[8] Four of these patients had normal CT scans. Follow-up studies were obtained in one-half of the group. Cerebral blood flow improved in the six patients showing clinical improvement and was unchanged in the one patient who did not recover. Similarly, another study (using SPECT and Xe-CT) reported three patients in whom delayed clinical deterioration correlated with decreased cerebral blood flow.[16]

Another method that may be quite sensitive to the pathophysiology underlying the development of delayed symptoms is magnetic resonance spectroscopy (MRS). In MRS, signal is obtained from metabolites that are present in very low concentrations (as opposed to MR imaging, in which most of the signal comes from water). The low amount of signal available demands acquisition from a relatively large volume (voxel). The signal is usually displayed as the spectrum of the amount of signal produced by each metabolite. In proton MRS of brain, signal is present from N-acetylaspartate (NAA, located primarily in neurons, a marker for neurons and axons), choline (Cho, principally phosphatidyl choline, a membrane constituent), and creatine (Cr, used as an internal standard because its level is usually stable). If an area is severely injured, there may also be a lactate peak. The absolute amount of signal in each spectral peak is highly dependent on the acquisition parameters, so for comparison purposes the signals of interest (NAA, Cho) are expressed relative to Cr. The Cho/Cr peak reflects membrane metabolism and has been found to be elevated during both degradation (demyelination) and rapid synthesis. The NAA/Cr peak reflects neuronal and axonal density.

Several small studies have found proton MRS to be quite sensitive to CO poisoning–related changes in white matter (see Figure 18–3).[19–21] In one patient, for example, NAA/Cr was below normal and Cho/Cr was elevated at the time of delayed onset of symptoms (which included bizarre behavior, urinary and fecal incontinence, and gait apraxia), yet both MR and cerebral blood flow measures were normal.[19] Abnormalities were visualized later on MR imaging, while the patient was still fully symptomatic. Cerebral blood flow measures were always normal. The MRS changes persisted for some time, returning toward normal in parallel with clinical recovery. In another study, spectral changes at delayed symptom onset were more severe in the patient who developed the more profound clinical symptoms. The two patients had similar levels of abnormality on MR imaging. Clinical recovery correlated with normalization of the spectra in both patients.[21] Thus, proton MRS may provide a much-needed measure of injury severity following CO exposure.

Although the common wisdom has been that most people who survive the initial insult will recover from CO poisoning within a year, recent studies have suggested long-lasting, perhaps permanent, more subtle impairments may occur rather frequently. Careful study of patients with only white matter lesions or only basal ganglia injury could shed valuable light on the functional significance of these areas as well as identify the best imaging techniques to discern injury in both the acute and delayed settings. Additionally, identification of neuropsychological deficits that may benefit from therapy or explain a downdrift in cerebral functioning can be invaluable.

References

1. Gale SD, Hopkins RO, Weaver LK, et al: MRI, quantitative MRI, SPECT, and neuropsychological findings following carbon monoxide poisoning. Brain Inj 1999; 13:229–243
2. O'Donnell P, Buxton PJ, Pitkin A, et al: The magnetic resonance imaging appearances of the brain in acute carbon monoxide poisoning. Clin Radiol 2000; 55:273–280
3. Henry JA: Carbon monoxide: not gone, not to be forgotten. J Accid Emerg Med 1999; 16:91–92
4. Turner M, Hamilton-Farrell MR, Clark RJ: Carbon monoxide poisoning: an update. J Accid Emerg Med 1999; 16:92–96
5. Pavese N, Napolitano A, De Iaco G, et al: Clinical outcome and magnetic resonance imaging of carbon monoxide intoxication: a long-term follow-up study. Ital J Neurol Sci 1999; 20:171–178
6. Hopkins RO, Weaver LK, Bigler ED: Longitudinal outcome following carbon monoxide poisoning (abstract). J Int Neuropsychol Soc 2000; 6:393
7. Dunham MD, Johnstone B: Variability of neuropsychological deficits associated with carbon monoxide poisoning: four case reports. Brain Inj 1999; 13:917–925
8. Choi IS, Cheon HY: Delayed movement disorders after carbon monoxide poisoning. Eur Neurol 1999; 42:141–144
9. Kesler SR, Hopkins RO, Blatter DD, et al: Verbal memory deficits associated with fornix atrophy in carbon monoxide poisoning. J Int Neuropsychol Soc 2001; 7:640–646
10. Porter SS, Hopkins RO, Weaver LK, et al: Corpus callosum atrophy and neuropsychological outcome following carbon monoxide poisoning. Arch Clin Neuropsychol 2002; 17:195–204

11. Jaffe FA: Pathogenicity of carbon monoxide. Am J Forensic Med Pathol 1997; 18:406–410
12. Turner M, Kemp PM: Isotope brain scanning with Tc-HMPAO: a predictor of outcome in carbon monoxide poisoning? J Accid Emerg Med 1997; 14:139–141
13. Tom T, Abedon S, Clark RI, et al: Neuroimaging characteristics in carbon monoxide toxicity. J Neuroimaging 1996; 6:161–166
14. Lee MS, Marsden CD: Neurological sequelae following carbon monoxide poisoning: clinical course and outcome according to the clinical types and brain computed tomography scan findings. Mov Disord 1994; 9:550–558
15. Murata T, Itoh S, Koshino Y, et al: Serial cerebral MRI with FLAIR sequences in acute carbon monoxide poisoning. J Comput Assist Tomogr 1995; 19:631–634
16. Sesay M, Bidabe AM, Guyot M, et al: Regional cerebral blood flow measurements with Xenon-CT in the prediction of delayed encephalopathy after carbon monoxide intoxication. Acta Neurol Scand Suppl 1996; 166:22–27
17. Kao CH, Hung DZ, Changlai SP, et al: HMPAO brain SPECT in acute carbon monoxide poisoning. J Nucl Med 1998; 39:769–772
18. Kao CH: Fan-beam Tc-99m HMPAO brain SPECT in acute carbon monoxide poisoning. Clin Nucl Med 1998; 23:382
19. Kamada K, Houkin K, Aoki T, et al: Cerebral metabolic changes in delayed carbon monoxide sequelae studied by proton MR spectroscopy. Neuroradiology 1994; 36:104–106
20. Sakamoto K, Murata T, Omori M, et al: Clinical studies on three cases of the interval form of carbon monoxide poisoning: serial proton magnetic resonance spectroscopy as a prognostic predictor. Psychiatry Res 1998; 83:179–192
21. Sohn YH, Jeong Y, Kim HS, et al: The brain lesion responsible for parkinsonism after carbon monoxide poisoning. Arch Neurol 2000; 57:1214–1218

Recent Publications of Interest

Prockop LD: Carbon monoxide brain toxicity: clinical, magnetic resonance imaging, magnetic resonance spectroscopy, and neuropsychological effects in 9 people. J Neuroimaging 2005; 15:144–149

Presents clinical, neuropsychological, magnetic resonance imaging, and magnetic resonance spectroscopy results on two groups of people (chronic exposure, acute exposure) exposed to carbon monoxide from a faulty heater. Of particular interest, magnetic resonance imaging was negative in several cases in which clear neuropsychological deficits were present.

Kwon OY, Chung SP, Ha YR, et al: Delayed postanoxic encephalopathy after carbon monoxide poisoning. Emerg Med J 2004; 21:250–251

Presents a case report of delayed postanoxic encephalopathy following carbon monoxide poisoning that was confirmed with diffusion-weighted magnetic resonance imaging.

Gorman D, Drewry A, Huang YL, et al: The clinical toxicology of carbon monoxide. Toxicology 2003; 187:25–38

Reviews the clinical toxicology of carbon monoxide, the present hypothesis proposed to explain its toxicity, and evidence-based management of patients with carbon monoxide poisoning.

Reprinted from Hurley RA, Hopkins RO, Bigler ED, et al: "Applications of Functional Imaging to Carbon Monoxide Poisoning." *Journal of Neuropsychiatry and Clinical Neurosciences* 13:157–160, 2001. Used with permission.

Chapter 19

BINSWANGER'S DISEASE

An Ongoing Controversy

ROBIN A. HURLEY, M.D.
HIDEKAZU TOMIMOTO, M.D.
ICHIRO AKIGUCHI, M.D.
RONALD E. FISHER, M.D., PH.D.
KATHERINE H. TABER, PH.D.

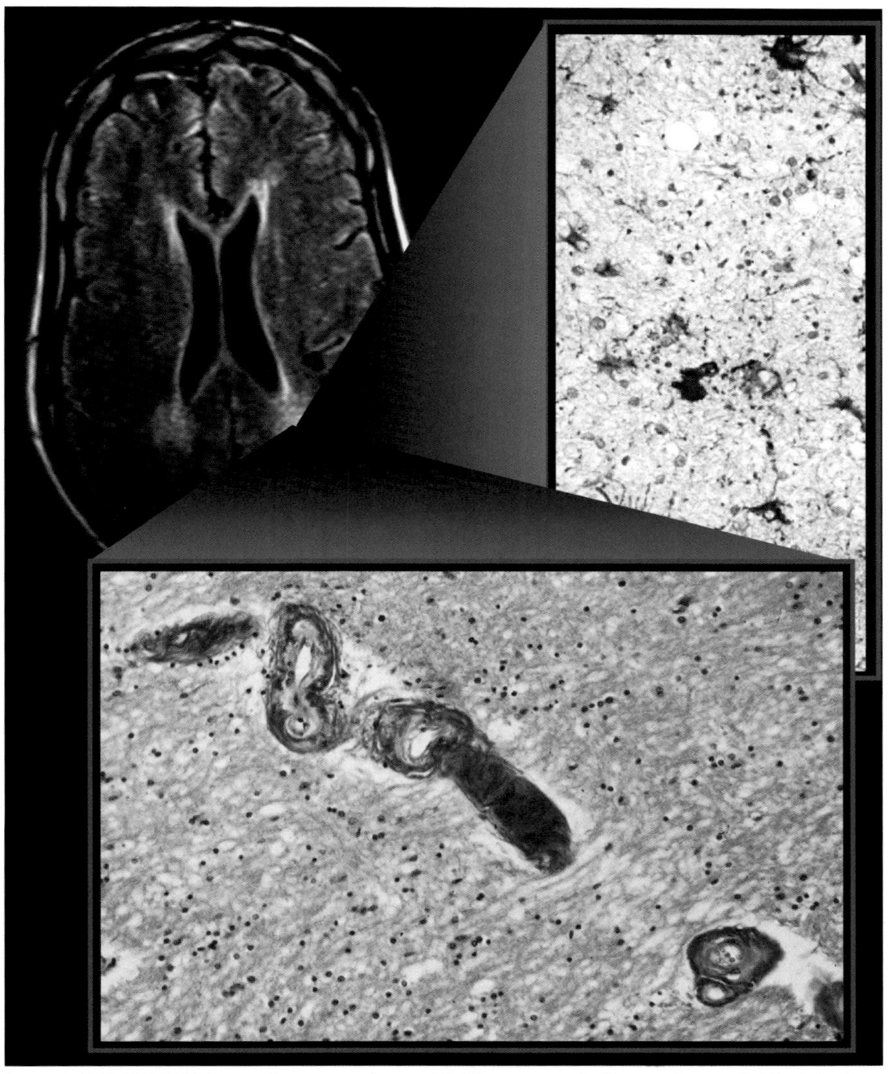

An axial FLAIR MR image from a patient with Binswanger's disease is overlaid with photomicrographs of the immunohistochemistry for glial fibrillary acidic protein (GFAP) staining (top) and Klüver-Barrera staining (bottom) of frontal white matter from a patient with Binswanger's disease.

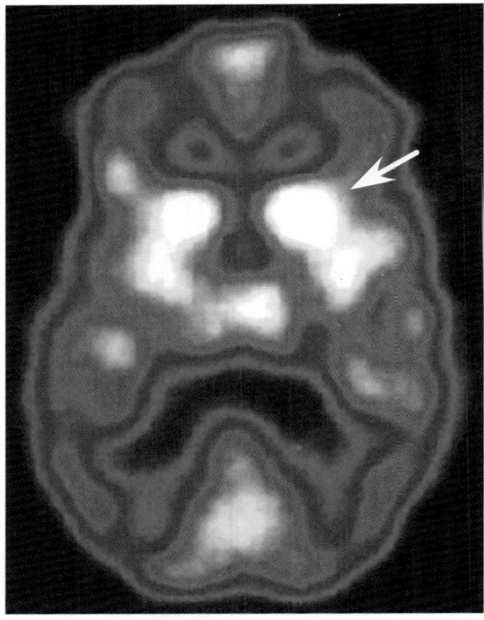

FIGURE 19–1. Transaxial slice of a SPECT (25 mCi of [^{99m}Tc]HMPAO) brain perfusion scan from a 57-year-old African-American male diagnosed with Binswanger's disease. Note the clearly increased uptake in the basal ganglia (arrow), consistent with the patient's long-standing history of torticollis. Cortical uptake is nearly normal except for a mild decrease in the parietal cortex bilaterally (not shown). The FLAIR magnetic resonance scan (see image at opening of chapter) showed multiple deep white matter and periventricular hyperintensities, particularly in the posterior areas. There was no lesion enhancement following contrast agent administration and no evidence of iron deposition or cerebral, cerebellar, or caudate atrophy. The patient presented for a first psychiatric hospitalization after wandering in the streets, wearing his pajamas, claiming that he was dying of AIDS, that his family was trying to kill him, and that if he raised his hands, the police would shoot him. Medical history indicated uncontrolled hypertension, idiopathic torticollis, and borderline hyperthyroidism. Investigative studies included negative rapid plasma reagin test, drug screen, and HIV serostatus. Thyroid function, B_{12}, folate, sedimentation rate, liver function, electrolytes, complete blood count, and cerebrospinal fluid studies were normal. He was also negative for oligoclonal bands, ceruloplasmin, and genetic markers of Huntington's disease. Neuropsychological testing revealed decreased cognitive tone, impaired concentration, slowed information processing, executive dysfunction, and visuoperceptual impairment (with normal verbal and visual memory)—suggesting cortical disconnection.

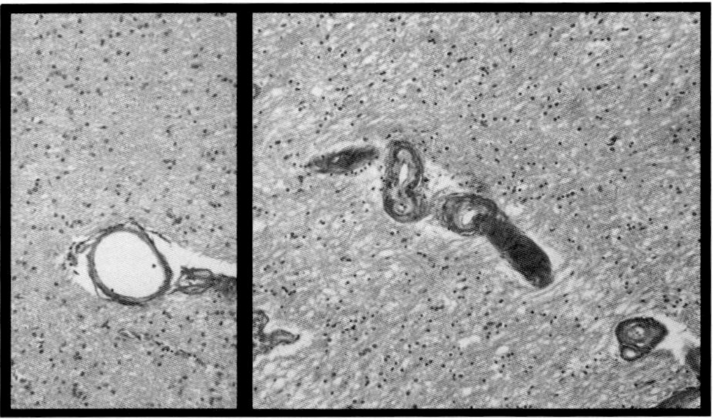

FIGURE 19–2. Photomicrographs of Klüver-Barrera staining in the frontal deep white matter from a nondiseased control brain (left) and one with Binswanger's disease (right). Note a marked proliferation of collagen fibrils (*blue*) in the adventitia and narrowing of the lumen in Binswanger's disease.

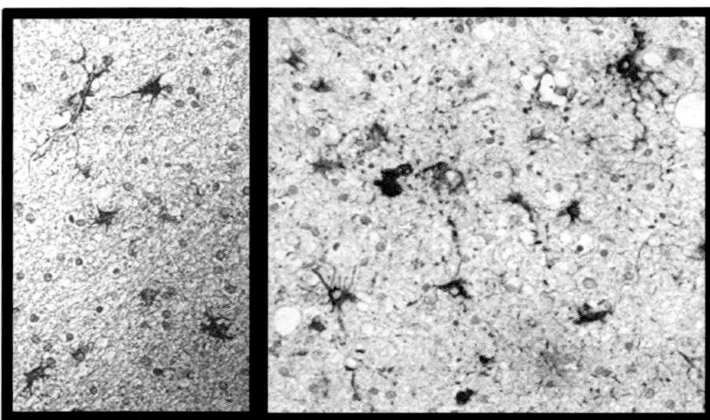

FIGURE 19–3. Photomicrographs of the immunohistochemistry for glial fibrillary acidic protein (GFAP) staining in the frontal deep white matter from a nondiseased control brain (left) and one with BD (right). Note that the astroglia (*brown*) show regressive changes such as swelling, vacuolation of the cell bodies, and disintegration of processes (recognizable as brown granules in the neuropil) in BD.

As the 19th century came to a close, Otto Binswanger, Alois Alzheimer, and Emil Kraepelin were defining the concept that dementia was a group of cognitive disorders with many underlying subtypes and pathophysiological causes. As the 20th century has ended, the descriptive criteria, incidence, and prevalence for many of these dementias continue to remain a controversy.[1] One subtype, labeled *Binswanger's disease* by Alzheimer in 1902, referred to arteriosclerotic subcortical white matter changes.[2] As time progressed, it became clear that subcortical white matter dementias varied in both pathology and clinical features. Recent authors propose differentiating patients with specific subcortical lacunar infarcts from those with only leukoaraiosis (LA; white matter rarefaction). Indeed, Pantoni and Garcia[2] state that the term *Binswanger's disease* "lacks medical significance or relevance," since Otto Binswanger's original case was probably neurosyphilis. Because this controversy is still unsettled, we have chosen to use here the historical term *Binswanger's disease* (BD).

Binswanger-type leukoencephalopathy (BD; LA; ischemic vascular leukoencephalopathy; progressive subcortical vascular encephalopathy; subcortical arteriosclerotic encephalopathy; periventricular leukoencephalopathy) is a slowly progressing vascular dementia with average onset by age 60. Approximately 4% of the general population and 35% of dementia patients show the characteristic lesions of BD on autopsy.[3] Clinical symptoms include frontal executive dysfunction, mild memory loss, psychosis, slowed thought processing, mood disorders, apathy, urinary incontinence, parkinsonian gait disturbance, and pseudobulbar palsy.[1,3,4] There may be signs of brain atrophy, including dilation of the ventricles and increased sulcal width (see image at opening of chapter and Figure 19–1). The lesions characteristic of BD are located in the periventricular and deep cerebral white matter. They may be large and confluent with smooth margins and be contiguous with the lateral ventricles, or they can occur in other subcortical locations as patchy or punctate lesions. The subcortical arcuate fibers (U-fibers) are usually spared.[5]

These lesions are believed to be due to repeated hypoxic-ischemic events in the long, thin end arterioles of the penetrating medullary arteries that supply the deep white matter.[5–7] The more superficial white matter interconnecting cortical areas (the U-fibers) is spared because of collateral supply. Vascular disease is present, including thickening of the walls (due to fibrohyalinosis) of these small arteries as well as fibroid necrosis and segmental arterial disorganization of large cerebral arteries and atherosclerosis (see Figure 19–2).[8] There is a strong association between the degree of wall thickening and the magnitude of white matter lesions.[9] There is evidence that changes in blood viscosity and coagulation state may be a factor in the development of lesions in BD. Thus, several intermediaries on the coagulation-fibrinolysis pathway have been shown to be elevated—including fibrinogen (which increases plasma viscosity), thrombin-antithrombin complex, prothrombin fragment F1+2, and D-dimer levels—in BD patients whose neurologic status had deteriorated within the previous 3 months, but not in stable BD patients.[10] Activation of this pathway can cause formation of microthrombi as well as microcirculatory disturbance, perhaps exacerbating development of lesions. Pathological changes within lesions include a reduction in the density of nerve fibers in the deep subcortical white matter, associated with rarefaction and astrocytic changes.[8,9] Axonal damage is present within BD lesions, as is decreased myelin. Activated microglia are present, perhaps as a response to chronic ischemia or to presence of damaged axons. Some astroglial cells may be swollen, with disintegration of processes, possibly in response to edema (see Figure 19–3).[11]

Diagnostic imaging using clinical magnetic resonance (MR) or computed tomography (CT) provides clear visualization of white matter lesions and areas of infarction. These areas have decreased density on CT and increased signal intensity on T_2-weighted MR images.[5] However, the appearance of these lesions is quite nonspecific with both of these techniques. Thus, areas of increased signal intensity on T_2-weighted MR images (sometimes referred to as "unidentified bright objects" or UBOs) are associated with a wide range of pathological conditions that can cause dilation of the perivascular spaces (état criblé), small areas of subcortical infarction (lacunae), or demyelination and gliosis.[2] Some studies have concluded that there is not a good correlation between lesion load and general cognitive measures, suggesting that the majority of these lesions may be clinically silent.[12] However, several studies suggest a close association between the extent and location of lesions and specific deficits related to the types of executive dysfunction commonly found in subcortical dementias, such as slowed thought processing.[13] It is likely that the discordant results arise from differences in patient populations, image analysis methods, and cognitive tests utilized. More extensive studies are needed to resolve this issue.

Alternative types of MR imaging show promise of being able to distinguish among some of these pathological conditions. One method is sensitive to interactions between free protons (unbound water in tissue) and bound protons (water bound to macromolecules such as those in myelin membranes).[14,15] This type of MR image, called a magnetization transfer (MT) image, may be able to differentiate white matter lesions of BD from those not accompanied by cognitive changes or due to other causes such as infarction.[14,15] Another method of MR imaging is sensitive to the speed of water diffusion. Diffusion-weighted MR imaging may be able to differentiate the white matter lesions in BD from those in Alzheimer's disease.[16] It may be that in future a combination of some of these newer methods of MR imaging will provide important information for differential diagnosis.

Functional brain imaging may provide more insight into the disease process in BD. Positron emission tomography studies indicate that cerebral blood flow and cerebral metabolic rate can be reduced in both cortex and white matter in BD patients compared with both normal control subjects and patients with white matter lesions but without dementia.[17–19] Oxygen extraction fraction is not elevated in either gray matter or white matter in these BD patients, suggesting that the areas are not at high risk for ischemia.[17,18] There are no histopathological abnormalities in the cortical areas with reduced blood flow and metabolic rate, so it is likely that these changes are secondary to damage to deep white matter and/or subcortical structures. In contrast, nondemented patients with white matter lesions have both decreased cerebral blood flow and increased oxygen extraction fraction in their deep white matter.[18] This suggests that these areas are maintaining a normal metabolic rate in the face of diminished blood supply, and thus might be at risk for ischemic damage. Thus, one might speculate that asymptomatic individuals are in an earlier stage of the process that will eventually be called BD when areas that affect cortical function (white matter or subcortical gray matter) are damaged. Although most of these studies have not reported a high correlation between degree of dementia and measures of cerebral blood flow, the most frequently used global screening measures are insensitive to deficits in executive function.

Only a few studies have used single-photon emission computed tomography (SPECT) to assess blood flow changes in vascular dementia, and even fewer to examine BD specifically. SPECT would not be expected to be more informative than standard diagnostic imaging (CT or MR) at directly demonstrating white matter lesions typical of BD, because white matter normally takes up very little radiotracer and is barely visible on a SPECT scan. However, SPECT is sensitive to the functional consequences of white matter and subcortical lesions. The most common finding early in BD is decreased perfusion in frontal cortex and basal ganglia (see Figure 19–1). As clinical symptoms increase in severity, more widespread perfusion deficits are found.[20,21] These results are consistent with evidence of subcortical infarcts on MR and CT imaging and loss of frontal lobe executive function on neuropsychological testing.[1] These SPECT studies used gamma cameras built prior to 1990. The higher resolution of the modern triple-headed cameras (as was used to collect the images shown here) may yield somewhat different results.

The poor correlation that has been found between several measures of pathology (lesion load, decreased cerebral blood flow) and degree of dementia indicates that the etiology of BD is still not clear. As pathological processes become better understood, they may provide insight into new potential treatments. At the present time the most promising treatment is the vasoactive drug nimodipine (a calcium channel blocker that inhibits contraction of vascular smooth muscle). Initial clinical trials have reported stable or improved cognitive function over periods of treatment as long as 1 year.[22,23] A different cerebral vasodilator, fasudil hydrochloride (a calcium antagonist that acts intracellularly), decreased dementia and returned cerebral metabolic measures (as monitored by phosphorus MR spectroscopy) to normal values in a patient with BD. Cerebral blood flow (as monitored by xenon CT) was not increased toward normal by the treatment.[18] The authors of the study suggest that the treatment was effective because of a direct effect on intracellular energy metabolism. A different approach targets the elevation in the levels of intermediaries on the coagulation-fibrinolysis pathway in BD. A recent study of a patient with BD and antiphospholipid syndrome reported improvement in gait disturbance and mental dysfunction with antithrombin (argatroban, a selective competitive inhibitor of thrombin) treatment.[24] An earlier study using a defibrinating agent (ancrod) was not successful.[25] Thus, although there is no clear treatment strategy for BD at the present time, the future looks promising.

References

1. Roman GC: A historical review of the concept of vascular dementia: lessons from the past for the future. Alzheimer Dis Assoc Disord 1999; 13 (suppl 3):S4–S8
2. Pantoni L, Garcia JH: The significance of cerebral white matter abnormalities 100 years after Binswanger's report: a review. Stroke 1995; 26:1293–1301
3. Santamaria OJ, Knight PV: Review: Binswanger's disease, leukoaraiosis and dementia. Age Ageing 1994; 23:75–81
4. Caplan LR: Binswanger's disease revisited. Neurology 1995; 45:626–633
5. Golomb J, Kluger A, Gianutsos J, et al: Nonspecific leukoencephalopathy associated with aging. Neuroimaging Clin N Am 1995; 5:33–44
6. Pantoni L, Garcia JH: Pathogenesis of leukoaraiosis: a review. Stroke 1997; 28:652–659
7. Roman GC: New insight into Binswanger disease (editorial). Arch Neurol 1999; 56:1061–1062
8. Ogata J: Vascular dementia: the role of changes in the vessels. Alzheimer Dis Assoc Disord 1999; 13 (suppl 3):S55–S58
9. Tomimoto H, Akiguchi I, Akiyama H, et al: Vascular changes in white matter lesions of Alzheimer's disease. Acta Neuropathol (Berl) 1999; 97:629–634
10. Tomimoto H, Akiguchi I, Wakita H, et al: Coagulation activation in patients with Binswanger disease. Arch Neurol 1999; 56:1104–1108
11. Akiguchi I, Tomimoto H, Suenaga T, et al: Alterations in glia and axons in the brains of Binswanger's disease patients. Stroke 1997; 28:1423–1429
12. Smith CD, Snowdon DA, Wang H, et al: White matter volumes and periventricular white matter hyperintensities in aging and dementia. Neurology 2000; 54:838–842
13. de Groot JC, de Leeuw FE, Oudkerk M, et al: Cerebral white matter lesions and cognitive function: the Rotterdam Scan Study. Ann Neurol 2000; 47:145–151
14. Hanyu H, Asano T, Sakurai H, et al: Magnetization transfer ratio in cerebral white matter lesions of Binswanger's disease. J Neurol Sci 1999; 166:85–90
15. Tanabe JL, Ezekiel F, Jagust WJ, et al: Magnetization transfer ratio of white matter hyperintensities in subcortical ischemic vascular dementia. AJNR Am J Neuroradiol 1999; 20:839–844
16. Hanyu H, Imon Y, Sakurai H, et al: Regional differences in diffusion abnormality in cerebral white matter lesions in patients with vascular dementia of the Binswanger type and Alzheimer's disease. Eur J Neurol 1999; 6:195–203
17. Yao H, Sadoshima S, Kuwabara Y, et al: Cerebral blood flow and oxygen metabolism in patients with vascular dementia of the Binswanger type. Stroke 1990; 21:1694–1699
18. Yao H, Sadoshima S, Ibayashi S, et al: Leukoaraiosis and dementia in hypertensive patients. Stroke 1992; 23:1673–1677

19. Sultzer DL, Mahler ME, Cummings JL, et al: Cortical abnormalities associated with subcortical lesions in vascular dementia: clinical and positron emission tomographic findings. Arch Neurol 1995; 52:773–780
20. Tohgi H, Chiba K, Sasaki K, et al: Cerebral perfusion patterns in vascular dementia of Binswanger type compared with senile dementia of Alzheimer type: a SPECT study. J Neurol 1991; 238:365–370
21. Shyu WC, Lin JC, Shen CC, et al: Vascular dementia of Binswanger's type: clinical, neuroradiological and 99mTc-HMPAO SPET study. Eur J Nucl Med 1996; 23:1338–1344
22. Parnetti L, Senin U, Carosi M, et al: Mental deterioration in old age: results of two multicenter, clinical trials with nimodipine: the Nimodipine Study Group. Clin Ther 1993; 15:394–406
23. Pantoni L, Carosi M, Amigoni S, et al: A preliminary open trial with nimodipine in patients with cognitive impairment and leukoaraiosis. Clin Neuropharmacol 1996; 19:497–506
24. Akiguchi I, Tomimoto H, Kinoshita M, et al: Effects of antithrombin on Binswanger's disease with antiphospholipid antibody syndrome. Neurology 1999; 52:398–401
25. Ringelstein EB, Mauckner A, Schneider R, et al: Effects of enzymatic blood defibrination in subcortical arteriosclerotic encephalopathy. J Neurol Neurosurg Psychiatry 1988; 51:1051–1057

Recent Publications of Interest

Starkstein SE, Jorge R, Capizzano AA: Uncommon causes of cerebrovascular dementia. Int Psychogeriatr 2005; 17 (suppl 1):S51–S64
Provides an update on the evidence for and against the concept of BD as a diagnostic entity.

Libon DJ, Price CC, Davis Garrett K, et al: From Binswanger's disease to leukoaraiosis: what we have learned about subcortical vascular dementia. Clin Neurospsychol 2004; 18:83–100
Provides an overview of the neuropathological, neuropsychological, and neuroradiological research on vascular dementias, including BD.

Bastos Leite AJ, Scheltens P, Barkhof F: Pathological aging of the brain: an overview. Top Magn Reson Imaging 2004; 15:369–389
Reviews the causes of dementia in the elderly and the application of various neuroimaging methods for differential diagnosis.

Reprinted from Hurley RA, Tomimoto H, Akiguchi I, et al: "Binswanger's Disease: An Ongoing Controversy." *Journal of Neuropsychiatry and Clinical Neurosciences* 12:301–304, 2000. Used with permission.

Chapter 20

NORMAL PRESSURE HYDROCEPHALUS

Significance of Magnetic Resonance Imaging in a Potentially Treatable Dementia

ROBIN A. HURLEY, M.D.
WILLIAM G. BRADLEY JR., M.D., PH.D.
HALEEMA T. LATIFI, M.D.
KATHERINE H. TABER, PH.D.

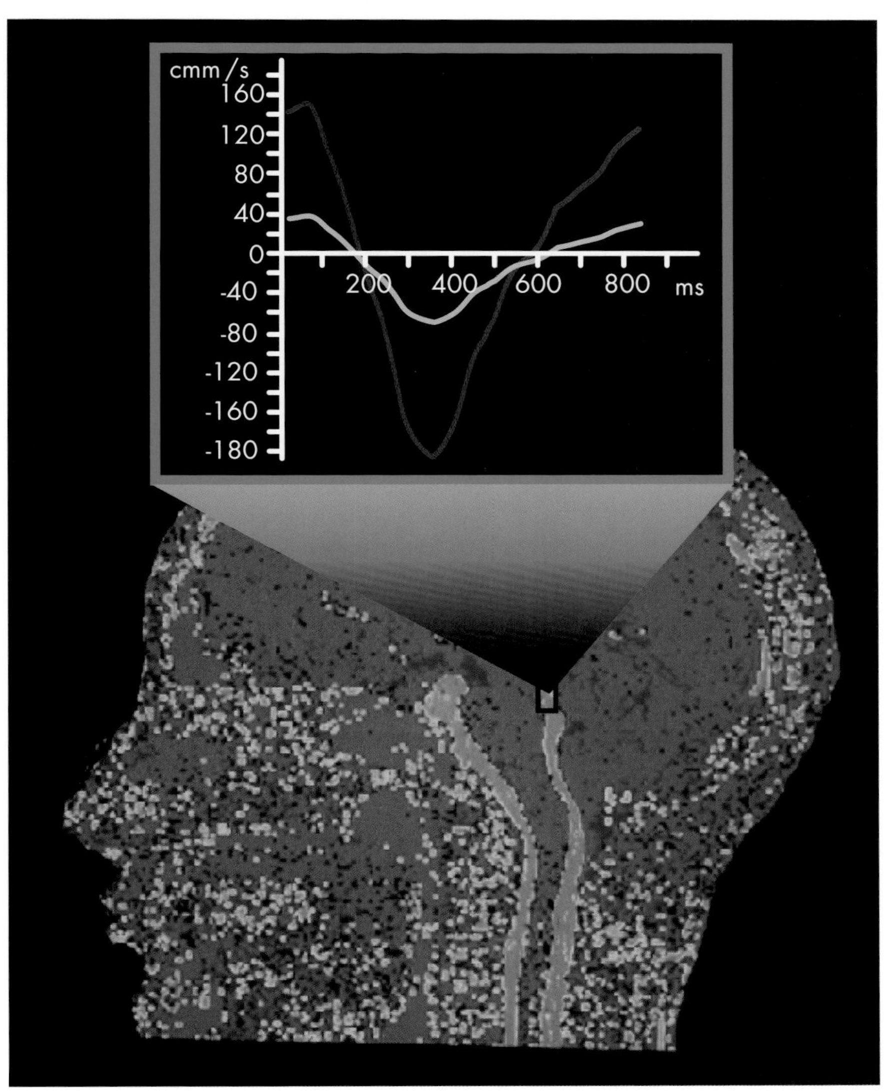

A sagittal phase-contrast flow study is overlaid with a graph of flow rate versus time.

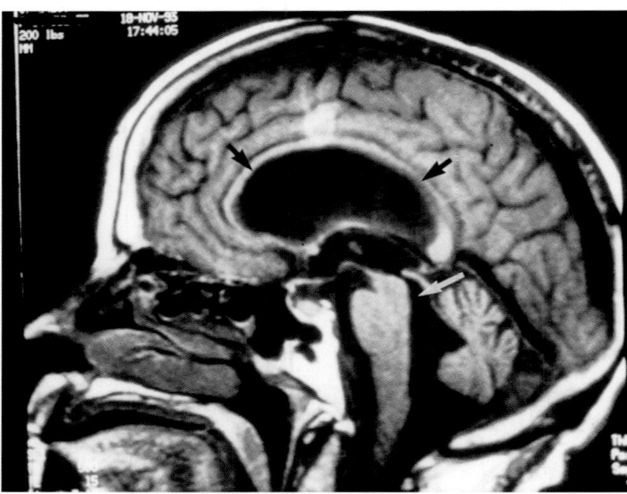

FIGURE 20–1. Sagittal T_1-weighted magnetic resonance scan from a 62-year-old woman with shunt-responsive normal pressure hydrocephalus shows the enlarged cerebral aqueduct (*white arrow*) and the classic upward bowing of the corpus callosum (*black arrows*) caused by the enlarged lateral ventricles. Note the flattening of the cortex against the inner table of the skull.

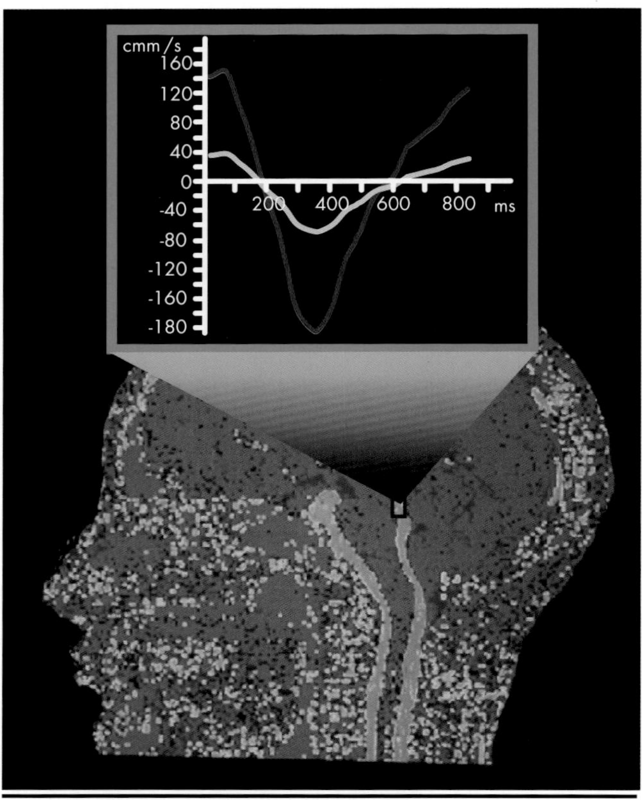

FIGURE 20–2. Sagittal magnetic resonance phase-contrast cerebrospinal fluid (CSF) flow study shows normal flow in the cerebral aqueduct (*black box*). Note the smaller width of the CSF spaces in this normal study compared with the image in Figure 20–1. The superimposed graph plots CSF volumetric flow rate (μL/s) versus time (ms) at the level of the aqueduct. (A microliter is equivalent to a cubic millimeter.) The area under the curve represents the CSF stroke volume in the aqueduct. The *yellow line* is from a normal study. The *red line* illustrates an increased CSF stroke volume (~82 μL). Stroke volumes greater than 42 μL are commonly found in patients with shunt-responsive normal pressure hydrocephalus.

Normal pressure hydrocephalus (NPH) was first proposed in 1965 as a form of communicating hydrocephalus that could result in a treatable dementia.[1,2] *Hydrocephalus* refers to dilation of the ventricles of the brain. It often results from an obstruction to the normal flow of cerebrospinal fluid (CSF), causing CSF to accumulate in the ventricles (obstructive hydrocephalus). In communicating hydrocephalus, CSF flow is not blocked within the ventricles, but it accumulates because it is not absorbed properly. In NPH, the CSF pressure is generally within normal values. The prevalence of NPH in the general population has not been quantified. Two European studies in small populations have roughly estimated that 1%–6% of all dementias are due to NPH and 0.41% of persons in the general population 65 years or older have the disease.[3,4] However, both groups felt that NPH is significantly underestimated because many cases go unreported and untreated.

NPH has a classic symptom triad of gait disturbance, urinary incontinence, and neuropsychological impairments that are most often labeled as dementia. This dementia of NPH has not been standardized with specific criteria. However, common symptoms include severe somnolence, fatigue, emotional lability, cognitive dulling (mild to severe), and memory impairments. These changes in memory can be mild or as severe as those of Korsakoff's syndrome. In fact, some authors define the memory disorder of NPH as a Korsakoff's amnesia (anterograde and retrograde memory deficits with confabulations).[5,6] Other disabilities include episodic mutism, hypokinesia, and catatonia. More rarely, cases of ultrarapid mood cycling, disinhibition, aggression, delusions, hallucinations, and depression have been reported.[7,8]

The gait disturbance of NPH has been traditionally classified as "apraxia," or cortical inability to direct movement. Recent computerized analyses of gait patterns have led some researchers to propose that the slowness of step, decreased step height, truncal flexion, and decreased pelvic rotation of NPH are more similar to Parkinson's disease than to a cortical motor disorder.[9] These descriptions and other case reports describing bradykinesia, rigidity, dystonias, and tremors have led to further examination of the pathogenesis of NPH.[10]

Although most cases of NPH are idiopathic, it can be associated with many conditions, including trauma, subarachnoid hemorrhage, prior intracranial surgery, and meningitis. There are two primary theories for the origin of NPH. The first is that it is an obstructive yet communicating type of hydrocephalus with a blockage of CSF resorption.[11] The other is that it results from weakening of the ventricular wall subsequent to periventricular white matter ischemic damage.[12]

Whatever the precipitating events, as the ventricles begin to enlarge, the surrounding white matter is pressed outward. The fibers of the corona radiata are damaged by the tangential shearing forces generated by the expansion and contraction of the brain during the cardiac cycle. In addition, cerebral blood flow may be impaired as vessels are stretched and compressed, resulting in ischemic damage. With continued ventricular expansion, the cortex is compressed against the inner table of the skull (see Figure 20–1).[1,11,12] With prolonged compression comes further cortical and subcortical damage (e.g., nigrostriatal axis impairment) and the appearance of symptoms.[10] Positron emission tomography (PET), xenon-enhanced computed tomography (xenon-CT), and single-photon emission computed tomography (SPECT) studies all indicate widespread cortical and subcortical hypometabolism and impaired cerebral blood flow.[13–15]

Diagnosis of NPH can be made based on the presence of all or a portion of the clinical triad (gait disturbance, dementia, urinary incontinence) on examination, combined with lumbar puncture and diagnostic imaging findings. In NPH, lumbar puncture reveals a mean CSF opening pressure within the range of normal variation (<180 mm H_2O or 13 mm Hg with the patient in the lateral decubitus position). If resistance to CSF outflow is tested with an infusion of isotonic Ringer-lactate solution, the outflow resistance will be increased.[16,17] Diagnostic imaging reveals ventricular enlargement without sulcal widening. Ventricular enlargement is generally most evident in the frontal and temporal horns of the lateral ventricles. The corpus callosum may be bowed upward and the cerebral gyri flattened against the inner table of the skull. Periventricular white matter lesions are often present. Magnetic resonance imaging (MRI) is preferred over computed tomography because of its higher resolution, better delineation of pathology, and sensitivity to CSF flow dynamics.

The direction of CSF flow through the cerebral aqueduct reverses during the cardiac cycle. Thus, it is caudal (into the fourth ventricle) during systole and rostral (into the third ventricle) during diastole. MRI is very sensitive to fluid motion. This normal movement of CSF results in a loss of signal (flow void) within the cerebral aqueduct. CSF flow in NPH is hyperdynamic, with an increase in the amount and velocity of CSF passing rostrally, then caudally, through the cerebral aqueduct with each cardiac cycle. This fluid movement is visualized on proton density–weighted MRI as an increased flow void in the cerebral aqueduct (that is, a flow void extending outside the aqueduct into the posterior part of the third ventricle and the anterior portion of the fourth ventricle).[18] When present, a hyperdynamic CSF flow void is a specific indicator of treatment responsiveness in NPH. However, *absence* of an increased flow void is not a reliable indicator that NPH is *not* present, since the appearance of the flow void is profoundly decreased by many of the commonly used MRI acquisition parameters (i.e., flow compensation and fast spin-echo techniques).

Therapeutic options for NPH are limited to surgical shunt placement, which dampens the pressure in the ventricular system during systole (peak pressure times). An indwelling catheter that includes a low- or medium-pressure one-way valve is inserted into one of the lateral ventricles. It commonly drains into the peritoneal cavity or the superior vena cava. Success rates range from 20% to 80%, with reports of symptom relief lasting up to 4 years.[5,19] However, postsurgical complications have been reported in up to 40% of patients.[19] Thus, identifying those patients most likely to benefit from shunting is of key importance. The most promising factors under investigation to predict shunt responsiveness include duration of presurgical symptoms (less than 6 months appears favorable) and onset of gait disturbance before dementia; temporary pre-shunt symptom relief from a CSF tap test (removal of 40 mL of CSF via lumbar puncture); and absence of significant cerebral vascular disease.[16,17,19] Cerebral blood flow greater than 20 mL per 100 g per min on xenon-CT, with impaired vascular response to acetazolamide in perivascular white matter only, has also been reported to indicate good response.[14] However, these results have not been replicated.

The recent development of phase-contrast CSF velocity imaging may provide a reliable method for identifying those patients with NPH who can be treated successfully. This method is a new MRI technique that allows quantification of CSF flow. Measurements are performed in the cerebral aqueduct, the narrowest portion of the ventricular system and therefore the location of highest CSF flow velocity.[20,21] Since CSF motion is pulsatile, the average of the volume of CSF moving caudally during systole and rostrally during diastole is calculated. This is defined as the CSF stroke volume. In the initial study with this technique, CSF stroke volumes above 42 μL were associated with a favorable response to shunting (see Figure 20–2).[21] This is a promising tool for screening patients with clinical symptoms of NPH and thus identifying a treatable dementia without risking postsurgical complications in patients who will not benefit.

References

1. Hakim S, Adams RD: The special clinical problem of symptomatic hydrocephalus with normal cerebrospinal fluid pressure: observations on cerebrospinal fluid hydrodynamics. J Neurol Sci 1965; 2:307–327
2. Adams RD, Fisher CM, Hakim S, et al: Symptomatic occult hydrocephalus with "normal" cerebrospinal fluid pressure. N Engl J Med 1965; 273:117–126
3. Casmiro M, Benassi G, Cacciatore FM, et al: Frequency of idiopathic normal pressure hydrocephalus (letter). Arch Neurol 1989; 46:608
4. Trenkwalder C, Schwarz J, Gebhard J, et al: Starnberg trial on epidemiology of parkinsonism and hypertension in the elderly. Arch Neurol 1995; 52:1017–1022
5. Larsson A, Wikkelsö C, Bilting M, et al: Clinical parameters in 74 consecutive patients shunt operated for normal pressure hydrocephalus. Acta Neurol Scand 1991; 84:475–482
6. Lindqvist G, Andersson H, Bilting M, et al: Normal pressure hydrocephalus: psychiatric findings before and after shunt operation classified in a new diagnostic system for organic psychiatry. Acta Psychiatr Scand Suppl 1993; 373:18–32
7. Nagaratnam N, Verma S, Nagaratnam K, et al: Psychiatric and behavioural manifestations of normal-pressure hydrocephalus. Br J Clin Pract 1994; 48(3):122–124
8. Schneider U, Malmadier A, Dengler R, et al: Mood cycles associated with normal pressure hydrocephalus. Am J Psychiatry 1996; 153:1366–1367
9. Sudarsky L, Simon S: Gait disorder in late-life hydrocephalus. Arch Neurol 1987; 44:263–267
10. Krauss JK, Regel JP, Droste DW, et al: Movement disorders in adult hydrocephalus. Mov Disord 1997; 12:53–60
11. Gleason PL, Black PM, Matsumae M: The neurobiology of normal pressure hydrocephalus. Neurosurg Clin N Am 1993; 4:667–675
12. Bradley WG Jr, Whittemore AR, Watanabe AS, et al: Association of deep white matter infarction with chronic communicating hydrocephalus: implications regarding the possible origin of normal-pressure hydrocephalus. Am J Neuroradiol 1991; 12:31–39
13. Tedeschi E, Hasselbalch SG, Waldemar G, et al: Heterogeneous cerebral glucose metabolism in normal pressure hydrocephalus. J Neurol Neurosurg Psychiatry 1995; 59:608–615
14. Tanaka A, Kimura M, Nakayama Y, et al: Cerebral blood flow and autoregulation in normal pressure hydrocephalus. Neurosurgery 1997; 40:1161–1165; discussion, 1165–1167
15. Shih WJ, Tasdemiroglu E: Reversible hypoperfusion of the cerebral cortex in normal-pressure hydrocephalus on technetium-99m-HMPAO brain SPECT images after shunt operation. J Nucl Med 1995; 36:470–473
16. Sand T, Bovim G, Grimse R, et al: Idiopathic normal pressure hydrocephalus: the CSF tap-test may predict the clinical response to shunting. Acta Neurol Scand 1994; 89:311–316
17. Boon AJ, Tans JTJ, Delwel EJ, et al: Dutch Normal-Pressure Hydrocephalus Study: the role of cerebrovascular disease. J Neurosurg 1999; 90:221–226
18. Bradley WG Jr, Whittemore AR, Kortman KE, et al: Marked cerebrospinal fluid void: indicator of successful shunt in patients with suspected normal-pressure hydrocephalus. Radiology 1991; 178:459–466
19. Caruso R, Cervoni L, Vitale AM, et al: Idiopathic normal-pressure hydrocephalus in adults: results of shunting correlated with clinical findings in 18 patients and review of the literature. Neurosurg Rev 1997; 20:104–107
20. Nitz WR, Bradley WG Jr, Watanabe AS, et al: Flow dynamics of cerebrospinal fluid: assessment with phase-contrast velocity MR imaging performed with retrospective cardiac gating. Radiology 1992; 183:395–405
21. Bradley WG Jr, Scalzo D, Queralt J, et al: Normal-pressure hydrocephalus: evaluation with cerebrospinal fluid flow measurements at MR imaging. Radiology 1996; 198:523–529

Recent Publications of Interest

Gallia GL, Rigamonti D, Williams MA: The diagnosis and treatment of idiopathic normal pressure hydrocephalus. Nat Clin Pract Neurol 2006; 2:375–381
Reviews the clinical presentation, radiographic findings, supplemental prognostic tests, differential diagnosis, surgical treatment, and outcomes of normal pressure hydrocephalus.

Relkin N, Marmarou A, Klinge P, et al: Diagnosing idiopathic normal-pressure hydrocephalus. Neurosurgery 2005; 57:S4–S16
Presents the recently developed evidence-based guidelines for the diagnosis of idiopathic normal pressure hydrocephalus.

Marmarou A, Bergsneider M, Relkin N, et al: Development of guidelines for idiopathic normal-pressure hydrocephalus: introduction. Neurosurgery 2005; 57:S1–S3
Presents the commonly used supplementary tests for diagnosis of normal pressure hydrocephalus and provides evidence-based guidelines for their use.

Reprinted from Hurley RA, Bradley WG Jr, Latifi HT, et al: "Normal Pressure Hydrocephalus: Significance of MRI in a Potentially Treatable Dementia." *Journal of Neuropsychiatry and Clinical Neurosciences* 11:297–300, 1999. Used with permission.

Chapter 21

Neuropsychiatric Presentation of Multiple Sclerosis

Robin A. Hurley, M.D.
Katherine H. Taber, Ph.D.
Jingwu Zhang, M.D., Ph.D.
L. Anne Hayman, M.D.

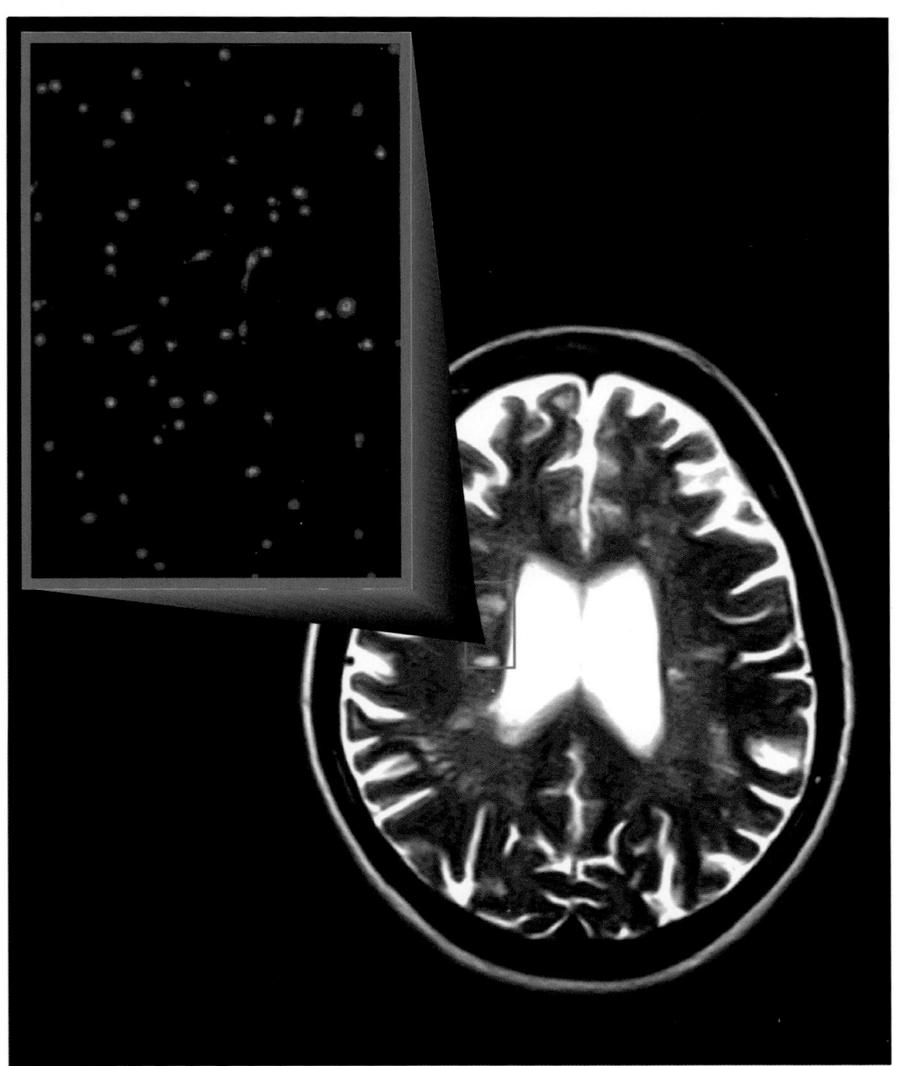

An axial magnetic resonance image from a patient with multiple sclerosis is overlaid with a representative photomicrograph showing lymphocyte infiltration in an area of plaque formation.

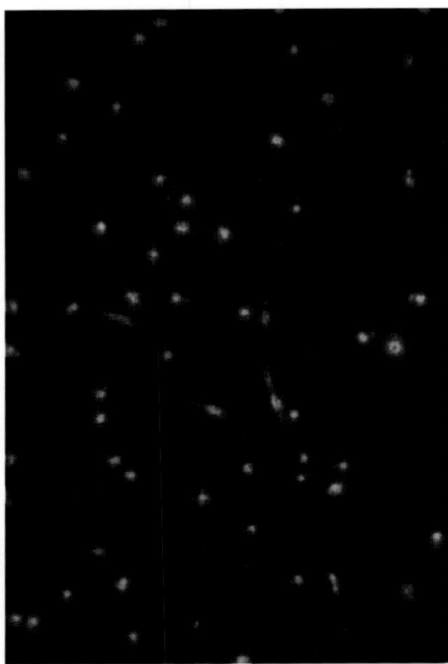

FIGURE 21–1. Monoclonal antibody labeling of CD4+T lymphocytes with fluorescent rhodamine staining (*orange*) of a postmortem MS brain specimen. These lymphocytes infiltrate the white matter of the central nervous system along the periventricular veins.

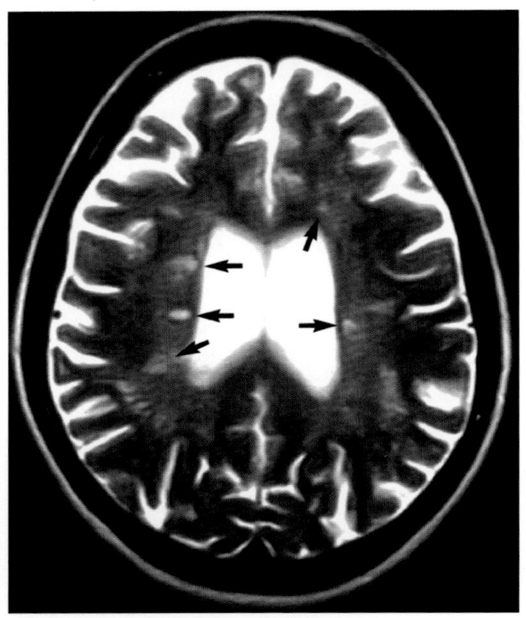

FIGURE 21–2. T_2-weighted axial magnetic resonance image of a 23-year-old woman with multiple sclerosis (MS). Note the characteristic ovoid high signal-intensity demyelinating lesions (arrows indicate the largest periventricular lesions). These are perpendicular to the cerebrospinal fluid (CSF)–filled spaces. Generalized brain atrophy is manifested by symmetric enlargement of the CSF spaces. The patient presented with a history of two past psychiatric hospitalizations (one at age 19 for mania and one at age 22 for depression), intractable insomnia, anxiety, depressed mood, suicidal ideas, bradykinesia, and bradyphrenia. She had none of the usual presenting symptoms of MS (i.e., visual disturbances, weakness, urinary or bowel incontinence, or swallowing and speaking difficulties). However, subsequent testing revealed classic findings of MS, including abnormal visual evoked potentials, positive CSF for oligoclonal bands, and an elevated immunoglobulin G synthesis and index rate.

Multiple sclerosis (MS) is a degenerative disorder of the central nervous system occurring, in the United States, in approximately 6–50 per 100,000 persons.[1] It commonly has a relapsing-remitting course.[2] Although neuropsychiatric symptoms have been reported in MS since the time of Cruveilhier and Charcot, in the 1800s, this possibility is often overlooked in the differential diagnosis of patients with new-onset psychiatric symptoms.[3] Slowed cognition, executive dysfunction, mania, depression, pathological crying, and personality changes have been reported in up to 66% of patients with MS and are, in many cases, the first symptoms for which the patient seeks medical attention.[4,5] Recent studies link these symptoms to the anatomical disease and not to the stress of chronic illness.[6,7]

The classic histopathology of MS is characterized by demyelination and inflammation surrounding venules and extending into the myelin sheath.[8] The infiltrating cells include T lymphocytes of predominantly the CD4 phenotype, activated macroglia, and plasma cells. Infiltration of these inflammatory cells and inflammatory cytokines produced in situ is directly associated with demyelination and plaque formation (see Figure 21–1). The histopathologic features of MS lesions are suggestive of a myelin-directed autoimmune process.[9]

Currently, magnetic resonance imaging (MRI) is the most sensitive tool available to document lesions in patients with a clinical diagnosis of MS and to predict progression to MS in patients who present with optic neuritis. An excellent recent review has summarized the significance of MRI in diagnosis and management of MS.[10] In brief, a combination of T_2-weighted MRI (for lesion identification) and contrast-enhanced T_1- weighted MRI (for detection of blood–brain barrier abnormality) is commonly used in clinical practice. The ability to track lesions over time using MRI can be very important in diagnosing MS. New enhancing lesions indicate probable MS.

Most MS lesions appear hyperintense on T_2-weighted MRI, an appearance that is nonspecific for MS. Occasional MS lesions are hypointense on T_2-weighted MRI, an appearance that has been attributed to the presence of nonheme iron deposition. Presence of multiple lesions, an ovoid shape, and periventricular location are considered characteristic of MS, as is involvement of the corpus callosum (see Figure 21–2). However, attempts to correlate lesion load based on standard T_2-weighted MRI with the clinical progression of MS have not been successful. Many patients have multiple lesions on MRI that are asymptomatic.

Newer MRI methods may further improve lesion detection. The fast spin echo (FSE) technique for acquiring T_2-weighted magnetic resonance images provides similar contrast but allows thinner sections that are contiguous. Addition of an inverting pulse (fluid-attenuated inversion recovery; FLAIR) to the T_2-weighted MRI provides a heavily T_2-weighted image in which the strong signal from cerebrospinal fluid (CSF) has been removed, allowing identification of MS lesions at the interfaces between CSF and brain. The combination of these two techniques (FSE-FLAIR) may be the best for detecting MS lesions, although not all studies agree.

MS lesions appear hypointense on T_1-weighted MRI. There is evidence suggesting that lesions seen on T_1-weighted MRI (sometimes referred to as "black holes") correlate more closely to the degree of disability and disease progression than those seen on T_2-weighted MRI. Lesions that enhance on T_1-weighted MRI following administration of a contrast agent are considered likely to be active, and this appearance correlates with the presence of macrophage infiltration. However, the relationship between blood–brain barrier abnormality and active disease is still considered controversial. The number of lesions that enhance will depend to some extent on the MRI methods used. More lesions will enhance if a higher dose (usually triple the standard dose) of contrast agent is used, if there is a delay (generally 15–60 minutes) between contrast agent administration and MRI, or if magnetization transfer is used in addition to contrast agent in order to decrease the signal from normal tissue.

Magnetic resonance spectroscopy (MRS) is being used to study the chemistry of MS lesions. These lesions have lower levels of *N*-acetylaspartate (NAA, a neuronal marker) than normal brain. NAA can also be decreased in areas without clearly identifiable lesions and may indicate presence of microscopic disease. There has been some success correlating changes in NAA with clinical disease classification, and it has been suggested that this may be a measure of axonal loss. Increased choline has been associated with enhancing lesions, whereas decreases may indicate chronic, nonenhancing plaques.

Some of the newer methods of acquiring or analyzing magnetic resonanc images may provide more information about the fundamental processes occurring in the tissue. Magnetization transfer MRI may be sensitive to structural change at the molecular level in MS. Analysis of the T_2 decay curve may provide insight into structural changes within the myelin bilayer. An increase in the self-diffusion of water within MS plaques has been found by using diffusion-weighted MRI, but the increase did not correlate with disability. These are exciting research tools that may eventually lead to a clearer understanding of the pathophysiology of MS and to treatment guidelines and protocols.

References

1. Rodgers J, Bland R: Psychiatric manifestations of multiple sclerosis: a review. Can J Psychiatry 1996; 41:441–445
2. White RF: Emotional and cognitive correlates of multiple sclerosis. J Neuropsychiatry Clin Neurosci 1990; 2:422–428
3. Finger S: A happy state of mind: a history of mild elation, denial of disability, optimism, and laughing in multiple sclerosis. Arch Neurol 1998; 55:241–250
4. Stenager E, Knudsen L, Jensen K: Psychiatric and cognitive aspects of multiple sclerosis. Semin Neurol 1990; 10:254–261
5. Beatty WW: Cognitive and emotional disturbances in multiple sclerosis. Neurol Clin 1993; 11:189–204
6. Pujol J, Bello J, Deus J, et al: Lesions in the left arcuate fasciculus region and depressive symptoms in multiple sclerosis. Neurology 1997; 49:1105–1110
7. Feinstein A: Depression associated with multiple sclerosis: an etiological conundrum. Can J Psychiatry 1995; 40:573–576
8. Ffrench-Constant C: Pathogenesis of multiple sclerosis. Lancet 1994; 343:271–275
9. Zhang J: Multiple sclerosis: perspectives on autoimmune pathology and prospect for therapy, in Current Neurology. Edited by Appel S. St. Louis, MO, Mosby–Year Book, 1995, pp 115–155
10. Grossman RI, McGowan JC: Perspectives on multiple sclerosis. AJNR Am J Neuroradiol 1998; 19:1251–1265

Recent Publications of Interest

Benedict RH, Zivadinov R: Predicting neuropsychological abnormalities in multiple sclerosis. J Neurol Sci 2006; 245:67–72

Found a significant correlation between results from the Multiple Sclerosis Neuropsychological Screening Questionnaire and neuropsychiatric impairment, whole-brain lesion burden, atrophy, secondary progressive course, and vocational disability.

Caramanos Z, Narayanan S, Arnold DL: 1H-MRS quantification of tNA and tCr in patients with multiple sclerosis: a meta-analytic review. Brain 2005; 128:2483–2506

Includes an excellent discussion of the various methodological approaches to proton magnetic resonance spectroscopy. It concludes that there is reasonably strong evidence that the NAA/Creatine ratio is a useful surrogate measure for tissue integrity.

Zhang J, Hutton G: Role of magnetic resonance imaging and immunotherapy in treating multiple sclerosis. Annu Rev Med 2005; 56:273–302

Provides an overview of recent progress in MS research including the clinical, pathologic, and immunologic as-

pects, the mechanism of action of currently available disease-modifying drugs, the role of magnetic resonance imaging in clinical management and clinical trials, and emerging treatments.

Polman CH, Reingold SC, Edan G, et al: Diagnostic criteria for multiple sclerosis: 2005 revisions to the "McDonald Criteria." Ann Neurol 2005; 58:840–846
Presents International Panel on the Diagnosis of Multiple Sclerosis's revisions to the McDonald Diagnostic Criteria.

Frohman EM, Stüve O, Havrdova E, et al: Therapeutic considerations for disease progression in multiple sclerosis: evidence, experience, and future expectations. Arch Neurol 2005; 62:1519–1530
Provides a guide to clinical management of MS including assessment of disease activity, defining breakthrough disease, and the effects of pharmacotherapies on disease progression.

Feinstein A: The neuropsychiatry of multiple sclerosis. Can J Psychiatry 2004; 49:157–163
Reviews the prevalence, expression, suggested etiologies, and treatment approaches for many of the neuropsychiatric symptoms that occur in patients with MS, including depression, bipolar disorder, psychosis, and cognitive dysfunction.

Reprinted from Hurley RA, Taber KH, Zhang J, et al: "Neuropsychiatric Presentation of Multiple Sclerosis." *Journal of Neuropsychiatry and Clinical Neurosciences* 11:5–7, 1999. Used with permission.

Part 3

Anatomy and Circuitry

Human consciousness, cognition, behavior, and emotion occur as incredibly complex processes by way of billions of neurons arrayed in multiple circuits. These higher-order processes are beginning to be understood through the work of 20th-century pioneers in the field. Structures of the brain once thought to have no influence on personality, judgment, or memory are now viewed as critical to normal functioning. This section of the book focuses on example structures and circuits that underlie these capabilities. As challenging as understanding this seems, the complexity is greatly increased by the fact that lesions in multiple places along a single circuit or in other circuits may give rise to similar clinical symptoms. For example, a lesion of the basal ganglia or thalamus may produce clinically indistinguishable presentations. Thus, it becomes imperative for the practicing neuropsychiatrist to have a basic understanding of cognitive and behavioral circuits.

The papers in this section describe known anatomical structures, circuits, or centrally active compounds (e.g., estrogen) that play important roles in neuropsychiatric disease or normal functioning. Circuitry information is presented in the context of both normal functioning and disease states. Imaging methods used to study these processes are discussed in each paper. When reviewing this section, the reader must be mindful that the current understanding of the human brain is only in its infancy. These circuits and structures contain many complexities that have yet to be fully understood or described. The papers can be read as a group or individually for a particular circuit of interest. At the conclusion of this section, the reader should have a basic understanding of the major neuroanatomical circuits that underlie human behavior and cognition and be able to appreciate how imaging contributes to their study.

Chapter 22

Functional Neuroanatomy of Sleep and Sleep Deprivation

Katherine H. Taber, Ph.D.
Robin A. Hurley, M.D.

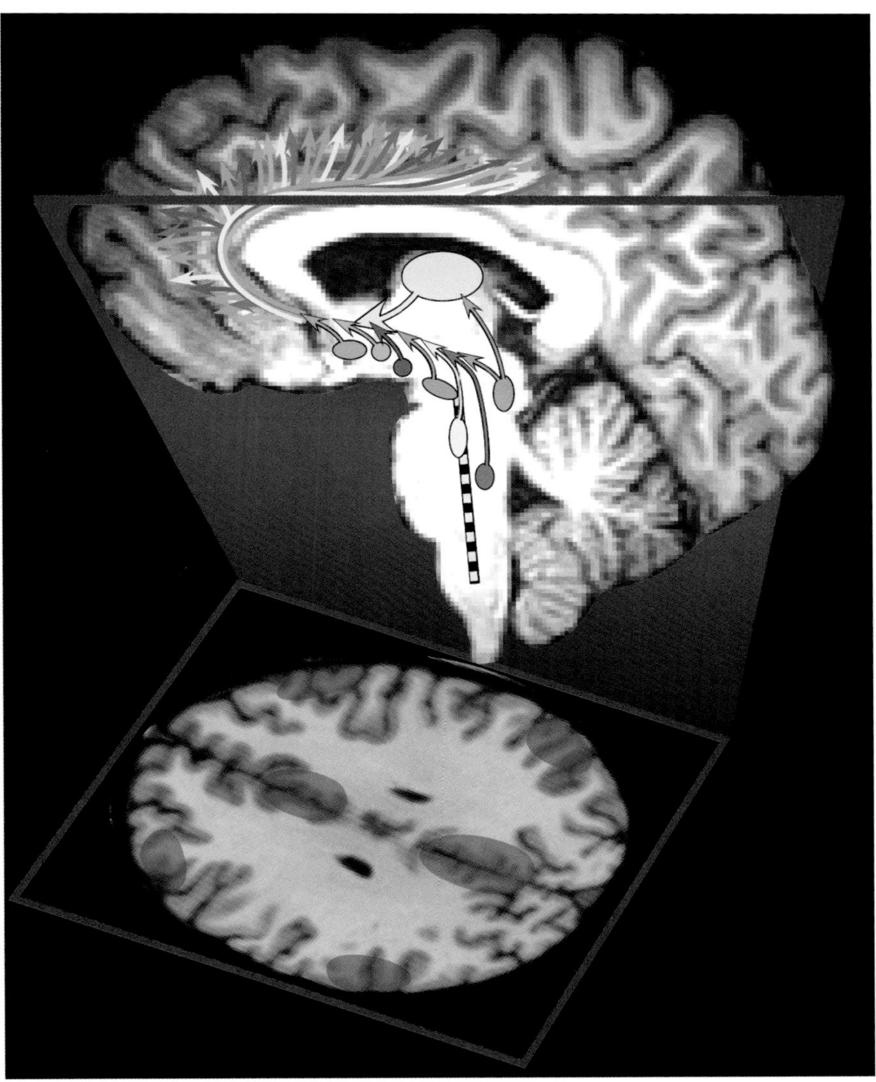

The structures and pathways that govern arousal are color-coded by neurotransmitter (see Figure 22–1) onto a midline sagittal magnetic resonance image (top). Areas in which regional cerebral blood flow is higher while awake than while asleep are indicated (*pink*) on an axial magnetic resonance image.

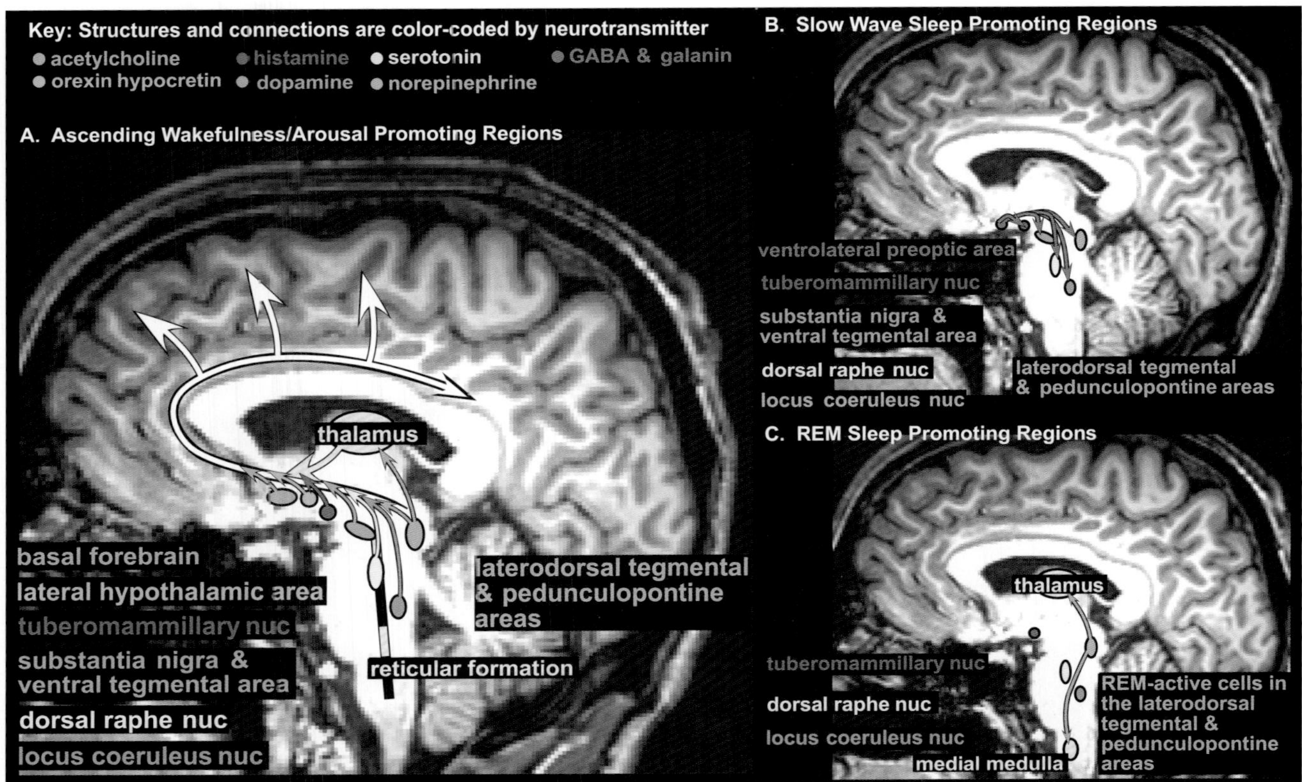

FIGURE 22–1. The brain regions that govern arousal and sleep are illustrated on a midline sagittal magnetic resonance image. Structures and pathways are color-coded by neurotransmitter.

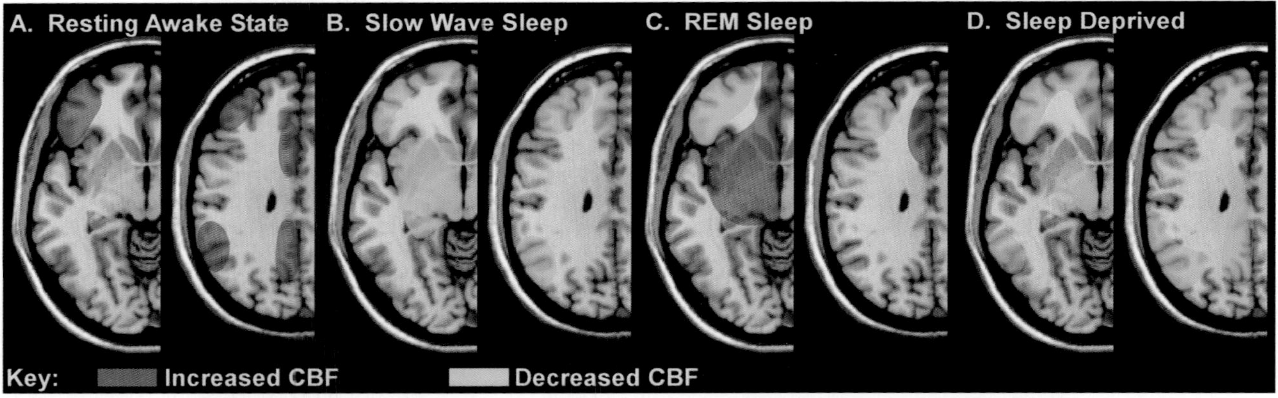

FIGURE 22–2. The activity level of the brain, as indicated by regional cerebral blood flow (CBF) imaging, varies with the state of consciousness and rest.[1,2] The areas most active in the 'control' resting waking state (lying still with the eyes closed) compared to sleeping are in prefrontal and parietal cortex (A). During slow wave sleep (SWS) several areas consistently exhibit decreased activity compared to wakefulness (B). When REM sleep is compared to SWS there are areas of increased activity (C, *pink*). There are areas of decreased activity when REM sleep is compared to the awake state (C, *blue*). Sleep deprivation is associated with decreases in several areas compared to the rested awake state (D).

Chronic sleep restriction is pervasive in society, with 40% of people in the United States reporting less than 7 hours of sleep most nights.[3] Sleep is undervalued, perhaps because the functions of sleep are not yet well understood.[4] The biological importance of sleep, on the other hand, is quite clear:

> Sleep has survived ubiquitously throughout all of mammalian evolution; some experiments have shown that animals cannot survive without sleep; and animals have made numerous behavioral and physiological accommodations to permit the survival of sleep in different habitats and life styles. Sleep persists in predators and prey; in carnivores and vegetarians; on the land and in the water (marine mammals); in most mammals as they lie down relaxed, in ruminants while they stand, in birds while they perch, and in dolphins which constantly swim; in hot and cold climates; in elephants and shrews; in sloths that hardly move and mice that hardly sit still; in the smartest and the dumbest of all mammalian species. These facts suggest a primary, essential, functional core to sleep. . .[5]

If sufficiently prolonged, sleep deprivation is deadly, indicating the critical role it plays in maintaining health.[5] Sleep appears to affect many processes in the body including energy metabolism, immune system function, learning/memory, appetite regulation, and gene expression.[6–16] Recent work suggests that sleep may enhance creativity by facilitating the mental restructuring that is critical to insight.[17] Sleep abnormalities are frequently associated with both primary psychiatric disorders and traumatic brain injuries.

Regulation of the sleep–waking cycle is complex.[18–21] Onset of sleep is governed by the interacting forces of the sleep drive, which steadily increases with duration of wakefulness, and circadian fluctuations in arousal level. The ascending arousal system is comprised of multiple ascending projections from brainstem, hypothalamus, thalamus, and basal forebrain (Figure 22–1A). There is interplay among many neurotransmitter systems to maintain the waking state, as recently reviewed.[18–21] Wakefulness-promoting actions of acetylcholine (midbrain, pons, and basal forebrain areas, Figure 22–1, *light orange*), dopamine (substantia nigra and ventral tegmental area, Figure 22–1, *green*), and norepinephrine (locus coeruleus nucleus, Figure 22–1, *purple*) are well known. Recent work indicates that serotonin (dorsal raphe nucleus, Figure 22–1, *yellow*), histamine (tuberomammillary nucleus, Figure 22–1, *red*), and orexin (also called hypocretin, lateral hypothalamic area, Figure 22–1, *blue*) also promote wakefulness. Sleep-promoting regions in the anterior hypothalamus (principally the ventrolateral preoptic area, Figure 22–1B, *pink*) utilize the neurotransmitters GABA and galanin to inhibit wake-promoting regions in the hypothalamus and brainstem during slow wave sleep (SWS, also called non-REM [NREM] sleep) (Figure 22–1B). Brainstem regions inhibited during wakefulness and NREM sleep become active during REM sleep (Figure 22–1C). Ascending projections from cholinergic neurons in the brainstem (laterodorsal tegmental and pedunculopontine areas, Figure 22–1C, *light orange*) activate the thalamus, which in turn activates the cortex. Descending projections from this area, utilizing other neurotransmitters in addition to acetylcholine, inhibit motor neurons, producing atonia (Figure 22–1C, *light orange*). Further complexity has been introduced by the recognition that sleep-promoting substances (somnogens) accumulate during wakefulness. Synthesis of adenosine (which appears to directly inhibit wake-promoting neurons), for example, increases during periods of high metabolic demand (e.g., prolonged wakefulness, seizures, ischemia). The wake-promoting effect of caffeine is probably due to its ability to block adenosine receptors.

In the waking state the electroencephalogram (EEG) is characterized by low amplitude fast activity (13–30 Hz, beta frequency band). Functional imaging studies indicate that during waking (as compared to sleeping) cerebral blood flow is high in the prefrontal and parietal cortices (Figure 22–2A).[1] With relaxation, particularly when the eyes are closed, slower activity (8–12 Hz, alpha frequency band) dominates the EEG. During the transition to sleep, EEG activity gradually decreases further. In deep (stage 3 and 4) sleep (SWS), the EEG is characterized by large amplitude slow activity (<2 Hz, delta frequency band) due to widespread synchronous rhythmic thalamocortical activity. Animal studies indicate that thalamic neurons become hyperpolarized and change their firing pattern to a delta rhythm because tonic activation by brainstem centers decreases. The heart and respiratory rates also slow and blood pressure decreases (increased parasympathetic tone). Functional imaging studies indicate that cerebral blood flow decreases compared to wakefulness, particularly in core subcortical structures such as the thalamus, basal forebrain, basal ganglia, and brainstem (Figure 22–2B).[1] Decreases have also been reported for the cerebellum, and ventromedial prefrontal (orbitofrontal and anterior cingulate), parietal, and mesiotemporal cortices. Several times during a normal night's sleep both the metabolic rate of the brain and EEG activity increase to levels similar to the waking state, accompanied by deep relaxation of the muscles. This state (paradoxical sleep, PS) is associated with vivid dreaming and rapid eye movements (REM). Functional imaging indicates that thalamus, pons, limbic/paralimbic areas, and occipital cortex (visual association cortex) are very active (high blood flow and/or metabolic rate), while frontal and parietal cortices are suppressed (Figure 22–2C).[1,22]

Decreases in both global and regional cerebral metabolism have been found following periods of sleep deprivation compared to the baseline rested state.[2,23,24] Only regional decreases in cerebral metabolic rate were found in the earliest study.[24] Following sleep deprivation, cerebral metabolism in thalamus, basal ganglia, cerebellum, and frontal and temporal cortex was decreased, whereas that in parietal cortex was increased (a visual vigilance task was performed during uptake in both conditions to standardize brain state). Decreased performance was positively correlated with decreased cerebral metabolic rate for thalamus and basal ganglia. More recent work has found globally decreased metabolism (~6%) with relative regional decreases (2%–11%) in multiple areas of cortex (a serial addition/subtraction task was performed during uptake).[2,23] During a period of 72 hours of sleep deprivation, the most consistent regional decreases (compared to the awake rested state) were in prefrontal, posterior parietal, and temporal cortices as well as thalamus and cerebellum (Figure 22–2D). Decreased performance was positively correlated with decreased metabolic rate for several prefrontal cortex regions and thalamus. These studies support the vulnerability of the thalamocortical circuits that are so critical for higher order cognitive functions to the effects of sleep deprivation.

The cognitive and emotional effects of sleep loss (generally quantified as sleep debt) have been studied using a variety of interventions, including total sleep deprivation, sleep restriction (<8 hours of sleep allowed per night), and sleep disruption (frequent awakenings during the sleep period). Comparison across studies is hampered by many factors, including differences in the method and duration of sleep disturbance employed and in the cognitive tasks used to evaluate performance deficits.[25] In addition, the common practice of averaging performance measures across groups may obscure differences, as there is a substantial range of sensitivity among individuals to the negative effects of sleep deprivation (trait-like differential vulnerability).[26]

Both sleep deprivation and sleep restriction have adverse effects on mood, cognitive performance, and motor function.[25,27] The most commonly used tasks in this research area are simple vigilance and continuous performance tasks, which are quite sensitive to sleep deprivation. Studies utilizing more complex tasks indicate that convergent, logical thinking is relatively insensitive to sleep deprivation, whereas divergent, flexible thinking is adversely affected. Although controversy exists, executive functions (working memory, divided attention, self-monitoring, risk assessment) seem to be particularly vulnerable, leading to the suggestion that the prefrontal areas of the brain are more sensitive to the effects of sleep disturbances.

Recent studies have shown that both acute sleep deprivation (~24 hour) and short-term chronic sleep restriction (<6 hours sleep per night for week) cause as much impairment on a simulated driving test as moderate alcohol consumption.[28–30] Similar results have been found in more naturalistic studies. Research utilizing medical residents has shown decrements in several tests of psychomotor performance following a 4-week period of heavy duty (mean work time ~90 hours per week) compared to following a similar period of normal duty (mean work time ~44 hours per week).[31] When alcohol was administered to residents following a period of normal duty, performance was impaired to an extent similar to following 4 weeks of heavy duty.[31]

Performance impairment is greater with total sleep deprivation than sleep restriction for a set number of hours of total sleep debt.[32–34] Thus, a single night of total sleep deprivation (8 hours of sleep debt) results in a greater impairment than four nights of mild (2 hours of sleep debt per night) or two nights of moderate (4 hours of sleep debt per night) sleep restriction.[33] One interpretation of this finding is that adaptation occurs to chronic sleep deprivation.[32] Another is that the critical factor is the number of hours of wakefulness beyond what is normal for the individual (cumulative wake extension time).[33] When analyzed from this perspective, the behavioral impairments due to total and partial sleep deprivation approximated a single near-linear model.[33,34] These results support the view that even mild chronic sleep restriction gradually but inexorably erodes performance. Interestingly, sleep deprivation studies indicate that subjects are often not aware of their level of sleep debt, as they do not necessarily experience daytime sleepiness.[33,35] Lack of insight increases the risk of accidents and sleep-related errors.[36] These results are worrisome, given the prevalence of chronic sleep restriction in the United States.[3]

The impact of sleep loss is potentially more devastating for the elderly, the medically compromised, and individuals with psychiatric disorders. Sleep disturbances are extremely common in this vulnerable population (estimates for insomnia range from 50%–80% in psychiatric illness), and are part of the diagnostic criteria for many psychiatric disorders.[37–39] Commonly related disorders include the sleep disorders themselves, such as narcolepsy and mood, anxiety, and substance use disorders. Of note is the recent evidence that sleep architecture can remain abnormal in patients with treated depressive episodes and is also found in nondepressed relatives of these patients.[37] Many patients who have achieved sobriety after significant substance abuse continue to have abnormalities in sleep (slow wave) for years after recovery.[37] Insomnia is also frequently present following traumatic brain injury (present in 30%–50% of patients with traumatic brain injury), and studies indicate that these symptoms may persist for many years.[39]

All major classes of psychotropic medications affect the neurotransmitters that modulate the sleep–wake cycle. For example, the selective serotonin reuptake inhibitors and tricyclic antidepressants decrease REM sleep and benzodiazepines increase the affinity of GABA receptors for GABA, thus increasing sleep. Clinicians often consider too much or too little "sleep" when choosing a psychopharmacologic intervention for a mood or other disorder. However, the secondary effects of these medications on neurotransmitter balance in sleep–waking functional anatomy and ultimately in the quality of resulting sleep have not, to date, been incorporated into standard treatment guidelines. The complexities of sleep–arousal neuroanatomy/neurochemistry and the relationship with stress, anxiety, and psychiatric disease have been an area of study for decades. Yet, there is still much more required to fully understand this complex system in order to design pharmacologic interventions for illness that will produce symptom relief and natural sleep, and have minimal side effects.

References

1. Maquet P: Functional neuroimaging of normal human sleep by positron emission tomography. J Sleep Res 2000; 9:207–231
2. Thomas M, Sing M, Belenky G, et al: Neural basis of alertness and cognitive performance impairments during sleepiness. I. Effects of 24 h of sleep deprivation on waking human regional brain activity. J Sleep Res 2000; 9:335–352
3. National Sleep Foundation: 2005 Sleep in America Poll. National Sleep Foundation; http://www.sleepfoundation.org/_content/hottopics/2005_summary_of_findings.pdf (accessed 12–9–2005)
4. Foster RG, Wulff K: The rhythm of rest and excess. Nat Rev Neurosci 2005; 6:407–414
5. Rechtschaffen A: Current perspectives on the function of sleep. Perspect Biol Med 1998; 41:359–390
6. Marshall L, Born J: Brain-immune interactions in sleep. Int Rev Neurobiol 2002; 52:93–131
7. Vgontzas AN, Chrousos GP: Sleep, the hypothalamic-pituitary-adrenal axis, and cytokines: multiple interactions and disturbances in sleep disorders. Endocrinol Metab Clin North Am 2002; 31:15–36
8. Spiegel K, Leproult R, L'hermite-Baleriaux M, et al: Leptin levels are dependent on sleep duration: relationship with sympathovagal balance, carbohydrate regulation, cortisol, and thyrotropin. J Clin Endocrinol Metab 2004; 89:5762–5771
9. Spiegel K, Tasali E, Penev P, et al: Brief communication: sleep curtailment in healthy young men is associated with decreased leptin levels, elevated ghrelin levels, and increased hunger and appetite. Ann Intern Med 2004; 141:846–850
10. Bryant PA, Trinder J, Curtis N: Sick and tired: Does sleep have a vital role in the immune system? Nat Rev Immunol 2004; 4:457–467
11. Cirelli C: A molecular window on sleep: changes in gene expression between sleep and wakefulness. Neuroscientist 2005; 11:63–74
12. Cirelli C: How sleep deprivation affects gene expression in the brain: a review of recent findings. Appl Physiol 2002; 92:394–400
13. Greene R, Siegel J: Sleep: a functional enigma. Neuromolecular Med 2004; 5:59–68
14. Rauchs G, Desgranges B, Foret J, et al: The relationship between memory systems and sleep stages. J Sleep Res 2005; 14:123–140
15. Stickgold R, Walker MP: Memory consolidation and reconsolidation: what is the role of sleep? Trends Neurosci 2005; 28:408–415
16. Gais B, Born J: Declarative memory consolidation: mechanisms acting during human sleep. Learn Mem 2004; 11:679–685
17. Wagner U, Gais S, Haider H, et al: Sleep inspires insight. Nature 2004; 427:352–355
18. España RA, Scammell TE: Sleep neurobiology for the clinician. Sleep 2004; 27:811–820
19. Stiller JW, Postolache TT: Sleep-wake and other biological rhythms: functional neuroanatomy. Clin Sports Med 2005; 24:205–235
20. Staunton H: Mammalian sleep. Naturwissenschaften 2005; 92:203–220
21. Zeman A, Reading P: The science of sleep. Clin Med 2005; 5:97–101
22. Nofzinger EA: Functional neuroimaging of sleep. Semin Neurol 2005; 25:9–18
23. Thomas ML, Sing HC, Belenky G, et al: Neural basis of alertness and cognitive performance impairments during sleepiness. II. Effects of 48 and 72 h of sleep deprivation on waking human brain activity. Thalamus Relat Syst 2003; 2:199–229
24. Wu JC, Gillin JC, Buchsbaum MS, et al: The effect of sleep deprivation on cerebral glucose metabolic rate in normal humans assessed with positron emission tomography. Sleep 1991; 14:155–162
25. Durmer JS, Dinges DF: Neurocognitive consequences of sleep deprivation. Semin Neurol 2005; 25:117–129
26. Van Dongen HP, Baynard MD, Maislin G, et al: Systematic interindividual differences in neurobehavioral impairment from sleep loss: evidence of trait-like differential vulnerability. Sleep 2004; 27:423–433
27. Harrison Y, Horne JA: The impact of sleep deprivation on decision making: a review. J Exp Psychol Appl 2000; 6:236–249
28. Arnedt JT, Wilde GJ, Munt PW, et al: How do prolonged wakefulness and alcohol compare in the decrements they produce on a simulated driving task? Accid Anal Prev 2001; 33:337–344
29. Powell NB, Schechtman KB, Riley RW, et al: The road to danger: the comparative risks of driving while sleepy. Laryngoscope 2001; 111:887–893
30. Maruff P, Falleti MG, Collie A, et al: Fatigue-related impairment in the speed, accuracy and variability of psychomotor performance: comparison with blood alcohol levels. J Sleep Res 2005; 14:21–27

31. Arnedt JT, Owens J, Crouch M, et al: Neurobehavioral performance of residents after heavy night call versus after alcohol ingestion. JAMA 2005; 294:1025–1033
32. Drake CL, Roehrs TA, Burduvali E, et al: Effects of rapid versus slow accumulation of 8 hours of sleep loss. Psychophysiology 2001; 38:979–987
33. Van Dongen HP, Maislin G, Mullington JM, et al: The cumulative cost of additional wakefulness: dose-response effects on neurobehavioral functions and sleep physiology from chronic sleep restriction and total sleep deprivation. Sleep 2003; 26:117–126
34. Van Dongen HP, Dinges DF: Sleep debt and cumulative excess wakefulness (letter). Sleep 2003; 26:249
35. Dement WC: Sleep extension: getting as much extra sleep as possible. Clin Sports Med 2005; 24:251–268
36. Carskadon MA: Sleep deprivation: health consequences and societal inpact. Med Clin North Am 2004; 88:767–776
37. Krahn LE: Psychiatric disorders associated with disturbed sleep. Semin Neurol 2005; 25:90–96
38. Spira AP, Friedman L, Flint A, et al: Interaction of sleep disturbances and anxiety in later life: perspectives and recommendations for future research. J Geriatr Psychiatry Neurol 2005; 18:109–115
39. Ouellet MC, Savard J, Morin CM: Insomnia following traumatic brain injury. Neurorehabil Neural Repair 2004; 18:187–198

Recent Publications of Interest

Shakhar K, Valdimarsdottir HB, Guevarra JS, et al: Sleep, fatigue, and NK cell activity in healthy volunteers: significant relationships revealed by within subject analyses. Brain Behav Immun 2007; 21:180–184

Measured natural killer cell activity (a measure of immune function), amount of sleep, and fatigue in healthy women at two times separated by ~1 month. Within-subjects analysis indicated that increased sleep and decreased fatigue were associated with improved immune system function.

Killgore WD, Balkin TJ, Wesensten NJ: Impaired decision making following 49 h of sleep deprivation. J Sleep Res 2006; 15:7–13

Compared risk-taking behavior (Iowa Gambling Task) prior to and following 49.5 hours of sleep deprivation in healthy normal subjects. Within-subjects analysis showed that increased levels of risk-taking were associated with sleep deprivation and that older subjects were more adversely affected. These results support the vulnerability of prefrontal cortex to sleep loss.

Wu JC, Gillin JC, Buchsbaum MS, et al: Frontal lobe metabolic decreases with sleep deprivation not totally reversed by recovery sleep. Neuropsychopharmacology 2006; 31:2783–2792

Assessed regional brain glucose utilization (PET) changes as a result of sleep deprivation and recovery sleep in healthy normal subjects. The results support previous studies indicating decreased metabolism in frontal and temporal cortices, thalamus, and striatum that was only partially reversed by recovery sleep.

Reprinted from Taber KH, Hurley RA: "Functional Neuroanatomy of Sleep and Sleep Deprivation." *Journal of Neuropsychiatry and Clinical Neurosciences* 18:1–5, 2006. Used with permission.

Chapter 23

Neural Underpinnings of Fear and Its Modulation

Implications for Anxiety Disorders

Lisa A. Miller, M.D.
Katherine H. Taber, Ph.D.
Glen O. Gabbard, M.D.
Robin A. Hurley, M.D.

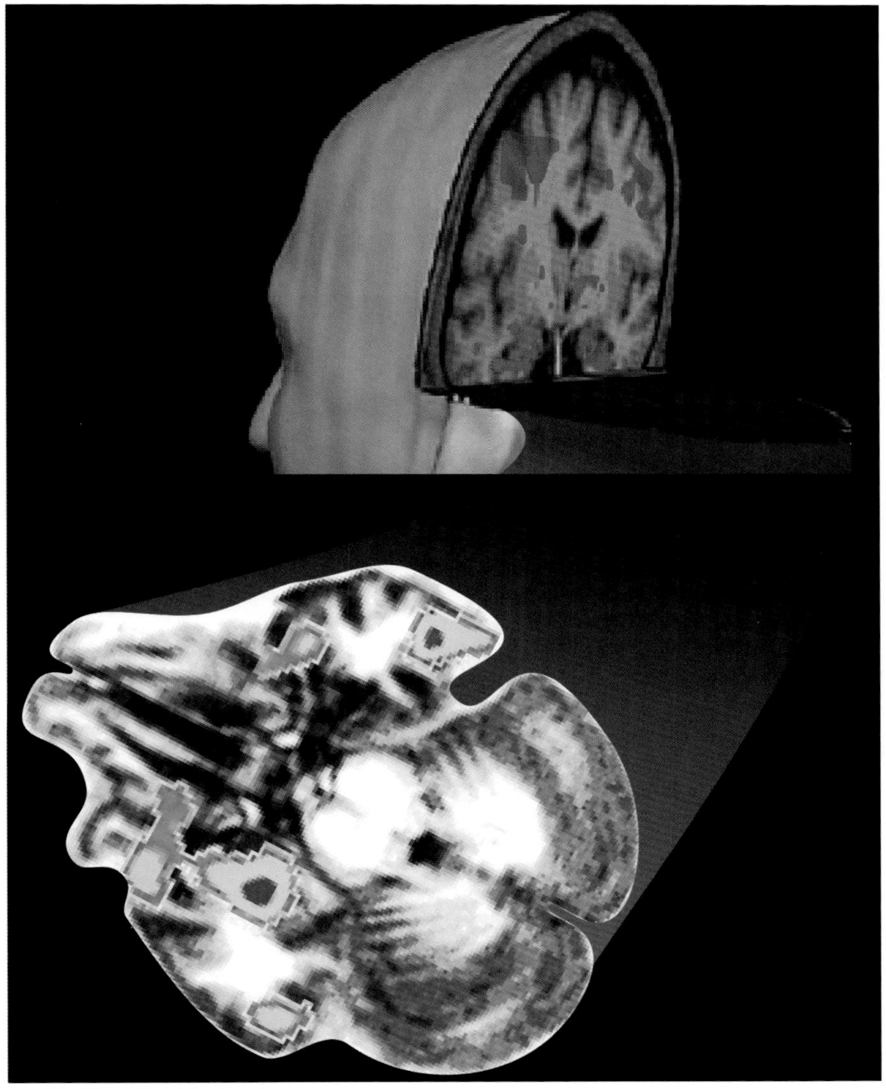

Statistical parametric map displaying regions of significant activation (as measured by functional magnetic resonance imaging) in patients with posttraumatic stress disorder (PTSD, *orange*) and controls (*purple*) superimposed on a three-dimensional reconstruction of magnetic resonance images. The amygdala was much more activated in the patients with PTSD. Adapted with permission.[1]

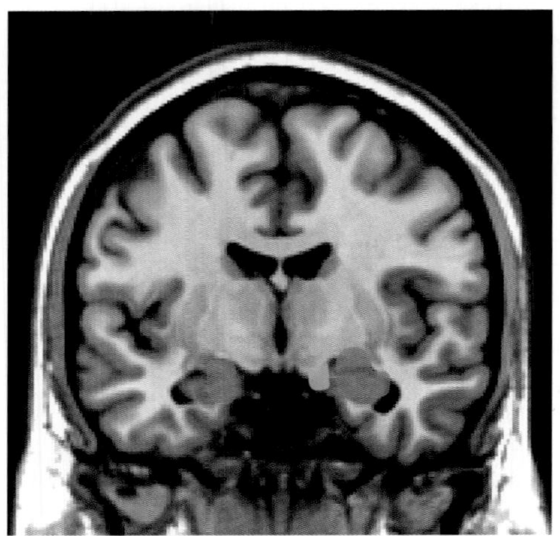

FIGURE 23–1. Combined results from two functional magnetic resonance imaging studies in normal subjects in which emotionally arousing images were presented extremely briefly prior to a longer presentation of a neutral image, resulting in masking of the briefly presented images. Although the subjects had no conscious awareness of the masked images, the amygdala was activated by both fearful faces[2] (*gold*) and angry faces[3] (*green*), but not by happy or neutral faces.

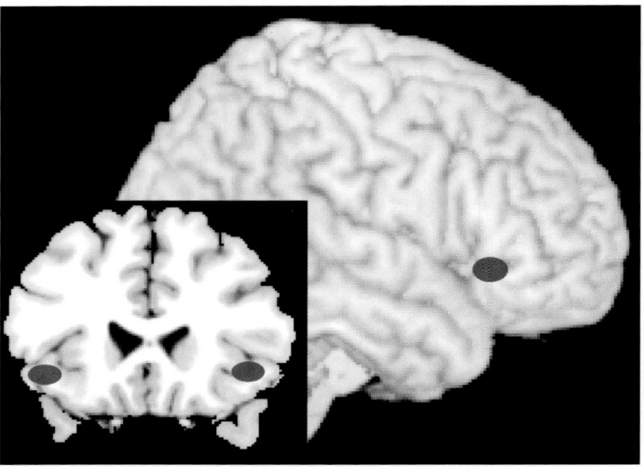

FIGURE 23–2. Combined results from two functional magnetic resonance imaging studies in normal subjects that support top-down modulation of emotions by prefrontal cortex.[4,5] Activation in the amygdala was strong with a simple matching task using emotionally arousing pictures (not shown). Tasks requiring conscious evaluation of the same pictures evoked stronger responses in ventral prefrontal cortex (*pink*) that correlated negatively with activity in the amygdala.

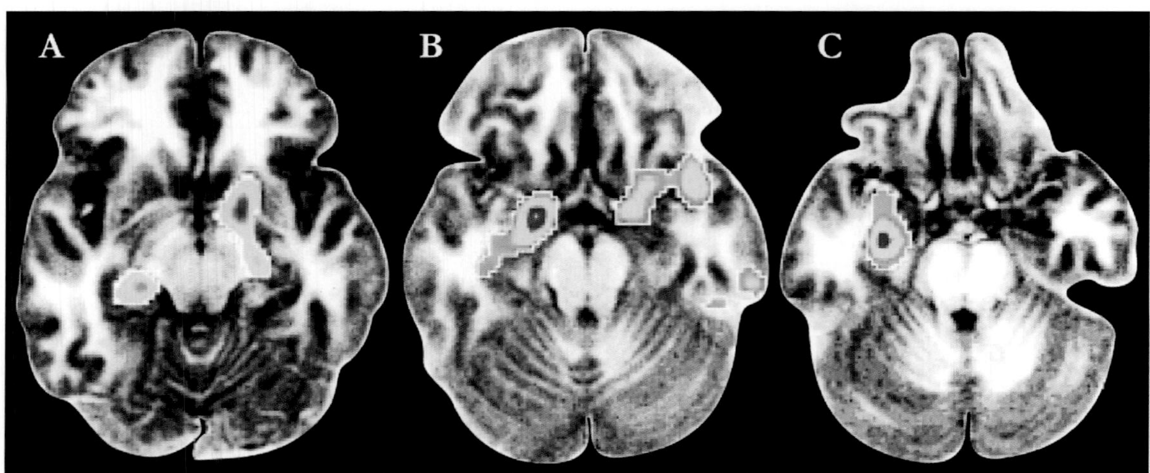

FIGURE 23–3. In patients with social phobia, a public speaking task results in increased regional cerebral blood flow (rCBF) (as measured by positron emission tomography) in many areas of the brain. Following successful treatment with either cognitive-behavioral group therapy (A) or citalopram (B), rCBF was reduced in amygdala, hippocampus, and surrounding cortical areas. When responders were compared to nonresponders (C), rCBF was decreased in dorsolateral prefrontal and anterior cingulate cortices, regardless of therapeutic intervention. Used with permission.[6]

Understanding how brain structures are functionally interrelated into networks is important to an understanding of psychiatric disorders and to interpreting the findings in functional neuroimaging studies. The recent emphasis on the neuroscience of emotions is of particular relevance. Current advances in the understanding of the neural circuitry of fear and how fear is modulated have widespread applications. Fear has a major influence upon memory, cognition, and behavior. Functional neuroimaging now allows researchers to probe the neural circuitry of both conscious and unconscious mental processes underlying fear and anxiety. It has also been used to assess functional brain changes in response to different modes of therapeutic intervention. Insights gained from such studies may contribute to advances in treatment of anxiety disorders, including therapies with greater specificity for underlying brain abnormalities.

Fear is defined as "an unpleasant, often strong emotion caused by anticipation or awareness of danger."[7] Feelings are conscious experiences that help in the identification of emotions.[8–10] When one feels afraid, one can identify the emotion of fear. "Not all feelings are emotions, but all (conscious) emotional experiences are feelings."[8] The current understanding of fear circuitry in humans is based on animal research studies, imaging studies of human subjects with pertinent brain lesions, and, more recently, on human functional neuroimaging. Studies of both normal and pathological fear states (e.g., anxiety disorders) are relevant.

The Amygdala and Fear

Activation of the amygdala is central to generation of the fear response. The amygdala, in turn, activates areas of the brain important to measurable neurobehavioral correlates of fear, including the hypothalamus (release of the flight/fight hormones) and brainstem (freezing, startle).[8,9,11,12] The amygdala also causes widespread brain activation via its connections to the basal forebrain as well as cholinergic and noradrenergic centers in the brainstem.[9] Activation of the amygdala is required for acquisition of learned fear responses.[8–10,13–15] Learned fear states may be associated with increased excitability in the amygdala.[16,17] Animal research supports the concept that the amygdala and hippocampus act together to form long-term memories of affectively laden information and events.[18] The hippocampus is believed to link information about physical contexts with the emotional context provided by the amygdala.[14] Researchers believe that the amygdala strengthens memory consolidation during times of strong emotion.[9,12,15,17,18] Some types of fear-related memory may be stored in the amygdala.

Several interconnected areas are important for recall (retrieval) of fear-related memories including the amygdala, hippocampus, and anterior cingulate.[16,19–22] Although controversial, there is evidence that, once recalled (reactivated), a memory must undergo a new consolidation process (reconsolidation) in order to be maintained in long-term memory.[23–25] Thus while reactivated the memory may become vulnerable (labile) to modification or disruption. The reconsolidation process may involve the same areas as retrieval, although the processes appear to be different. The amygdala is also central to extinction of conditioned fear, whereby the fear response is weakened by multiple exposures to the conditioning context without the painful or frightening event.[15,22,26] Extinction does not remove the conditioned fear, but rather suppresses it by new learning.[22,26] The amygdala is activated during both acquisition and extinction of conditioned fear in humans.[22,27–29] Long-term storage of extinction-related memory to some extent depends upon modulation of the amygdala by medial prefrontal cortex (PFC).[15,17,22,29]

Current research indicates that external sensory information reaches the amygdala by two pathways. All sensory input is first relayed to the thalamus. Two divergent pathways emerge from the thalamus. Direct pathways from the thalamus (thalamoamygdalar) can activate the amygdala very rapidly, on the basis of crude thalamic appraisals of sensory stimuli indicating potential danger (i.e., a long and thin object might be a snake). This reflexive activation of the amygdala has been referred to as "bottom-up" regulation of emotion.[30] The thalamoamygdalar route appears to operate at an unconscious level and can mediate fear conditioning independently of cortical input.[8,9,15]

Several lines of evidence from human studies support the existence of this pathway. The amygdala is activated by emotionally salient stimuli even when presented to the blind hemifield in a patient with an extensive left visual cortex lesion.[31,32] Various methods for presenting unconscious visual stimuli have been used in conjunction with functional imaging, including backward masking or binocular rivalry to suppress conscious awareness in normal subjects.[2,33,34] Most studies have reported activation of the amygdala during the suppressed condition to a range of emotionally salient images, supporting the existence of the direct pathway (Figure 23–1). Conditioned responses can also be established with masked stimuli that activate the amygdala.[35] Studies in which attention to fearful or threatening stimuli was manipulated found that the amygdala was activated even when the stimuli were not attended to.[36,37] One study found that the amygdala responded to a broader range of stimuli during the "unattended" condition.[37] These studies support the concept that the amygdala has limited specificity when relying on information from the subcortical route (thalamoamygdalar pathways) and that this limited specificity reflects a trade-off between speed of processing and specificity.

Researchers believe that thalamoamygdalar pathways facilitate automatic, reflexive responses to a potentially aversive situation before it registers in conscious awareness.[8,38,39] The faster, imprecise, unconscious thalamoamygdalar pathway can activate the amygdala rapidly, which could mean the difference between life and death.

However, such rapid amygdalar activation of a cascade of fear responses (e.g., release of epinephrine, norepinephrine, and cortisol) may overwhelm the capacity for conscious cognitive appraisals, which occur via prefrontal cortical networks.[38]

Fear may enhance or interfere with attention, learning, and social judgments.[8,10,12,40] Damasio emphasizes the importance of intuition in decision making.[41] Studies in human subjects support the concept that unconscious mental processes influence conscious cognitions and feelings.[42,43] For example, studies employing subliminal emotional priming have demonstrated that test subjects liked or disliked a neutral stimulus (i.e., a Chinese ideogram or polygon) depending upon whether the stimulus was subliminally (unconsciously) primed by facial expressions of anger, fear, disgust, or happiness. Learned conscious and subliminal fear responses bias cognition and affective style.[13]

Alternatively, sensory input from the thalamus may reach the amygdala by *indirect* pathways involving sensory cortices. The sensory cortices, in conjunction with other brain regions such as the hippocampus and parahippocampal, association, and prefrontal cortices, assign significance to sensory stimuli based upon context and prior experience.[9] Sensory information reaches the amygdala more slowly by this pathway, but conveys highly refined appraisals. These connections are reciprocal, allowing mutual regulatory influences.[8] Both the sensory cortices and amygdala are believed to relay information to PFC. Sensory information is not thought to enter conscious awareness unless processed in PFC networks concerned with conscious perception. The vast majority of sensory stimuli do not enter conscious awareness.

Modulation by Prefrontal Cortex

In neuropsychiatry, the PFC is commonly divided into three main divisions: the medial PFC (containing the anterior cingulate and paracingulate cortices), the orbital PFC, and the dorsolateral PFC. Medial PFC functions relevant to fear include attention to the emotional states of the self and others, guidance of response selection by emotional states, and suppression of fear-related behavioral responses as situations change.[15,19,22] Orbital PFC functions relevant to fear include modulation of behavioral and visceral responses associated with fear-related situations as situations change and modulation of emotional responses by correcting associations when they become inappropriate.[19,44] Dorsolateral functions relevant to fear are believed to include involvement in working memory, response preparation, and response selection.[44]

The amygdala has reciprocal connections with orbital and medial PFC and is indirectly connected to the dorsolateral PFC. Orbital and medial PFC appear to exert a predominantly inhibitory influence upon the amygdala by activation of inhibitory interneurons (top-down modulation).[13,15,22] Several recent functional magnetic resonance imaging (fMRI) studies in normal subjects support top-down modulation of emotions by these areas of PFC. One group has compared patterns of brain activation while subjects perform tasks requiring conscious evaluation of emotionally arousing pictures versus simple matching tasks using the same pictures (Figure 23–2).[4,5] When the two conditions were compared, stronger activation of the ventral PFC (Brodmann's area [BA] 44/45 and 47) by the more complex evaluative tasks was associated with decreased activation of the amygdala. During the simple matching tasks, which evoked less activation of the ventral PFC, stronger activation of the amygdala was demonstrated. Autonomic reactivity as monitored by changes in skin conductance correlated with activation of the amygdala. A similar inverse correlation between activity in the amygdala and ventral PFC was also found in a study using subliminal priming with emotionally arousing stimuli.[3] In addition, both a gender-decision task and an emotion-identification task evoked less activation in the amygdala and more in ventral PFC than passive viewing of the same images.[45]

Modulation of the amygdala by the PFC may be one of the biological mechanisms that underlie the effectiveness of cognitive behavioral therapy (CBT) in anxiety disorders.[10,46,47] Similarities exist between extinction (in which a learned fear response is replaced or overlaid by new learning) and CBT.[10,47,48] Two small studies have employed functional imaging to monitor the brain's response to symptom provocation in patients with phobias (spider and social phobias) prior to and following therapeutic interventions (CBT was utilized in both studies and compared to treatment with citalopram in one).[6,49] In both studies patients who responded successfully to therapy exhibited decreased activity in limbic-related areas. In the study of patients with spider phobia, activation (measured by fMRI) in dorsolateral PFC (BA 10) and the parahippocampal gyrus during exposure to film excerpts depicting spiders was no longer found following successful completion of CBT.[49] Similarly, in the study of patients with social phobia, those who responded well to either CBT or citalopram had decreased regional cerebral blood flow (rCBF) (measured by positron emission tomography [PET]) in the amygdala and hippocampus as well as periamygdaloid, parahippocampal, and rhinal cortices while performing a public speaking task (Figure 23–3).[6] In addition, the decrease in blood flow in the amygdala prior to and following treatment correlated with long-term clinical outcome. Both authors note that these results indicate that CBT is able to modify the abnormal neural functioning underlying anxiety disorders, perhaps by deconditioning or habituating contextual fear.

There is experimental evidence that extinction of fear can be facilitated by manipulation of neurotransmitters, specifically via the *N*-methyl-D-aspartate (NMDA) glutamate receptor.[50] In animal studies administration of D-4-amino-3-isoxazolidone (D-cycloserine, DCS) after extinction trials enhanced extinction. DCS is a partial agonist for the NMDA receptor, acting at the strychnine-insensitive glycine-recognition site. Efficacy of this approach for enhancing treatment of phobia was recently tested in a small double-blind placebo-controlled study.[51] Patients with acrophobia were randomly assigned to receive a high dose of DCS (500 mg), a low dose (50 mg), or placebo prior to two sessions of virtual reality therapy separated by 1–2 weeks. Presence of DCS did not affect level of fear exhibited during the first session, indicating no direct anxiolytic effect. During the second session and at follow-up 1 week and 3 months later, the patients who received DCS prior to therapy sessions exhibited significantly reduced fear of heights. These findings suggest that DCS may be a useful adjunct to therapeutic interventions for disorders in which fear-related learning is an important component.

Converging evidence supports the theory that genetic differences may influence development and/or expression of anxiety disorders. Increased reactivity of the amygdala has been demonstrated in individuals with a polymorphism in the promoter region of the serotonin transporter gene.[52,53] Presence of this polymorphism has been associated with susceptibility to fear conditioning as well as increased expression of anxiety and affective illness.[54–56] In patients with social phobia its presence is associated with both greater symptom severity and amygdala excitability.[53] It has been suggested that it may be associated with greater vulnerability to life stress.[57] These results are consistent with studies supporting a genetic component to all three phases of fear conditioning (acquisition, habituation, extinction).[58] It is likely that there is lifelong interaction between biological factors (e.g., genetic) and environment in the establishment and remodeling of networks involving fear and fear memory.

Functional imaging has demonstrated hyperexcitability of the amygdala in various anxiety disorders. Often an inverse relationship exists between activity in the amygdala and areas in PFC.[47] Recent studies illustrate this for social phobia and posttraumatic stress disorder (PTSD). Patients with social phobia exhibited increased rCBF (measured by PET) in the amygdala/periamygdaloid cortex during a public speaking task compared with controls.[59] At the same time, rCBF in orbital PFC decreased in the patients and increased in the controls. In another study, activation of the amygdala (measured by fMRI) did not differ between patient and control groups when viewing fearful or neutral faces (compared to happy faces).[40] However, the patients demonstrated significantly greater activation than controls in the amygdala and nearby cortex when viewing contemptuous or angry faces, indicating specificity related to their disorder. Larger than normal activations in the amygdala have also been measured in patients with social phobia during all phases of aversive conditioning (habituation, conditioning, extinction).[60] Patients with PTSD have also exhibited increased reactivity of the amygdala (measured by PET or fMRI).[1,61,62] Furthermore, measures of PTSD symptom severity were positively correlated with rCBF in the amygdala and inversely correlated with rCBF in the medial PFC in one study.[62] Regional CBF in the two areas was inversely related.

Conclusion

The study of fear-related learning and the modulation of fear are highly relevant to understanding and treatment of anxiety-based psychiatric disorders. Functional neuroimaging is proving to be a powerful technique in this area. The presence of both conscious and unconscious processing of fear has implications for both the development and treatment of anxiety disorders. Biological differences, such as individual differences in reactivity and tonic activation of the amygdala and prefrontal cortex, may contribute to individual differences in anxiety, learning of stimulus–threat contingencies, and expression of cue-specific fear, and perhaps vulnerability to stressors. In addition, functional imaging may also have the potential to predict sustained response to therapeutic interventions in anxiety disorders.

References

1. Hendler T, Rotshtein P, Yeshurun Y, et al: Sensing the invisible: differential sensitivity of visual cortex and amygdala to traumatic context. Neuroimage 2003; 19:587–600
2. Whalen PJ, Rauch SL, Etcoff NL, et al: Masked presentations of emotional facial expressions modulate amygdala activity without explicit knowledge. J Neurosci 1998; 18:411–418
3. Nomura M, Ohira H, Haneda K, et al: Functional association of the amygdala and ventral prefrontal cortex during cognitive evaluation of facial expressions primed by masked angry faces: an event-related fMRI study. Neuroimage 2004; 21:352–363

4. Hariri AR, Bookheimer SY, Mazziotta JC: Modulating emotional responses: effects of a neocortical network on the limbic system. Neuroreport 2000; 11:43–48
5. Hariri AR, Mattay VS, Tessitore A, et al: Neocortical modulation of the amygdala response to fearful stimuli. Biol Psychiatry 2003; 53 494–501
6. Furmark T, Tillfors M, Marteinsdottir I, et al: Common changes in cerebral blood flow in patients with social phobia treated with citalopram or cognitive-behavioral therapy. Arch Gen Psychiatry 2002; 59:425–433
7. Merriam Webster I: Merriam Webster's Collegiate Dictionary. Springfield, MA, Merriam-Webster, 1997
8. LeDoux JE: The Emotional Brain: The Mysterious Underpinnings of Emotional Life. New York, Simon & Schuster, Inc, 1996
9. LeDoux JE: Emotion circuits in the brain. Annu Rev Neurosci 2000; 23:155–184
10. LeDoux JE: Synaptic Self: How Our Brains Become Who We Are. New York, Penguin, Putman, Inc, 2002
11. Adolphs R: The neurobiology of social cognition. Curr Opin Neurobiol 2001; 11:231–239
12. McIntyre CK, Power AE, Roozendaal B, et al: Role of the basolateral amygdala in memory consolidation. Ann NY Acad Sci 2003; 985:273–293
13. Davidson RJ: Anxiety and affective style: Role of prefrontal cortex and amygdala. Biol Psychiatry 2002; 51:68–80
14. Fanselow MS, Gale GD: The amygdala, fear, and memory. Ann NY Acad Sci 2003; 985:125–134
15. Maren S, Quirk GJ: Neuronal signalling of fear memory. Nat Rev Neurosci 2004; 5:844–852
16. Maren S: Neurobiology of Pavlovian fear conditioning. Annu Rev Neurosci 2001; 24:897–931
17. Quirk GJ, Gehlert DR: Inhibition of the amygdala: Key to pathological states? Ann NY Acad Sci 2003; 985:263–272
18. Pape HC, Stork O: Genes and mechanisms in the amygdala involved in the formation of fear memory. Ann NY Acad Sci 2003; 985:92–105
19. Charney DS: Neuroanatomic circuits modulating fear and anxiety behaviors. Acta Psychiatr Scand 2003; 108:38–50
20. Frankland PW, Bontempi B, Talton LE, et al: The involvement of the anterior cingulate cortex in remote contextual fear memory. Science 2004; 304:881–883
21. Izquierdo I, Cammarota M: Neuroscience. Zif and the survival of memory. Science 2004; 304:829–830
22. Sotres-Bayon F, Bush DEA, LeDoux JE: Emotional perseveration: An update on prefrontal-amygdala interactions in fear extinction. Learn Mem 2004; 11:525–535
23. Nader K: Memory traces unbound. Trends Neurosci 2003; 26:65–72
24. Lee JL, Everitt BJ, Thomas KL: Independent cellular processes for hippocampal memory consolidation and reconsolidation. Science 2004; 304:839–843
25. Duvarci S, Nader K: Characterization of fear memory reconsolidation. J Neurosci 2004; 24:9269–9275
26. Bouton ME: Context and behavioral processes in extinction. Learn Mem 2004; 11:485–494
27. LaBar KS, Gatenby JC, Gore JC, et al: Human amygdala activation during conditioned fear acquisition and extinction: A mixed-trial fMRI study. Neuron 1998; 20:937–945
28. Morris JS, Dolan RJ: Dissociable amygdala and orbitofrontal responses during reversal fear conditioning. Neuroimage 2004; 22:372–380
29. Phelps EA, Delgado MR, Nearing KI, et al: Extinction learning in humans: Role of the amygdala and vmPFC. Neuron 2004; 43:897–905
30. Berntson GG, Sarter M, Cacioppo JT: Ascending visceral regulation of cortical affective information processing. Eur J Neurosci 2003; 18:2103–2109
31. de Gelder B, Vroomen J, Pourtois G, et al: Non-conscious recognition of affect in the absence of striate cortex. Neuroreport 1999; 10:3759–3763
32. Morris JS, de Gelder B, Weiskrantz L, et al: Differential extrageniculate and amygdala responses to presentation of emotional faces in a cortically blind field. Brain 2001; 124:1241–1252
33. Morris JS, Ohman A, Dolan RJ: A subcortical pathway to the right amygdala mediating unseen fear. Proc Natl Acad Sci USA 96:1680–1685
34. Williams MA, Mattingley JB: Unconscious perception of non-threatening facial emotion in parietal extinction. Exp Brain Res 2004; 154:403–406
35. Morris JS, Buchel C, Dolan RJ: Parallel neural responses in amygdala subregions and sensory cortex during implicit fear conditioning. Neuroimage 2001; 13:1044–1052
36. Vuilleumier P, Armony JL, Driver J, et al: Effects of attention and emotion on face processing in the human brain: an event-related fMRI study. Neuron 2001; 30:829–841
37. Anderson AK, Christoff K, Panitz D, et al: Neural correlates of the automatic processing of threat facial signals. J Neurosci 2003; 23:5627–5633
38. Goleman D: Emotional Intelligence: Why It Can Matter More Than IQ. New York, Random House, 1995
39. Dolan RJ, Vuilleumier P: Amygdala automaticity in emotional processing. Ann NY Acad Sci 2003; 985:348–355
40. Stein MB, Goldin PR, Sareen J, et al: Increased amygdala activation to angry and contemptuous faces in generalized social phobia. Arch Gen Psychiatry 2002; 59:1027–1034
41. Damasio AR: Descartes' Error: Emotion, Reason, and the Human Brain. New York, Avon, 1994
42. Winkielman P, Berridge K: Irrational wanting and subrational liking: How rudimentary motivational and affective processes shape preferences and choices. Political Psychology 2003; 24:657–680
43. Winkielman P, Berridge K: Unconscious emotion. Curr Dir Psychol Sci 2004; 13:120–123
44. Stuss DT, Knight RT: Principles of Frontal Lobe Function. New York, Oxford University Press, 2002
45. Lange K, Williams LM, Young AW, et al: Task instructions modulate neural responses to fearful facial expressions. Biol Psychiatry 2003; 53:226–232
46. Anand A, Shekhar A: Brain imaging studies in mood and anxiety disorders: special emphasis on the amygdala. Ann NY Acad Sci 2003; 985:370–388
47. Rauch SL, Shin LM, Wright CI: Neuroimaging studies of amygdala function in anxiety disorders. Ann NY Acad Sci 2003; 985:389–410
48. Davis M, Walker DL, Myers KM: Role of the amygdala in fear extinction measured with potentiated startle. Ann NY Acad Sci 2003; 985:218–232
49. Paquette V, Levesque J, Mensour B, et al: "Change the mind and you change the brain": effects of cognitive-behavioral therapy on the neural correlates of spider phobia. Neuroimage 2003; 18:401–409

50. Richardson R, Ledgerwood L, Cranney J: Facilitation of fear extinction by D-cycloserine: Theoretical and clinical implications. Learn Mem 2004; 11:510–516
51. Ressler K, Rothbaum B, Tannenbaum L, et al: Cognitive enhancers as adjuncts to psychotherapy. Arch Gen Psychiatry 2004; 61:1136–1144
52. Hariri AR, Mattay VS, Tessitore A, et al: Serotonin transporter genetic variation and the response of the human amygdala. Science 2002; 297:400–403
53. Furmark T, Tillfors M, Garpenstrand H, et al: Serotonin transporter polymorphism related to amygdala excitability and symptom severity in patients with social phobia. Neurosci Lett 2004; 362:189–192
54. Lesch KP, Bengel D, Heils A, et al: Association of anxiety-related traits with a polymorphism in the serotonin transporter gene regulatory region. Science 1996; 274:1527–1531
55. Osher Y, Hamer D, Benjamin J: Association and linkage of anxiety-related traits with a functional polymorphism of the serotonin transporter gene regulatory region in Israeli sibling pairs. Mol Psychiatry 2000; 5:216–219
56. Garpenstrand H, Annas P, Ekblom J, et al: Human fear conditioning is related to dopaminergic and serotonergic biological markers. Behav Neurosci 2001; 115:358–364
57. Caspi A, Sugden K, Moffitt TE, et al: Influence of life stress on depression: Moderation by a polymorphism in the 5-HTT gene. Science 2003; 301:386–389
58. Hettema JM, Annas P, Neale MC, et al: A twin study of the genetics of fear conditioning. Arch Gen Psychiatry 2003; 60:702–708
59. Tillfors M, Furmark T, Marteinsdottir I, et al: Cerebral blood flow in subjects with social phobia during stressful speaking tasks: A PET study. Am J Psychiatry 2001; 158:1220–1226
60. Veit R, Flor H, Erb M, et al: Brain circuits involved in emotional learning in antisocial behavior and social phobia in humans. Neurosci Lett 2002; 328:233–236
61. Rauch SL, Whalen PJ, Shin LM, et al: Exaggerated amygdala response to masked facial stimuli in posttraumatic stress disorder: A functional MRI study. Biol Psychiatry 2000; 47:769–776
62. Shin LM, Orr SP, Carson MA, et al: Regional cerebral blood flow in the amygdala and medial prefrontal cortex during traumatic imagery in male and female Vietnam veterans with PTSD. Arch Gen Psychiatry 2004; 61:168–176

Recent Publications of Interest

Quirk GJ: Extinction: new excitement for an old phenomenon. Biol Psychiatry 2006; 60:317–318

Reviews the evidence from animal studies implicating medial prefrontal cortex in extinction of conditioned fear. Pharmacologic agents that strengthen extinction learning and therefore have potential therapeutic applications are discussed briefly.

Hofmann SG, Meuret AE, Smits JA, et al: Augmentation of exposure therapy with D-cycloserine for social anxiety disorder. Arch Gen Psychiatry 2006; 63:298–304

Performed a randomized, placebo-controlled trial comparing the efficacy of short-term exposure therapy with and without prior administration of D-cycloserine for social anxiety disorder. The preliminary results (1 month) are consistent with previous studies that have found the combination to significantly enhance the effectiveness of exposure therapy.

Reprinted from Miller LA, Taber KH, Gabbard GO, et al: "Neural Underpinnings of Fear and Its Modulation: Implications for Anxiety Disorders." *Journal of Neuropsychiatry and Clinical Neurosciences* 17:1–6, 2005. Used with permission.

Chapter 24

RABIES AND THE CEREBELLUM

New Methods for Tracing Circuits in the Brain

KATHERINE H. TABER, PH.D.
PETER L. STRICK, PH.D.
ROBIN A. HURLEY, M.D.

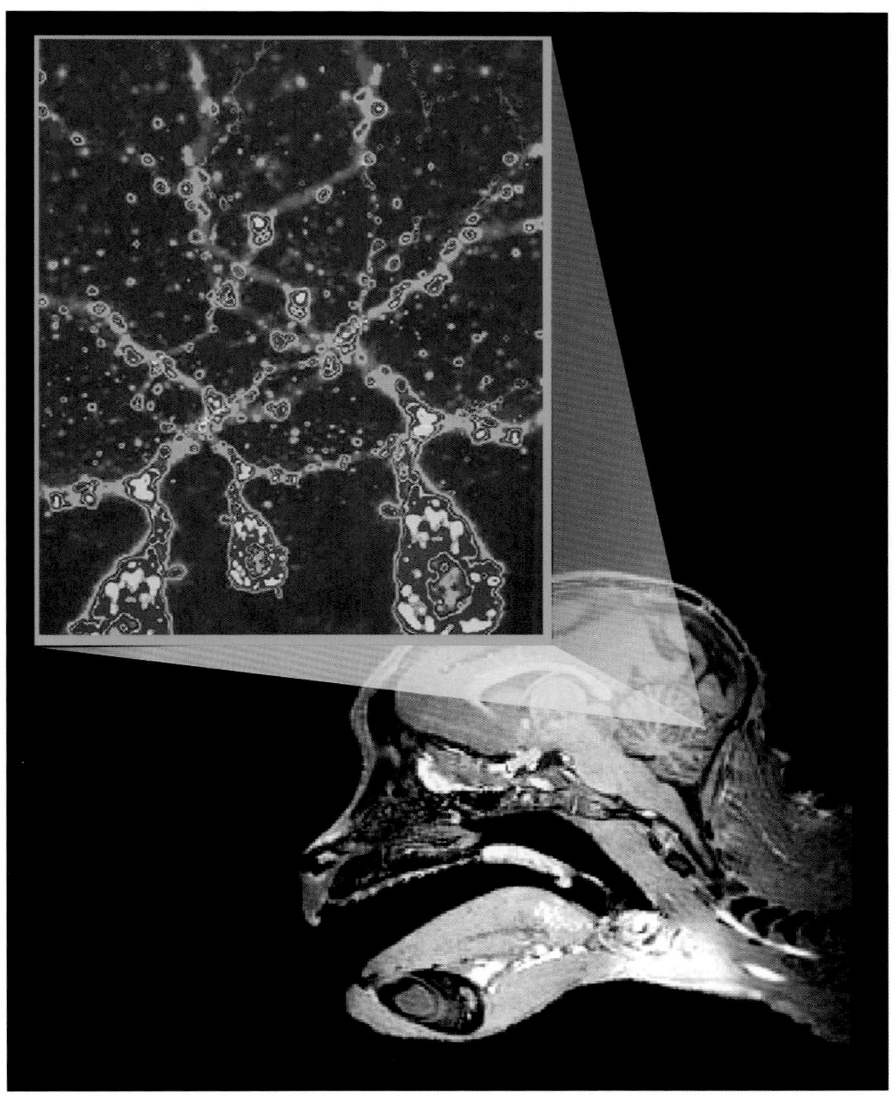

Sagittal T_1-weighted magnetic resonance image of a *Cebus* monkey and pseudocolored micrograph of cerebellar Purkinje cells immunohistochemically labeled for rabies virus.

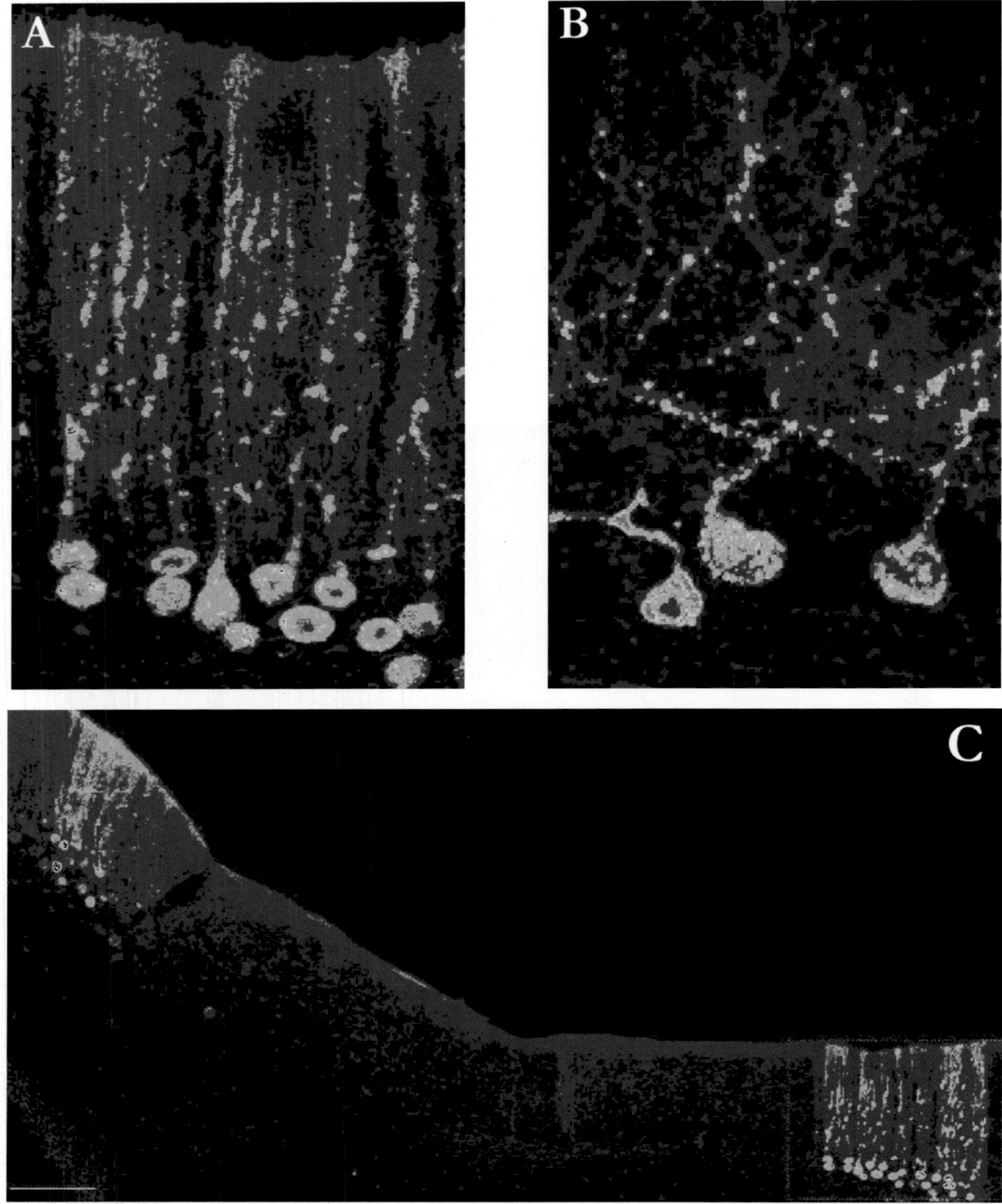

FIGURE 24–1. Cerebellar neurons immunohistochemically labeled for the transneuronally transported rabies virus 4 days after injection of virus into cerebral cortex are shown in transverse (A) and sagittal (B) planes of section. A lower magnification transverse section (C) shows the highly localized nature of the staining. Adapted with permission.[1]

Core to current neuropsychiatry is the concept that parallel circuits originating in multiple areas of the cerebral cortex underlie much of human behavior. Emotion, memory, and behavior are widely studied in relation to circuits that begin and end in either the frontal lobes or the limbic system.[2] The cerebellum was not traditionally incorporated into these circuits. As case reports and series emerge from the literature noting nonmotor symptoms in patients with isolated cerebellar lesions, the cerebellar role in cognition, mood, and behavior is becoming more visible.

In the past, the anatomy of brain circuits was inferred by combining case reports, imaging data, autopsy results, and many experimental animal studies in which anterograde and retrograde tracing techniques were used to label neurons and their projections. Recently, exciting new virus-based tracers have been introduced that are able to cross the synapse and

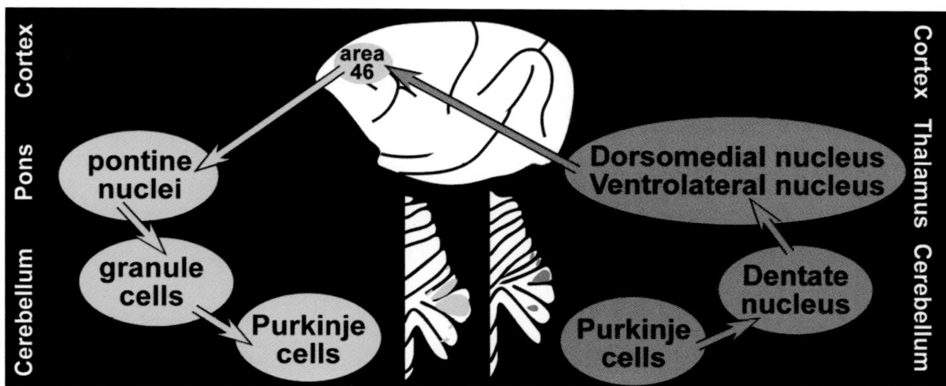

FIGURE 24–2. Retrograde transneuronal transport of rabies virus has been used to delineate the cerebrocerebellar circuit. Comparison of results from anterograde and retrograde tracers indicates that extremely similar areas within the cerebellum are labeled. It is therefore likely, although not proven, that the circuits are truly reciprocal.

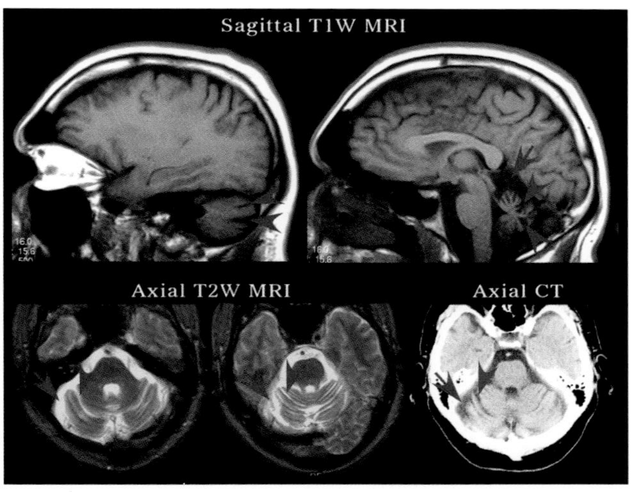

FIGURE 24–3. The patient is a middle-aged male with history of cognitive impairment, reported seizures, multiple minor head injuries without loss of consciousness, and limited alcohol and polysubstance use (cocaine, amphetamine) in the distant past. Once a successful business owner, he is now struggling to complete activities of daily living independently. Current symptoms include low frustration tolerance, poor concentration, and declining cognition. On examination, he was slightly disinhibited with poor concentration, decreased memory skills, child-like affect, and inability to shift sets. He exhibited a wide-based gait with mild truncal ataxia. No focal abnormalities or cortical atrophy was present on neuroimaging. The only brain abnormality found by MRI and computed tomography (CT) was prominent cerebellar atrophy, as indicated by widened cisterns (arrows) and widened cerebellar sulci (arrowheads).

thus allow specific labeling of neurons in sequence for the first time. With these new methods it is now possible to trace neuronal connections across several synapses, allowing mapping of parallel circuits in unprecedented detail. These studies provide strong evidence for the segregated nature of parallel frontosubcortical circuits and support the addition of the cerebellum to these pathways. Very importantly, they are beginning to open a window to the functional topography of the cerebellar cortex and the deep cerebellar nuclei.

Corticocerebellar Circuits and Virus-Based Tracers

Most studies delineating neuronal connections within the brain are done in animals. The rapid progress made in the past few decades in identifying these connections has been primarily based on the use of anterograde and retrograde tracers such as horseradish peroxidase and the dextran amines.[3] These substances have made it possible to probe the fine structure of the brain, but are limited to labeling of single neurons. Circuits are inferred by combining the results of multiple experiments. With the recent development of tract-tracing methodology based upon the use of neurotropic viruses, it is now possible to directly visualize neurons that are linked together in a circuit. These viruses are taken up into neurons where they replicate and pass from neuron to neuron at synaptic connections in a time-dependent manner. The apparent rate of transport is to some extent dependent on the rate of viral replication and the time required for *trans*-synaptic passage of the virus. Neurons infected with virus are identified using conventional immunohistochemical labeling with antibodies to the virus. Evidence to date supports the view that virus transport is not restricted to particular types of synapses, but rather labels both excitatory and inhibitory connections.[4] By appropriate selection of survival time after injection, multisynaptic pathways can be labeled with great precision. For example, by 2 days after injection of rabies (retrograde tracer) into primary motor cortex (M1), neurons in the ventrolateral nucleus of the thalamus were labeled. By 3 days, label was also found in the dentate nucleus of the cerebellum. At 4 days, it was present in cerebellar Purkinje cells. By 5 days, cerebellar granule cells were labeled (Figure 24–1).[5]

In primates, commonly used viruses are herpes simplex virus type 1 (HSV1) and rabies. HSV1 is transported in either the anterograde (H129 strain) or retrograde (McIntyre-B strain) direction, depending upon the strain used.[6] At longer survival times HSV1 causes neuronal lysis.[4] There is the potential that release of the virus into the extracellular space could complicate interpretation of the labeling pattern. Glial proliferation is also seen, as well as occasional glial labeling, although these do not seem to present major problems.[4] Rabies virus is particularly useful because it specifically infects neurons (glial infection is quite rare) and it does not cause cellular lysis.[5] Several strains of rabies have been evaluated. Although the rates of transport varied, all were transported only in the retrograde direction. Theoretically, both viruses could be combined in a single experiment in order to define an entire circuit. Unfortunately, the presence of HSV1 inhibits uptake and transport of the rabies virus, so they cannot be used together.[1] Coadministration of other tracers, such as wheat germ agglutinin (WGA), may also interfere with uptake of the rabies virus.

It has been known for many years that the cerebellum receives input (via the corticopontocerebellar pathways) from multiple cortical regions, including motor, premotor, posterior parietal, cingulate, and prefrontal cortices.[7] Now it has been demonstrated that the cerebellum projects (via the dentatothalamocortical pathways) back to these same areas. A series of studies in nonhuman primates utilizing neurotropic viruses (rabies and HSV1) to demonstrate the parallel segregated nature of these reciprocal connections was recently reviewed.[1] In brief, rabies virus (CVS-11 strain, retrograde tracer) or HSV1 (H129 strain, anterograde tracer) was injected into either M1 or the dorsolateral area (46) of prefrontal cortex (PFC). Labeled cells were confined to specific areas of the cerebellum. M1 injections labeled clusters of neurons in lobules IV–VIII, while area 46 injections labeled clusters of neurons in Crus I and Crus II (Figure 24–2). Comparison of results with the two tracers (anterograde and retrograde) indicated that extremely similar areas within the cerebellum were labeled. Thus it is likely, although not proven, that the circuits are truly reciprocal.

The overall structure of the corticocerebellar pathways is a three-neuron chain in each direction, beginning and ending at the pyramidal cells in the cortex and Purkinje cells in the cerebellum (Figure 24–2). Older studies in nonhuman primates using standard anterograde and retrograde tracers indicate that the corticopontine projections from the PFC arise primarily from the dorsolateral and dorsomedial regions, with little or no contribution from ventromedial, ventrolateral, or orbital areas.[7,8] Recently, it has been demonstrated that the cerebellum projects back to PFC via the thalamus.[9,10] Neurons within the cerebellar dentate nucleus were labeled following injections of HSV1 (McIntyre-B strain, retrograde tracer) into dorsolateral and dorsomedial PFC (areas 46 and 9). No label was found in the dentate following injections into ventrolateral or orbital PFC (ventral area 46 and lateral area 12). Different regions within both the dentate nucleus and the thalamus were labeled following injections into each of these areas, confirming the segregated nature of these circuits.[9–11] Thus, the functional topography of the cerebellum—how the cerebral cortex maps onto the cerebellum—is starting to be defined.

Cognitive and Behavioral Symptomatology

As individuals and groups of patients with similar diagnoses are studied, the clinical evidence for the cerebellar influence on cognition, emotion, and to a lesser extent personality and behavior is beginning to emerge. Several recent reviews have summarized the literature regarding this evidence.[12–14] Rapoport et al. remind the reader that more than 50% of all the brain's neurons are located in the cerebellum, yet, it contains only 10% of the total brain weight.[12] This group proposes that the cerebellum has a "balancing, integrating, and stabilizing" effect on nonmotor functions including affect, mood, and cognition. Schmahmann reviews the history of the study of the cerebellum as well as continuing to develop evidence for the "cerebellar cognitive affective syndrome" (CCAS).[13] He describes CCAS as the psychopathology evident after a cerebellar lesion, most commonly after a posterior lobe lesion. He proposes the cerebellar influence on cognition and behavior to be an "oscillation dampener maintaining function automatically around a homeostatic baseline."

A common method utilized in matching neuroanatomy to function is to study patients with new psychopathology following acquisition of a lesion or after a new neurological condition is diagnosed (Figure 24–3). Schmahmann and Sherman used in-depth neurological and neuropsychological testing to evaluate a series of 20 patients with cerebellar pathology.[15] All 20 demonstrated some level of cognitive, visuospatial, or psychiatric symptomatology. The authors proposed that a common syndrome appears after lesions to the cerebellum (most commonly and intensely after lesions to the posterior cerebellum and vermis). CCAS consists of a quadrad of executive dysfunction, visual-spatial deficits, personality changes, and linguistic abnormalities. The executive dysfunction includes problems with planning and judgment, set-shifting, and working memory. Other deficits include disinhibition, flat affect, visuospatial disorganization, and dysprosodia. The quadrad together creates a general reduction in overall intellectual functioning/cognition. The patient group was diagnostically hetereogeneous, but with no history of previous psychopathology. The authors excluded patients with clinical or magnetic resonance imaging (MRI) (MRI, T_1- or T_2-weighted images) evidence of pathology outside of the cerebellum. However, the patients were imaged before more sensitive MRI techniques such as the fluid attenuated inversion recovery (FLAIR) sequence were commonly used. Additionally, only three patients in the study had functional imaging (two with single-photon emission tomography [SPECT] and one with positron emission tomography [PET]). All three had abnormal scans with cortical, basal ganglia, or thalamic hypoperfusion. The authors attribute this to diaschisis, a previously observed phenomenon where hypoperfusion may occur distant from the site of injury.

Executive dysfunction has also been confirmed in several recent studies of patients with focal cerebellar lesions (infarct, tumor, hematoma). In one study, 13 of 15 patients with isolated cerebellar infarcts demonstrated abnormal performance in categorical fluency, naming, attention, language, or visuospatial abilities, when matched against comparison subjects.[16] Most (14/15) had superior cerebellar or posterior inferior cerebellar artery infarcts. The one patient with an anterior inferior artery infarct was one of the two with no cognitive deficits on testing. MRI was obtained to rule out noncerebellar lesions. The MRI sequences used were not documented. SPECT was performed in 10 of the 15. Six demonstrated basal ganglia or frontoparietal hypometabolism (the proposed mechanism was diaschisis). Another study compared patients with either isolated brainstem (45 patients) or cerebellar (37 patients) infarcts (identified from a stroke registry).[17] In unblinded testing, both groups had similar levels of frontal/executive dysfunction to patients with cerebral lesions in addition to either brainstem or cerebellar damage. One more study compared patients with either cerebellar (18 patients) or brainstem (4 patients) infarcts to comparison subjects.[18] The patients with cerebellar infarcts, although without symptoms on neurological examination, had more neuropsychiatric symptoms (working memory and cognitive flexibility) than patients with brainstem lesions. Unexpectedly, visuospatial deficits inversely correlated with employment at 12 months. The patients who were unable to successfully return to previous jobs complained of headache, anxiety, memory problems, fatigue, and irritation. The complexity of these jobs was not described, but the authors noted that disability accommodations were attempted prior to the patients' failing to function in the work environment. Deficits in working memory and specific aspects of attention were also found in another study of patients with focal cerebellar lesions.[19] These studies support a role for cerebellum in modulating cognitive function.

Another group retrospectively reviewed the charts of 133 patients with cerebellar degeneration or spinocerebellar ataxia (SCA).[20] In cases where only cerebellar pathology was found (74 patients), 18% had cognitive impairment and approximately 20% had depression. The extent and uniformity of the patient assessments are unclear. This same group prospectively compared 31 patients with degenerative cerebellar disease (CD), 21 patients with Huntington's chorea, and 29 comparison subjects.[21,22] Results paralleled the retrospective study, with 19% of the CD patients diagnosed with cognitive impairment. Other significant data from the study included an overall rate of 77% of the CD patients having psychiatric pathology (57.7% mood disorder and 25.8% personality change). Limitations of the study included incorporation of patients whose pathology extended outside of the cerebellum, no MRI or functional imaging examinations to exclude patients with basal ganglia pathology, and use of the Mini-Mental State Examination (MMSE) as the diagnostic tool for the cognitive impairment. The follow-up study examined the same patients with a more in-depth neuropsychological battery and confirmed the previous results. The patients with CD had significant executive dysfunction, but minimal loss of new learning or memory.[22]

Cerebellar neurological impairments in children are less defined, with fewer studies available. One retrospective chart review of 15 children with cerebellar tumors found 37% to have expressive language deficits; 37% to have visual-spatial deficits; and 33% to have verbal memory deficits coinciding with visual-spatial or language dysfunction.[23] Thirty-two percent had significant affective dysregulation, with all of these having extensive lesioning of the vermis. Fifty-six percent of those with severe vermal lesions (5/9) had the classic postoperative resolving mutism. The authors noted that the younger children in the study tended to perform better on the testing than the older ones and that some children's clinical presentation was much worse that the scores indicated. Possible explanations for this included the retrospective aspect of the study, testing difficulties in young children, neural plasticity, or developmental stage at time of surgery.

Although controversial, there is evidence for abnormal vermal size in several psychiatric conditions, including attention deficit hyperactivity disorder, autism, and schizophrenia. For example, a recent study examined 155 neuroleptic-naive patients with schizophrenia and compared them with 155 matched subjects.[24] One-fifth of the patients had focal cerebellar neurological signs. These were associated with higher rates of cognitive impairment, smaller total cerebellar volume on MRI, more severe negative symptoms, and poorer psychosocial functioning. A recent case report proposes a key role for the cerebellum in development of a variant of schizophrenia.[14]

In summary, there is growing clinical evidence for the involvement of the cerebellum in neuropsychological function. However, the specific cognitive deficits evident on testing are still quite variable from patient to patient. Both cognitive deficits and noncognitive psychopathology have been reported in patients with traumatic brain injury, tumors, strokes, or degenerative atrophies (e.g., SCAs) of the cerebellum. Numerous single-case reports are published, but few studies exist with large numbers of patients. Several factors make it difficult to draw firm conclusions. Oftentimes the patients in the existing reports are diagnostically heterogeneous. Studies have included patients whose pathology extends outside the cerebellum (e.g., pons or basal ganglia). In addition, secondary processes such as acute hydrocephalus are sometimes present that might have caused or influenced the presentation of the neuropsychiatric pathology. Finally, vascular conditions commonly associated with stroke generally have widespread effects in the brain. Thus, caution is needed when considering the evidence for cerebellar influence on nonmotor functions.

Functional Imaging

Functional imaging provides another line of evidence suggesting the participation of the cerebellum in cognitive/emotional functioning due to its engagement along with frontal areas during many tasks (e.g., making of moral judgments, processing of negative emotions, learning to solve the Tower of London task or a pegboard puzzle).[25–28] A developmental study of the areas involved in generating voluntary inhibition of responses found that adults, unlike children and adolescents, demonstrated activity in the lateral cerebellar cortex and dentate nuclei.[29] The authors suggest that the cerebellum may be important for the maturation of voluntary response suppression mediated by prefrontal areas. Cerebellar activation was also found in an attention shifting task which the authors attributed to response reassignment rather than attentional switching.[30] The results of the previous study suggest that an alternative explanation is engagement of the cerebellum in order to suppress the inappropriate response.

Three studies have used neurophysiological measures to assess the influence of the cerebellum on frontal lobe functioning. Two used low-resolution electromagnetic tomography (LORETA) to assess cortical function in patients with atrophy limited to the cerebellar cortex.[31,32] In one, the intracerebral distribution of both spontaneous electrical activity (measured by electroencephalogram [EEG]) and the midlatency auditory evoked potential (MLR) was measured.[31] Patients had decreased activity in the $\alpha 2$ band of the EEG over the left inferior frontal gyrus (Brodmann's area [BA] 45) and the P1 component of the MLR was decreased in the superior frontal gyrus (BA 9). In the other, event-related potentials (ERPs) were used to measure frontal lobe activation during a continuous performance task in which a motor response was either performed ("Go") or inhibited ("No Go") depending upon a cue.[32] Performance did not differ between the groups, but patients had significantly less frontal lobe activation during the No Go condition. In the third study, the relative activity of the left and right PFC (as measured by qualitative EEG) were compared prior to and following repetitive transcranial magnetic stimulation (rTMR) of the cerebellum in normal individuals (five patients).[33] A shift in activity in the fast gamma frequency band occurred such that activity was significantly higher in the right PFC than the left following stimulation of the medial cerebellum, a reversal of the baseline pattern. Intriguingly, subjects gave unsolicited reports of increased alertness and elevated mood following the stimulation. All of these studies suggest that frontal lobe function is influenced by the cerebellum.

Conclusion

This summary and synthesis of recent literature focused on the connections between cerebellum and prefrontal cortex. The cerebellum may also influence cognitive and emotional behavior through other pathways. Older animal studies indicate possible connections of the cerebellum with several critical brainstem centers, including the dorsal raphe and locus coeruleus, in addition to its well-known connections with the hypothalamus.[21] It is likely that future neuroimaging investigations will continue to uncover the vital role of the cerebellum in prefrontal functioning.

References

1. Kelly RM, Strick PL: Cerebellar loops with motor cortex and prefrontal cortex of a nonhuman primate. J Neurosci 2003; 23:8432–8444
2. Hurley RA, Black D, Stip E, et al: Surgical treatment of mental illness. J Neuropsychiatry Clin Neurosci 2000; 12:421–424
3. Lanciego JL,Wouterlood FG: Neuroanatomic tract-tracing methods beyond 2000: what's now and next. J Neurosci Methods 2000; 103:1–2

4. Hoover JE, Strick PL: The organization of cerebellar and basal ganglia outputs to primary motor cortex as revealed by retrograde transneuronal transport of herpes simplex virus type 1. J Neurosci 1999; 19:1446–1463
5. Kelly RM, Strick PL: Rabies as a transneuronal tracer of circuits in the central nervous system. J Neurosci Methods 2000; 103:63–71
6. Zemanick MC, Strick PL, Dix RD: Direction of transneuronal transport of herpes simplex virus 1 in the primate motor system is strain-dependent. Proc Natl Acad Sci USA 1991; 88:8048–8051
7. Schmahmann JD, Pandya DN: The cerebrocerebellar system. Int Rev Neurobiol 1997; 41:31–60
8. Schmahmann JD, Pandya DN: Anatomic organization of the basilar pontine projections from prefrontal cortices in rhesus monkey. J Neurosci 1997; 17:438–458
9. Middleton FA, Strick PL: Cerebellar projections to the prefrontal cortex of the primate. J Neurosci 2001; 21:700–712
10. Middleton FA, Strick PL: Basal ganglia and cerebellar loops: motor and cognitive circuits. Brain Res Rev 2000; 31:236–250
11. Dum RP, Li C, Strick PL: Motor and nonmotor domains in the monkey dentate. Ann N Y Acad Sci 2002; 978:289–301
12. Rapoport M, van Reekum R, Mayberg H: The role of the cerebellum in cognition and behavior: A selective review. J Neuropsychiatry Clin Neurosci 2000; 12:193–198
13. Schmahmann JD: Disorders of the cerebellum: ataxia, dysmetria of thought, and the cerebellar cognitive affective syndrome. J Neuropsychiatry Clin Neurosci 2004; 16:367–378
14. Turner R, Schiavetto A: The cerebellum in schizophrenia: A case of intermittent ataxia and psychosis—clinical, cognitive, and neuroanatomical correlates. J Neuropsychiatry Clin Neurosci 2004; 16:400–408
15. Schmahmann JD, Sherman JC: The cerebellar cognitive affective syndrome. Brain 1998; 121:561–579
16. Neau JP, Arroyo-Anllo E, Bonnaud V, et al: Neuropsychological disturbances in cerebellar infarcts. Acta Neurol Scand 2000; 102:363–370
17. Hoffmann M, Schmitt F: Cognitive impairment in isolated subtentorial stroke. Acta Neurol Scand 2004; 109:14–24
18. Malm J, Kristensen B, Karlsson T, et al: Cognitive impairment in young adults with infratentorial infarcts. Neurology 1998; 51:433–440
19. Gottwald B, Mihajlovic Z, Wilde B, et al: Does the cerebellum contribute to specific aspects of attention? Neuropsychologia 2003; 41:1452–1460
20. Liszewski CM, O'Hearn E, Leroi I, et al: Cognitive impairment and psychiatric symptoms in 133 patients with diseases associated with cerebellar degeneration. J Neuropsychiatry Clin Neurosci 2004; 16:109–112
21. Leroi I, O'Hearn E, Marsh L, et al: Psychopathology in patients with degenerative cerebellar diseases: a comparison to Huntington's disease. Am J Psychiatry 2002; 159:1306–1314
22. Brandt J, Leroi I, O'Hearn E, et al: Cognitive impairments in cerebellar degeneration: A comparison with Huntington's disease. J Neuropsychiatry Clin Neurosci 2004; 16:176–184
23. Levisohn L, Cronin-Golomb A, Schmahmann JD: Neuropsychological consequences of cerebellar tumour resection in children. Cerebellar cognitive affective syndrome in a paediatric population. Brain 2000; 123:1041–1050
24. Ho BC, Mola C, Andreasen NC: Cerebellar dysfunction in neuroleptic naive schizophrenia patients: clinical, cognitive, and neuroanatomic correlates of cerebellar neurologic signs. Biol Psychiatry 2004; 55:1146–1153
25. Kim SG, Ugurbil K, Strick PL: Activation of a cerebellar output nucleus during cognitive processing. Science 1994; 265:949–951
26. Moll J, Eslinger PJ, Oliveira-Souza R: Frontopolar and anterior temporal cortex activation in a moral judgment task. Ara Neuropsiquiatr 2001; 59:657–664
27. Beauchamp MH, Dagher A, Aston JAD, et al: Dynamic functional changes associated with cognitive skill learning of an adapted version of the Tower of London task. Neuroimage 2003; 20:1649–1660
28. Lee GP, Meador KJ, Loring DW, et al: Neural substrates of emotion as revealed by functional magnetic resonance imaging. Cogn Behav Neurol 2004; 17:9–17
29. Luna B, Thulborn KR, Munoz DP, et al: Maturation of widely distributed brain function subserves cognitive development. Neuroimage 2001; 13:786–793
30. Bischoff-Grethe A, Ivry RB, Grafton ST: Cerebellar involvement in response reassignment rather than attention. J Neurosci 2002; 22:546–553
31. Arai M, Tanaka H, Pascual-Marqui RD, et al: Reduced brain electric activities of frontal lobe in cortical cerebellar atrophy. Clin Neurophysiol 2003; 114:740–747
32. Tanaka H, Harada M, Arai M, et al: Cognitive dysfunction in cortical cerebellar atrophy correlates with impairment of the inhibitory system. Neuropsychobiology 2003; 47:206–211
33. Schutter DJLG, van Honk J, d'Alfonso AAL, et al: High frequency repetitive transcranial magnetic over the medial cerebellum induces a shift in the prefrontal electroencephalography gamma spectrum: a pilot study in humans. Neurosci Lett 2003; 336:73–76

Recent Publications of Interest

Zhu JN, Yung WH, Kwok-Chong Chow B, et al: The cerebellar-hypothalamic circuits: potential pathways underlying cerebellar involvement in somatic-visceral integration. Brain Res Brain Res Rev 2006; 52:93–106
Reviews the bidirectional pathways directly and indirectly connecting hypothalamus and cerebellum, and the evidence supporting the hypothesis that cerebellum participates in integration of motor, visceral, and behavioral responses.

Hoshi E, Tremblay L, Feger J, et al: The cerebellum communicates with the basal ganglia. Nat Neurosci 2005; 8:1491–1493

Used the rabies virus transneuronal retrograde tracer to demonstrate the presence in nonhuman primates of a two-neuron pathway from the deep nuclei of the cerebellum, primarily the dentate nucleus, to the putamen (via the thalamus). The origin of this pathway is widespread in the dentate nucleus, encompassing both motor and nonmotor areas. The authors note that the density of dentate neurons labeled after virus injections into globus pallidus was on the same order as previous studies have found after injections into cortical areas, suggesting that cerebellum may have a substantial influence on processing in the basal ganglia.

Reprinted from Taber KH, Strick PL, Hurley RA: "Rabies and the Cerebellum: New Methods for Tracing Circuits in the Brain." *Journal of Neuropsychiatry and Clinical Neurosciences* 17:133–138, 2005. Used with permission.

Chapter 25

CONVERSION HYSTERIA

Lessons From Functional Imaging

DEBORAH N. BLACK, M.D.
ANDREEA L. SERITAN, M.D.
KATHERINE H. TABER, PH.D.
ROBIN A. HURLEY, M.D.

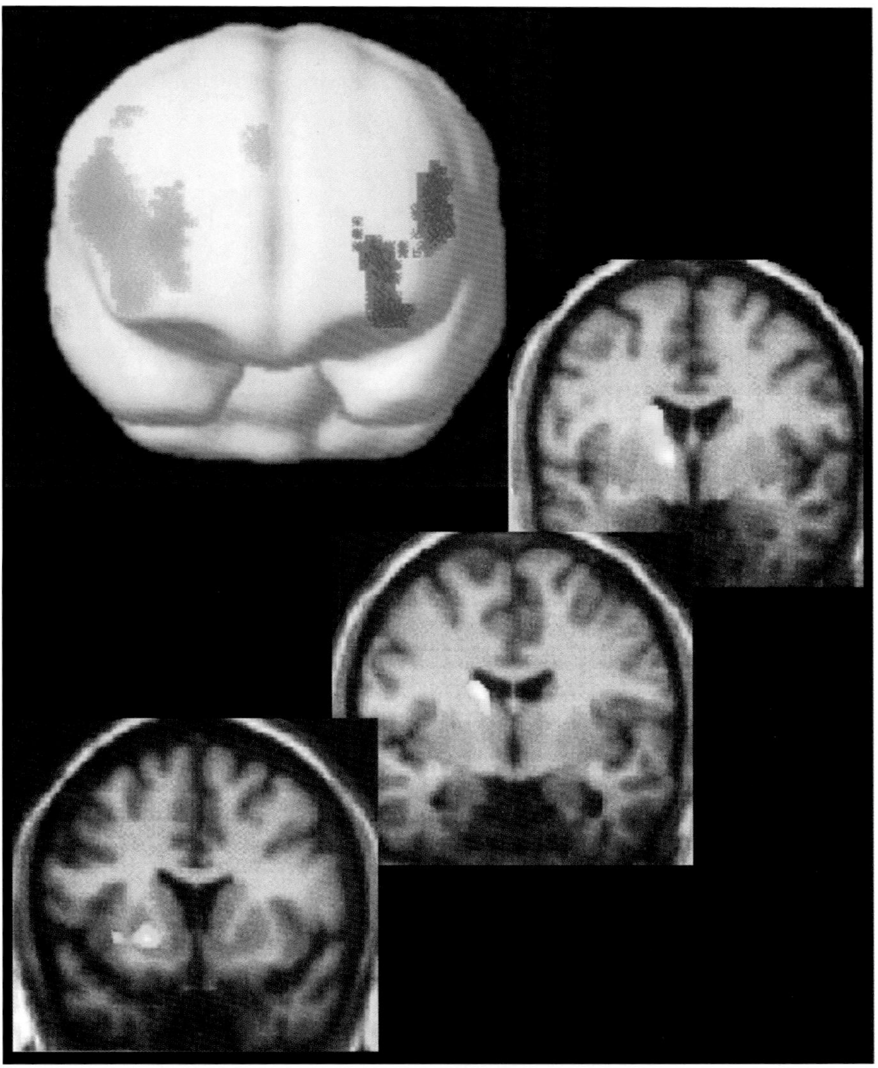

A three-dimensional reconstruction of a magnetic resonance (MR) data set (upper image) from a normal individual is used to illustrate areas of altered regional cerebral blood flow (rCBF) during attempted movement in patients with hysterical paresis (*red*) compared to normal individuals feigning paresis (*green*). Areas of decreased rCBF (compared with normal individuals) in patients with hysterical sensorimotor loss undergoing vibratory stimulation are overlaid on representative coronal MR images.

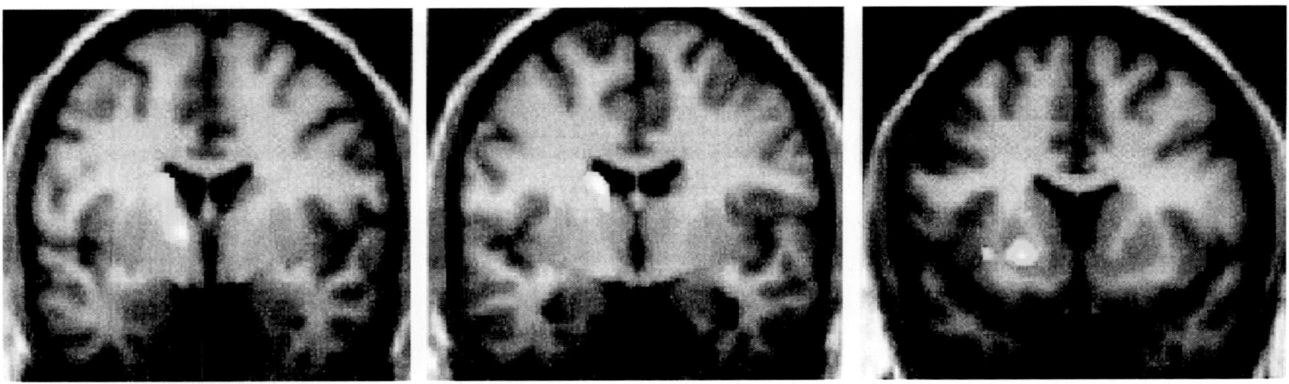

FIGURE 25–1. Regional cerebral blood flow (rCBF) was imaged with single-photon emission computed tomography during vibratory stimulation of both limbs in seven patients with hysterical sensorimotor loss prior to and after recovery. Decreased rCBF was found contralateral to the affected limb in thalamus, basal ganglia, and ventrolateral prefrontal cortex (BA 11, BA 44/45) prior to recovery, as indicated on coronal magnetic resonance images. Used with permission of Oxford University Press.[1]

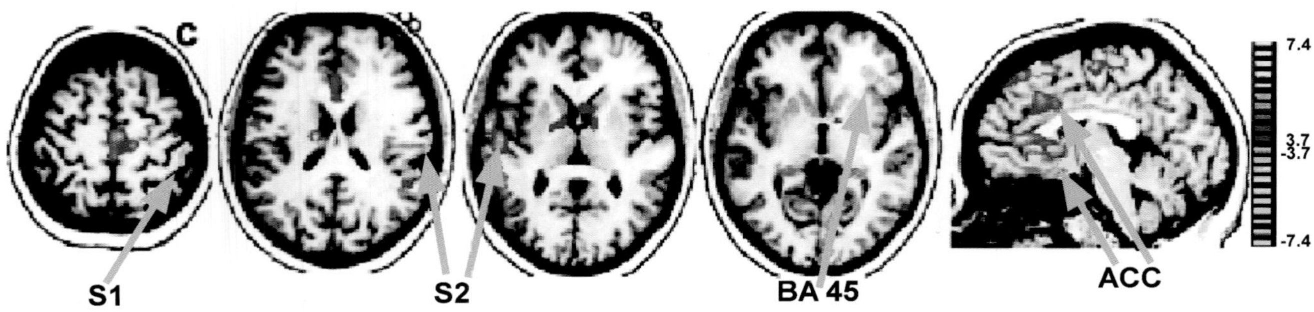

FIGURE 25–2. Functional magnetic resonance imaging. Sensory stimulation of the affected limb in four patients with nondermatomal somatosensory deficits failed to activate or deactivated contralateral brain regions normally activated by touch, including primary and secondary somatosensory cortex (S1, S2), the thalamus, posterior region of the anterior cingulate cortex, and ventrolateral prefrontal cortex (BA 44/45). In contrast, activation was found in rostral anterior and perigenual cingulate cortex (ACC). Significance is indicated by the z-score color bar. Used with permission.[2]

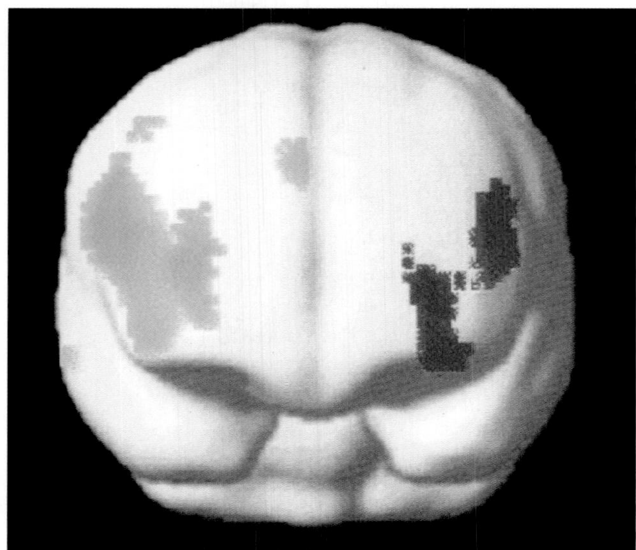

FIGURE 25–3. (left) Positron emission tomography was used to measure regional cerebral blood flow (rCBF) in 3 subjects with hysterical motor paresis while moving the affected limb as compared to healthy individuals moving normally or feigning limb weakness (see image at opening of chapter). rCBF was decreased in the left dorsolateral prefrontal cortex (*red*, BA 9/46) in the patients and the right anterior prefrontal cortex (*green*, BA 10) in the feigners compared with healthy individuals moving normally. Used with permission.[3]

Hysteria, or conversion disorder, has been described since antiquity. The term *hysteria,* based on the Egyptian theory of the wandering uterus, is credited to Hippocrates.[4] In 1859, Briquet described the *personnalité hystérique*.[5] The great French neurologist, Charcot, used hypnosis to elucidate and manipulate the clinical signs of the disorder. In the 20th century, Freud[6] proposed that an unconscious conflict is symbolically converted into a somatic symptom. To acknowledge this historical legacy, the terms *hysteria* and *conversion* will be used interchangeably in this paper.

Formerly considered a dissociative disorder, conversion disorder is classified in DSM-IV-TR as a somatoform disorder along with somatization (Briquet's syndrome), pain disorder, hypochondriasis, and body dysmorphic disorder.[7] Psychogenic disorders of memory and personal identity are classified as dissociative disorders.[7] Both somatoform disorders and dissociative disorders are considered disorders of unconsciousness (i.e., not under voluntary control, unlike factitious disorder and malingering). Conversion disorder shares high comorbidity with anxiety, depression, and personality disorders.

The symptoms of hysteria can affect any aspect of elementary neurological function, including involuntary movements or paralysis, nonepileptic seizures, mutism, urinary retention, hallucinations, pain, blindness, deafness, and analgesia. Inconsistencies on examination suggest this diagnosis. These include simultaneous contraction of muscular agonists and antagonists, fluctuating weakness, nonanatomical sensory loss, tunnel vision, and astasia-abasia. Some patients show a curious *la belle indifférence* toward their neurological handicap.[7] Brain imaging, electroencephalography, and sensory evoked potentials are normal. Although Slater[8] found that more than one-half of patients with hysteria would develop clear signs of neurologic disorder within 10 years of diagnosis, his claim has been contested recently.[9] Nevertheless, a diagnosis of conversion disorder does not rule out neurologic disease, and a diagnosis of neurologic disease does not rule out conversion disorder.[10]

Neuropsychological Studies

Pierre Janet[11] proposed that conversion disorder is a deficit of selective attention toward the pathological symptom. Janet emphasized the parallel between dissociation after overwhelming psychological trauma and hypnotically induced alteration in consciousness. In psychoanalytical terms, conversion is the symbolic transformation of a dangerous emotion (aggression, rage, sexual excitement) into a somatic symptom, representing a compromise between the undesirable affect and the defense against it. Roelofs et al.[12] reported more physical and sexual abuse and maternal unavailability in patients with conversion disorder compared to 50 patients with affective disorder, lending support to the proposed role of early emotional trauma in conversion disorder.

Ludwig[13] proposed that "selective corticofugal inhibition of afferent stimulation" operates in hysteria to exclude a somatic function from consciousness. C. Miller Fisher considered hysteria a delusion of somatic disability with lack of insight.[14] Flor-Henry et al.[15] reported bifrontal and right posterior hemispheric cognitive dysfunction in 10 patients with hysteria compared to normal subjects, patients with psychotic depression, and patients with schizophrenia. Impairment of the dominant (left) hemisphere was more severe, reflected in subtle verbal imprecision, affective incongruity, and defective processing of endogenous somatic percepts, analogous to schizophrenia. Sackeim et al.[16] showed that hysterically blind subjects, as well as subjects rendered blind by hypnosis, performed either better or worse than chance on visual recognition tasks, indicating that their choices were visually guided even if they were not consciously aware of seeing. Implicit visual processing may thus be disconnected from conscious awareness of vision.[16]

Perception is powerfully influenced by emotion and motivational state, which serve to enhance attention to salient stimuli.[17] Much of the preconscious processing of emotional stimuli involves connections between the amygdala-hippocampus and insular, orbital, and cingulate cortices, which link perception, emotional state, and memory.[17] The right hemisphere is theorized to be the locus of neural networks subserving attention to intra- and extrapersonal space, body schema, and personal identity.[18] Injury to this right hemispheric network is consistently associated with defects in emotion and feeling, as well as with anosognosia and neglect.[19] *La belle indifférence* may be a subtle form of neglect related to right hemisphere dysfunction. The right hemisphere may impart a negative bias to emotional experience.[20] These observations support Damasio's[21] hypothesis that hysteria involves defective mapping of the body state.

Functional Neuroimaging

There are to date few neuroimaging studies of hysteria. All of the studies described below are limited by small population size (the largest study includes only seven patients); heterogeneous patient populations (e.g., motor versus sensory symptoms, nonepileptic seizures or combined epileptic and nonepileptic seizures); duration of the deficit (acute versus chronic); and presence of comorbid disorders such as depression or chronic pain. Overall they suggest variable alterations in the activity of specific cortical and subcortical areas may underlie conversion disorder, particularly prefrontal and parietal cortices, thalamus, and basal ganglia. To facilitate comparison of results, the studies have been grouped by state (resting, activated) and duration of deficit (acute, chronic).

Initial Sensory Processing

An important finding in conversion disorder, as noted above, is that electrophysiological tests indicate that sensory and motor pathways are intact. Thus the question to be resolved is at what stage(s) does processing become abnormal. Magnetoencephalography (MEG) is a noninvasive electrophysiological technique that uses superconducting electrodes to measure the neuromagnetic fields generated by the brain's electrical activity. Hoechstetter et al [22] used MEG to record activity in primary (S1) and secondary (S2) somatosensory cortices in three patients with unilateral psychogenic motor and sensory loss (two acute, one chronic) in response to tactile stimulation of the index finger of the affected and unaffected hands. Sixteen healthy subjects served as controls. S2 is activated about 30–50 msec after S1 and is involved in the early attentive processing of tactile stimuli. Both the patients and normal controls showed normal responses in both the contralateral S1 and bilateral S2 areas, regardless of the stimulated side. This is consistent with previous studies indicating that the early components of somatosensory evoked potentials are normal in conversion disorder and suggests that the altered processing that underlies the failure to perceive the stimulation occurs at a later stage of sensory integration than the initial activity in S2.[23,24]

Resting (Baseline) State of the Brain

One study assessed the resting state of the brain in acute conversion disorder. Yazici and Kostakoglu[25] utilized ^{99m}Tc-HMPAO single-photon emission computed tomography (SPECT) to measure regional cerebral blood flow (rCBF) in five patients with astasia-abasia (2 week–1 month duration). The authors found decreased perfusion (0.72–0.88 of normal) involving only the left temporal lobe in two patients, left temporal and parietal lobes in one, bilateral temporal lobes in one, and only the left parietal lobe in one. The authors note that the finding of left hemispheric involvement in all patients supports previous neuropsychological studies indicating more severe impairments of the dominant hemisphere in conversion disorder. They suggest that the bilateral perfusion deficit found in one patient may have reflected the persistence of conversion symptoms in the left leg during imaging. However, all patients had bilateral symptoms at the time of imaging. The role of left hemisphere impairment in conversion is controversial; other authors have found a higher incidence of left-sided motor and sensory deficits in patients with conversion disorder, hence implicating the right hemisphere.[26,27] A weakness of this study is that areas of abnormality were identified primarily by calculating the ratio between ipsilateral and contralateral regions of interest, with decreases of 10% or more considered significant. Thus more subtle or bilateral decreases may have been missed.

Response of the Brain to Sensory Stimulation

Two SPECT studies found altered patterns of rCBF in response to sensory stimulation of the affected area during the acute stage of conversion disorder as compared to recovery. Tiihonen et al.[28] used left median nerve stimulation in a single patient with left hemiparesis and paresthesia and comorbid major depressive disorder. Median nerve stimulation is expected to increase contralateral parietal lobe rCBF. During the acute episode there was mild hyperperfusion (7.2%) in the frontal lobe and hypoperfusion (7.5%) in the parietal lobe contralaterally. After recovery (6 weeks later) rCBF in the contralateral parietal lobe was greater than ipsilateral. The results were interpreted as suggesting inhibition of somatosensory cortex by frontal cortex during the acute episode.

Vuilleumier et al.[1] applied simultaneous vibratory stimulation to both affected and normal limbs of seven patients during the acute stage of illness (less than 2 months; all patients displayed variable unilateral motor and sensory loss) and again 2–4 months later. By the second examination, four patients had completely recovered and three were still symptomatic. Two very different data analysis approaches were utilized, statistical parametric mapping (SPM) and scaled subprofile modeling (SSM). For SPM, analysis of covariance was applied on a voxel by voxel basis in order to identify areas that were significantly different in activation between conditions. In contrast to the previous study, no significant asymmetries in cortical rCBF were noted when rCBF was compared between the resting and stimulated state of acutely symptomatic patients. Comparison of rCBF in the stimulated state while patients were symptomatic and following recovery (four patients) indicated decreased rCBF in the contralateral thalamus and basal ganglia that returned to normal. For SSM a type of principal component analysis was performed in order to identify networks of brain areas that changed together (covaried). Of particular interest was the grouping of contralateral thalamus, caudate, and ventral lateral prefrontal cortex (Brodmann's area [BA] 44/45, BA 11), supporting the results of the SPM analysis (Figure 25–1). In addition, most (3/4) of the patients who recovered had a moderate increase in rCBF in dorsolateral prefrontal cortex on the right (contralateral for two, ipsilateral for one), resulting in the appearance of hypoactivation of the left dorsolateral prefrontal cortex similar to that reported by Spence in patients with chronic symptoms (to be discussed below).[3] An intriguing finding in the three patients with persisting deficits was that they had less activity in contralateral subcortical areas, particularly the caudate, at the first examination. Thus a finding of lower activation in these areas may predict poor recovery. The authors note that overall their findings support previous theories that attentional or motivational influences can modulate thalamus or basal ganglia to alter sensorimotor processes in conversion disorder. This is a salient study, as it points to involvement of subcortical structures in conversion disorder pathogenesis. The basal ganglia and thalamus participate in fronto-subcortical loops that modulate motor intention and sensory awareness under the influence of motivational state conveyed by reciprocal connections with the amygdala and orbitofrontal cortex.[29] These findings suggest disruption of sensory processing, movement, motivation, and attention at multiple nodes of a widely distributed network.

A third study used functional magnetic resonance imaging (fMRI) to look at patterns of activation in response to sensory stimulation in chronic conversion disorder.[2] Both innocuous (brush) and noxious (pressure) stimulation of either the affected (unperceived stimuli) or normal (perceived stimuli) limb were used in four patients with chronic pain and nondermatomal somatosensory deficits (NDSD).[2] All had variable motor loss in the affected limb, as well. Unperceived stimuli failed to activate areas that were activated by perceived stimulation, notably: anterior insula, thalamus, caudal anterior cingulate cortex, and ventrolateral prefrontal cortex (BA 44/45). This is similar to the network identified in the previous study. Unperceived stimuli were also associated with deactivation in primary and secondary somatosensory cortex (S1, S2), posterior parietal cortex, and prefrontal cortex. Interpretation of deactivations in fMRI studies is presently controversial. Finally, unperceived (but not perceived) stimuli activated the rostral and perigenual anterior cingulate cortex (Figure 25–2), an area not yet implicated in studies of patients with acute symptoms. The authors suggest conversion disorder may be a functional deafferentation due to active inhibition of somatosensory processing by limbic areas concerned with emotion and attention. This interpretation is compatible with that suggested by Tiihonen et al.[28] and with Ludwig's[13] hypothesis that "selective corticofugal inhibition of afferent stimulation" operates in hysteria to exclude a somatic function from consciousness.

Response of the Brain to Attempted Movement

Two studies using positron emission tomography (PET) found alterations in rCBF during attempted movement of the affected limb as compared to during movement of the normal limb in patients with chronic hysterical paralysis. Marshall et al.[30] studied a single patient with hysterical left hemiparesis of 2.5 years' duration. Voluntary movement of the unaffected right leg was associated with the expected increased rCBF bilaterally in dorsolateral prefrontal cortex, inferior parietal cortex, and cerebellum as well as contralateral primary sensorimotor and premotor cortex. Also as expected, preparation to move the normal limb increased rCBF in the same network, with the exception of primary sensorimotor cortex. In contrast, both preparation to move and attempted movement of the affected limb failed to increase rCBF in contralateral primary sensorimotor cortex, although cerebellum was activated. In addition, rCBF increased in contralateral anterior cingulate and orbitofrontal cortices. The authors note that both these areas have been found to be important for suppression of inappropriate motor responses. These results are similar to the previous study, and consistent with the functional disconnection hypothesis postulated above, with limbic-affiliated regions inhibiting or disconnecting cortical areas subserving motor planning and execution.

Spence et al.[3] used PET to elucidate the distinction between hysterical and feigned paralysis. They studied two patients with hysterical left arm monoparesis of 10 and 12 months' duration and one with hysterical right arm monoparesis of 6 months' duration. All three exhibited relatively decreased rCBF in the left dorsolateral prefrontal cortex during attempted movement of the limb in comparison to both controls and healthy individuals simulating paralysis by pretending difficulty with moving a limb (feigners). In contrast, decreased rCBF was found in the right anterior prefrontal cortex in feigners compared to both controls and patients (Figure 25–3). The comparison done in the previous study (activations associated with normal movement versus attempted movement within a subject) was not reported. Since the left dorsolateral prefrontal cortex is involved in the programming and selection of motor patterns, dysfunction in the patients was interpreted as an abnormality of the higher components of volition.

Response of the Brain During Hypnotically Induced Paralysis

Halligan et al.[31] used PET to study rCBF in a right-handed subject with hypnotically induced paralysis of the left leg. When the subject was asked to move the "paralyzed" leg, rCBF increased in the contralateral orbitofrontal and anterior cingulate cortices but not in the motor cortex. These results, virtually identical to those obtained by Marshall et al.,[30] support the hypothesis of prefrontal inhibition of motor and sensory cortex and suggest that hypnotic paralysis may be a good model of hysterical paralysis, as proposed 100 years ago by Janet.[11] These two studies also lend themselves to an alternative interpretation. Instead of inhibition of motor and sensory cortex by limbic-affiliated regions, disconnection of intention from awareness may take place at the level of attention, producing a psychic blindness for sensation and movement analogous to anosognosia.

These studies, although they are preliminary in nature and involve small numbers of patients with different constellations and durations of symptoms, combine to support the hypothesis that conversion disorder is the result of dynamic reorganization of neural circuits that link volition, movement, and perception. Disruption of this network may occur at the stage of preconscious motor planning, modality-specific attention, or right fronto-parietal networks subserving self-recognition and the affective correlate of self hood.[32] Activation of the anterior cingulate during conversion motor paralysis[30,31] and hysterical anesthesia[2] may reflect hyperattention to pain[2,33] or a site where inhibitory limbic input is conveyed to the motor cortex.[30,31] Alternatively, the anterior cingulate may be the "hidden observer"[34] whose activity reflects subliminal awareness of the conflict between intended action and outcome.[35–37]

Binding

The literature on binding may lend neurophysiological support to neuroimaging observations suggesting abnormal functional connectivity in conversion disorder. *Binding* refers to transient oscillatory hypersynchrony lasting hundreds of milliseconds among neurons in thalamus, posterior heteromodal association cortex, and anterior brain areas involved in memory, motivation, and planning.[38] Rapid integration of activity among these distributed neural populations is achieved through iterative and highly parallel signaling at a frequency of 40 Hz. With respect to working memory, for example, reentrant interactions between frontal and parietal regions facilitate "the integration of the activity of spatially segregated brain regions into a coherent, multimodal neural process that is stable enough to permit decision-making and planning."[38] Similar processes probably underlie conscious visual perception[39] and the conscious experience of free will.[40] In an auditory-visual associative learning paradigm, subjects who acquired awareness of the contingency schedule showed metabolic activation in a distributed network involving lateral prefrontal cortex, primary auditory and visual cortex, and medial cerebellum. As learning progressed, temporal coherence (binding) among these regions increased, suggesting that the involvement of prefrontal cortex, in interaction with other brain regions, is crucial for awareness.[41] Functional dysconnectivity, whether due to a structural brain lesion such as multiple sclerosis or head trauma, or to a sudden shift in neural state related to early adverse experience,[42] may disrupt conscious perception and voluntary control of movement.[38]

Brown and Marsden proposed that a primary role for the basal ganglia is to facilitate the binding of sensorimotor and dorsolateral prefrontal cortices and supplementary and cingulate motor areas in a coherent sequence of motor activity and thought. Slowness of voluntary movement, dystonia, and co-contraction of muscle agonists and antagonists are clinical hallmarks of basal ganglia dysfunction.[43] Bradykinesia, dystonia, and co-contraction of agonists and antagonists also occur in conversion disorder and may likewise reflect dysfunction of frontal-subcortical circuits.

Conclusion

A growing body of neuroimaging studies is beginning to propose possible biological explanations for hysteria. The mapping of the brain in conversion disorder has implications for the conscious experience of self and the disruption of selfhood in dissociative identity disorder and schizophrenia.[44] Performing larger studies that control for comorbidities such as depression,[1] incorporating broader deficits (e.g., blindness), imaging limbic brain areas (e.g., the insula and amygdala), using novel techniques such as MEG,[22] and studying patients at different phases of their illness[1] are all necessary in order to develop a more detailed understanding of this biology.

References

1. Vuilleumier P, Chicherio C, Assal F, et al: Functional neuroanatomical correlates of hysterical sensorimotor loss. Brain 2001; 124:1077–1090
2. Mailis-Gagnon A, Giannoylis I, Downar J, et al: Altered central somatosensory processing in chronic pain patients with "hysterical" anesthesia. Neurology 2003; 60:1501–1507
3. Spence SA, Crimlisk HL, Cope H, et al: Discrete neurophysiological correlates in prefrontal cortex during hysterical and feigned disorder of movement. Lancet 2000; 355:1243–1244
4. Veith I: Hysteria; The History of a Disease. Chicago: University of Chicago Press, 1965
5. Briquet P: Traité Clinique et Thérapeutique de L'Hystérie. Paris: J.B. Baillière et Fils, 1859
6. Freud S: Dora: An Analysis of a Case of Hysteria. New York: Touchstone, 1905
7. American Psychiatric Association: Diagnostic and Statistical Manual of Mental Disorders, 4th Edition, Text Revision. Washington DC: American Psychiatric Association, 2000
8. Slater E: Diagnosis of hysteria. British Medical Journal 1965; 1:1395–1399
9. Crimlisk HL, Kailash B, Cope H, et al: Slater revisited: 6 year follow up study of patients with medically unexplained motor symptoms. British Medical Journal 1998; 316 (7131):582–586
10. Marsden CD: Hysteria—a neurologist's view. Psychological Medicine 1986; 16:277–288
11. Janet P: The mental state of hystericals; a study of mental stigmata and mental accidents. New York: Putnam, 1901
12. Roelofs K, Keijsers GP, Hoogduin KA, et al: Childhood abuse in patients with conversion disorder. Am J Psychiatry 2002; 159:1908–1913

13. Ludwig AM: Hysteria: a neurobiological theory. Arch Gen Psychiatry 1972; 27:771–777
14. Fisher CM: Hysteria: a delusional state. Medical Hypotheses 1999; 53:152–156
15. Flor-Henry P, Fromm-Auch D, Tapper M, et al: A neuropsychological study of the stable syndrome of hysteria. Biol Psychiatry 1981; 16:601–626
16. Sackeim HA, Nordlie JW, Gur RC: A model of hysterical and hypnotic blindness: cognition, motivation, and awareness. J Abnorm Psychol 1979; 88:474–489
17. Dolan RJ: Emotion, cognition, and behavior. Science 2002; 298:1191–1194
18. Mesulam MM: Principles of Behavioral and Cognitive Neurology, 2nd ed. New York: Oxford University Press, 2000
19. Starkstein SE, Fedoroff JP, Price TR, et al: Anosognosia in patients with cerebrovascular lesions. A study of causative factors. Stroke 1992; 23:1446–1453
20. Ross ED, Homan RW, Buck R: Differential hemispheric lateralization of primary and social emotions. Neuropsychiatry Neuropsychol Behav Neurol 1994; 7:1–19
21. Damasio A: Looking for Spinoza: Joy, Sorrow and the Feeling Brain. New York: Harcourt, 2003
22. Hoechstetter K, Meinck HM, Henningsen P, et al: Psychogenic sensory loss: magnetic source imaging reveals normal tactile evoked activity of the human primary and secondary somatosensory cortex. Neurosci Lett 2002; 323:137–140
23. Fukuda M, Hata A, Niwa SI, et al: Event-related potential correlates of functional hearing loss: reduced P3 amplitude with preserved N1 and N2 components in a unilateral case. Psychiatry Clin Neurosci 1996; 50:85–87
24. Lorenz J, Kunze K, Bromm B: Differentiation of conversive sensory loss and malingering by P300 in a modified oddball task. NeuroReport 1998; 9:187–191
25. Yazici KM, Kostakoglu L: Cerebral blood flow changes in patients with conversion disorder. Psychiatry Res 1998; 83:163–168
26. Devinsky O, Mesad S, Alper K: Nondominant hemisphere lesions and conversion nonepileptic seizures. J Neuropsychiatry Clin Neurosci 2001; 13:367–373
27. Pascuzzi RM: Nonphysiological (functional) unilateral motor and sensory syndromes involve the left more often than the right body. J Nerv Ment Dis 1994; 182:118–120
28. Tiihonen J, Kuikka J, Viinamäki H, et al: Altered cerebral blood flow during hysterical paresthesia. Biol Psychiatry 1995; 37:134–137
29. Cummings JL: Frontal-subcortical circuits and human behavior. Arch Neurol 1993; 50:873–880
30. Marshall JC, Halligan PW, Fink GR, et al: The functional anatomy of a hysterical paralysis. Cognition 1997; 64:B1–8
31. Halligan PW, Athwal BS, Oakley DA, et al: Imaging hypnotic paralysis: implications for conversion hysteria. Lancet 2000; 355:986–987
32. Damasio A: The Feeling of What Happens: Body and Emotion in the Making of Consciousness. New York: Harcourt, 1999
33. Ploghaus A, Tracey I, Gati JS, et al: Dissociating pain from its anticipation in human brain. Science 1999; 284:1979–1981
34. Bob P: Subliminal processes, dissociation and the 'I'. J Anal Psychol 2003; 48:307–316
35. Fink GR, Marshall JC, Halligan PW, et al: The neural consequences of conflict between intention and the senses. Brain 1999; 122:497–512
36. Paus T: Primate anterior cingulate cortex: where motor control, drive and cognition interface. Nat Rev Neurosci 2001; 2:417–424
37. Matsumoto K, Tanaka K: Conflict and cognitive control. Science 2004; 303:969–970
38. Tononi G, Edelman GM: Consciousness and complexity. Science 1998; 282:1846–1851
39. Rees G, Kreiman G, Koch C: Neural correlates of consciousness in humans. Nat Rev Neurosci 2002; 3:261–270
40. Haggard P, Clark S, Kalogeras J: Voluntary action and conscious awareness. Nat Neurosci 2002; 5:382–385
41. McIntosh AR, Rajah MN, Lobaugh NJ: Interactions of prefrontal cortex in relation to awareness in sensory learning. Science 1999; 284:1531–1533
42. van der Kolk BA: Trauma, neuroscience, and the etiology of hysteria: An exploration of the relevance of Breuer and Freud's 1893 article in light of modern science. J Am Acad Psychoanal 2000; 28:237–262
43. Brown P, Marsden CD: What do the basal ganglia do? Lancet 1998; 351:1801–1804
44. Frith C: The role of the prefrontal cortex in self-consciousness: the case of auditory hallucinations. Philos Trans R Soc Lond B Biol Sci 1996; 351:1505–1512

Recent Publications of Interest

Burgmer M, Konrad C, Jansen A, et al: Abnormal brain activation during movement observation in patients with conversion paralysis. Neuroimage 2006; 29: 1336–1343

Compared brain activation (fMRI) in normal individuals and patients with dissociative hand paralysis during two conditions, while observing movement and while performing (or attempting to perform) the same movement. The authors note that their results support the importance of preconscious processes in this disorder and suggest that these may be appropriate therapeutic targets.

Stone J, Smyth R, Carson A, et al: Systematic review of misdiagnosis of conversion symptoms and "hysteria." BMJ 2005; 331:989

Reviewed the literature (1965–2003) on misdiagnosis of organic disorders as conversion disorders. They found that the mean rate decreased from 29% in the 1950s to 4% in the 1970s and beyond, suggesting that improved diagnostic accuracy was not due to the introduction of improved diagnostic imaging.

Reprinted from Black DN, Seritan AL, Taber KH, et al: "Conversion Hysteria: Lessons From Functional Imaging." *Journal of Neuropsychiatry and Clinical Neurosciences* 16:245–251, 2004. Used with permission.

Chapter 26

THE LIMBIC THALAMUS

KATHERINE H. TABER, PH.D.
CHRISTOPHER WEN, M.D.
ASRA KHAN, M.D.
ROBIN A. HURLEY, M.D.

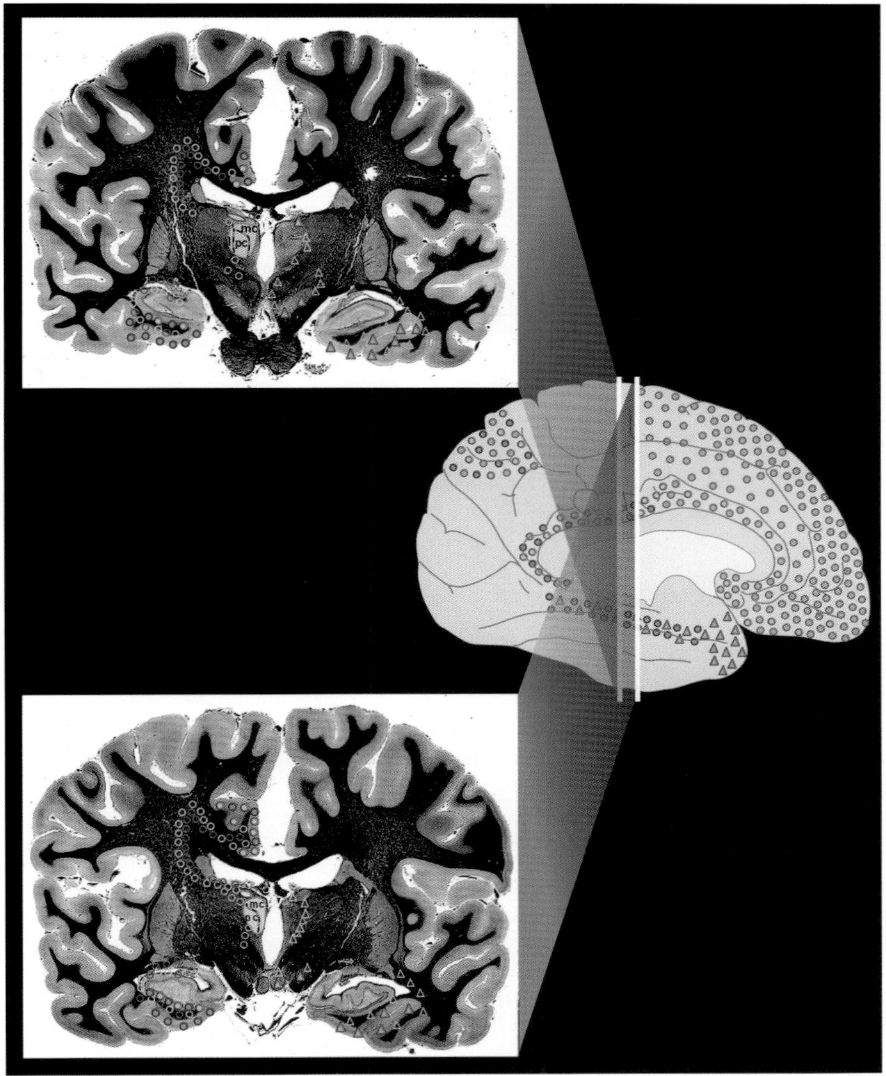

The principal cortical and subcortical connections of the medial dorsal (*orange*), anterior (*blue*), and lateral dorsal (*pink*) nuclei of the thalamus are color-coded onto a drawing of the medial cortical surface (right image) and two coronal myelin-stained brain slices (left images). The approximate locations of the coronal sections are indicated by vertical *white lines* on the medial illustration of the brain.

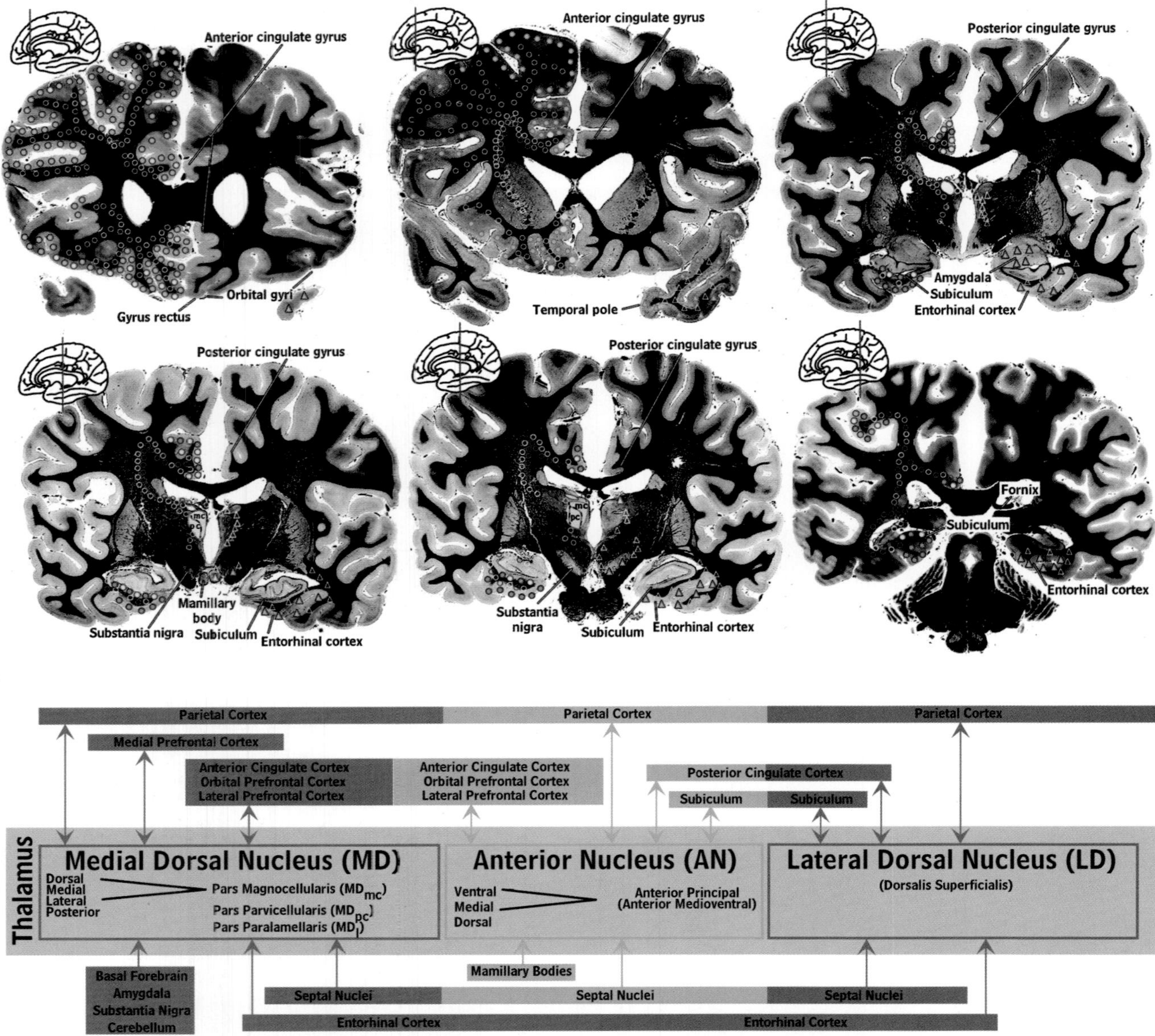

FIGURE 26–1. The principal cortical and subcortical connections of the medial dorsal (*orange*), anterior (*blue*), and lateral dorsal (*pink*) nuclei of the thalamus are color-coded onto images of coronal myelin-stained brain slices and summarized into a color-coded circuit diagram. Reciprocal connections are indicated by color-coded circles. Afferents are indicated by color-coded triangles. The approximate locations of fibers of passage are indicated by open symbols. Each thalamic nucleus is filled with the appropriate color on the left side of brain slices. Subdivisions and usual abbreviations for each nucleus are summarized in the circuit diagram. Some anatomic structures are labeled for orientation. The approximate location of each coronal section is indicated by a vertical line on the adjacent medial illustration of the brain.

The thalamus has been referred to as the "Grand Central Station" of the brain because virtually all incoming information relays through it en route to the cortex. In turn, virtually all areas of the cortex project to divisions of the thalamus. Thus, knowledge of thalamic anatomy and connections is critical in understanding thalamic influence on cortical function and in the interpretation of functional brain imaging studies. The multiple systems for naming the divisions of the thalamus make the literature challenging.[1,2] In addition, the illustrations used in traditional texts do not easily translate into the format of clinical imaging reports. The purpose of this paper is to bypass these obstacles by summarizing and synthesizing the complex functional anatomy of the portions of the human thalamus related to memory, emotion, and arousal. Color-coding is used to facilitate identification of the relevant nuclei and their connections. Clinical images are provided to assist in translating the anatomical knowledge to the bedside.

This communication is intended as a general guide, since both the connections and the functions of these nuclei are not completely understood. While some clinically based tracing of connections has been done, most of what is known comes from experimental studies. To assure the closest possible match to human functional anatomy, only the results from human and primate studies have been used in this synthesis. In the future, imaging techniques that allow functional anatomy to be studied in vivo in humans will provide the data needed to further refine these maps. In particular, the advent of much higher resolution magnetic resonance imaging will make fine mapping of pathway degeneration possible.[3] Diffusion tensor imaging also shows promise for both pathway tracing and perhaps identification of individual thalamic nuclei in vivo.[1,4] It is clear that the size and boundaries of both cortical projection areas and thalamic nuclei vary across individuals.[2,5,6] Detailed studies that will eventually provide probabilistic maps of cortical functional divisions (i.e., Brodmann's areas) are underway.[2]

Thalamic nuclei that are generally agreed to be involved in memory, emotion, and arousal are filled with color on the left side of the coronal brain sections in Figure 26–1. They are the medial dorsal nucleus (*orange*), the anterior nucleus (*blue*), and the lateral dorsal nucleus (*pink*).[7,8] These nuclei have intimate interconnections with cortical and subcortical areas (indicated by colored symbols on the coronal brain sections in Figure 26–1) that are considered part of the limbic system of the brain and deemed the *limbic thalamus*.[9] They have also been termed the *visceral thalamus* because they are vital for maintenance of circadian rhythms and for the generation of normal sleep patterns. Some authors also include the midline, intralaminar, and medial pulvinar nuclei in the limbic thalamus because of their projections to the cingulate cortex.[10–13]

The nomenclature, nuclear divisions, and subdivisions of the thalamus vary among medical specialties, a potential source of confusion when reading the literature of different fields. Two commonly used systems are summarized within the circuit diagram in Figure 26–1. Recognition of the various internal divisions of thalamic nuclei is increasingly important. The tracing of circuits within the brain has progressed to the point that function can be attributed, at least on a tentative basis, at this finer level of localization.[14,15] A summary of the major connections of these nuclei is color-coded onto surface drawings of the cortex (see image at opening to this chapter) and images of coronal myelin-stained brain slices (Figure 26–1). Connections within both the left and right hemisphere are thought to be very similar. Connections with brainstem nuclei are not included as they are not currently thought to be specifically involved in limbic function.

Medial Dorsal Nucleus

Medial dorsal nucleus (MD) has major reciprocal connections with orbital, medial prefrontal, lateral prefrontal, and anterior cingulate cortices.[10,11,16–30] Reciprocal connections with supplementary motor and parietal cortices as well as the frontal eye fields have also been reported.[10,11,18–21,26–28] It receives input from temporal polar, entorhinal, and primary olfactory cortices as well as much of the basal forebrain. This includes the septal nuclei, ventral pallidum, nucleus basalis of Meynert, and diagonal band of Broca.[10,16,20,24,25,31–38] The amygdala, substantia nigra, and cerebellum also project to MD.[19,20,24,36,38–42] These connections and the effects of injury to this region indicate a role in memory (perhaps specifically in retrieval of episodic memory), mood, motivation, and the sleep–waking cycle. It has been proposed that the connections of the MD segregate into at least three major functional circuits.[14,15,43] The dorsal portion of the magnocellular part of MD (MD_{mc}) has reciprocal connections with anterior cingulate cortex and is involved in motivation. The ventral portion of MDmc has reciprocal connections with orbitofrontal cortex and is involved in inhibition of inappropriate behavior. The parvicellular portion of MD (MD_{pv}) has reciprocal connections with dorsolateral prefrontal cortex and is involved in mediation of executive functions.

Anterior Nucleus

Anterior nucleus (AN) has major reciprocal connections with anterior and posterior cingulate cortices and the subiculum-presubiculum portion of the hippocampal complex.[9–11,16,18,25,28,34,44–48] Lesser connections with orbital frontal, dorsolateral prefrontal, and parietal cortices have also been reported.[10,18,26–28,30,34,39,45,46,49] AN also receives major input from the mamillary complex.[8,50] It may also receive a projection from the septal nuclei.[16,36] These connections and the effects of injury to this region indicate a role in memory, modulation of the sleep–waking cycle, and directed attention.

Lateral Dorsal Nucleus

Lateral dorsal nucleus (LD) has major reciprocal connections with posterior cingulate and parietal cortices as well as the subiculum-presubiculum and entorhinal cortex portions of the hippocampal complex.[8,10,11,26,27,34,48–52] It may also receive a projection from the septal nuclei.[16,36] A role in integration of motivation and/or attention with sensory processes has been suggested.[10,53]

Pathology

A common source of injury to the thalamus is vascular insult. Most vascular lesions are fairly large, affecting all or part of multiple nuclei as well as associated tracts. As a result, there is a great deal of overlap in symptoms related to infarction or hemorrhage from a particular artery that can serve the anterior and medial thalamus.[54–58] Injury to the left is associated with deficits in language, verbal intellect, and verbal memory. Right-sided injury is associated with deficits in visuospatial and nonverbal intellect and visual memory as well as delirium. Medial thalamus appears to be particularly important for temporal aspects of memory. Bilateral injury is associated with severe memory impairment (thalamic amnesia) as well as dementia. Some researchers attribute the memory deficits to destruction of the tracts connecting limbic structures to AN and MD (mammillothalamic tract, amygdalofugal tract). Injury to the anterior and medial thalamus can also result in disturbances of autonomic functions, mood, and the sleep–waking cycle.[59,60] Symptoms usually lessen with time, but commonly significant impairment remains.

The limbic areas of thalamus are vulnerable to nonvascular insults. Korsakoff's syndrome results from thiamine deficiency (often as a result of alcoholism). It is characterized by both anterograde and retrograde amnesia, particularly for recent events, and confusion (acutely). These symptoms have been attributed variously to involvement of the mamillary bodies, MD, and AN.[3,61–63] Fatal family insomnia is a prion disease characterized by severe neuronal degeneration in AN and MD.[64] Pathways are not affected. This degeneration is not visible on either computed tomography or magnetic resonance imaging, but is associated with anterior thalamic hypometabolism in some cases.[65,66] There may also be widespread cortical hypometabolism. Clinically there is progressive impairment of the sleep–waking cycle, progressing to total loss of sleep as well as autonomic dysfunction and gradual loss of hormonal circadian rhythms.[67,68] Prior to death the patient becomes stuporous. The clinical features may be a direct result of neuronal injury in AN and MD or may result from disconnection of the hypothalamus, and limbic and prefrontal cortices.[68]

Conclusion

The functional anatomy of the thalamus is both complicated and clinically important because multiple types of information pass through it on the way to the cortex. Thus, injury or dysfunction within the thalamus can alter functioning of other areas, as shown by remote alterations in cerebral blood flow and metabolism.[69–76] Conversely, injury remote from the thalamus can cause thalamic dysfunction or degeneration.[77–80] Knowledge of the functional anatomy of the thalamus should prove useful in evaluating diminished cortical functions caused by thalamic lesions. This includes, but is not limited to, patients undergoing functional imaging. It will promote understanding of thalamic lesions and hypometabolism caused by anterograde and/or retrograde degeneration following cortical injury. Additionally, it will aid in the detection of radiographically subtle, clinically significant lesions; in the planning of rehabilitation and psychiatric treatment; and in the planning of magnetic resonance imaging–guided thalamic surgery.

References

1. Wiegell MR, Tuch DS, Larsson HB, et al: Automatic segmentation of thalamic nuclei from diffusion tensor magnetic resonance imaging. Neuroimage 2003; 19:391–401
2. Amunts K, Schleicher A, Burgel U, et al: Broca's region revisited: cytoarchitecture and intersubject variability. J Comp Neurol 1999; 412:319–341
3. Yamada K, Shrier D, Rubio A, et al: MR imaging of the mamillothalamic tract. Radiology 1998; 207:593–598
4. Taber KH, Pierpaoli C, Rose SE, et al: The future for diffusion tensor imaging in neuropsychiatry. J Neuropsychiatry Clin Neurosci 2002; 14:1–5
5. Rajkowska G, Goldman-Rakic PS: Cytoarchitectonic definition of prefrontal areas in the normal human cortex: II. Variability in locations of areas 9 and 46 and relationship to the Talairach Coordinate System. Cereb Cortex 1995; 5:323–337
6. Uylings HB, Sanz Arigita E, de Vos K, et al: The importance of a human 3D database and atlas for studies of prefrontal and thalamic functions. Prog Brain Res 2000; 126:357–368
7. Armstrong E: Limbic thalamus: anterior and mediodorsal nuclei, in The Human Nervous System. Edited by Paxinos G. San Diego, Academic Press, 1990, 469–481

8. Bentivoglio M, Kultas-Ilinsky K, Ilinsky I: Limbic thalamus: structure, intrinsic organization, and connections, in Neurobiology of Cingulate Cortex and Limbic Thalamus: A Comprehensive Handbook. Edited by Vogt BA, Gabriel M. Boston, Birkhauser, 1993, 71–122
9. Yakovlev PI, Locke S, Koskoff DY, et al: Limbic nuclei of thalamus and connections of limbic cortex. Arch Neurology 1960; 3:620–641
10. Yeterian EH, Pandya DN: Corticothalamic connections of paralimbic regions in the rhesus monkey. J Comp Neurol 1988; 269:130–146
11. Vogt BA, Pandya DN, Rosene DL: Cingulate cortex of the rhesus monkey: I. Cytoarchitecture and thalamic afferents. J Comp Neurol 1987; 262:256–270
12. Schmahmann JD, Pandya DN: Anatomic investigation of projections from thalamus to posterior parietal cortex in the rhesus monkey: a WGA-HRP and fluorescent tracer study. J Comp Neurol 1990; 295:299–326
13. Van der Werf YD, Witter MP, Groenewegen HJ: The intralaminar and midline nuclei of the thalamus. Anatomical and functional evidence for participation in processes of arousal and awareness. Brain Res Brain Res Rev 2002; 39:107–140
14. Mega MS, Cummings JL, Salloway S, et al: The limbic system: an anatomic, phylogenetic, and clinical perspective [see comments]. J Neuropsychiatry Clin Neurosci 1997; 9:315–330
15. Burruss JW, Hurley RA, Taber KH, et al: Functional neuroanatomy of the frontal lobe circuits. Radiology 2000; 214:227–230
16. Powell EW: Limbic projections to the thalamus. Exp Brain Res 1973; 17:394–401
17. Tanaka DJ: Thalamic projections of the dorsomedial prefrontal cortex in the rhesus monkey (Macaca mulatta). Brain Res 1976; 110:21–38
18. Goldman-Rakic PS, Porrino LJ: The primate mediodorsal (MD) nucleus and its projection to the frontal lobe. J Comp Neurol 1985; 242:535–560
19. Ilinsky IA, Jouandet ML, Goldman-Rakic PS: Organization of the nigrothalamocortical system in the rhesus monkey. J Comp Neurol 1985; 236:315–330
20. Russchen FT, Amaral DG, Price JL: The afferent input to the magnocellular division of the mediodorsal thalamic nucleus in the monkey, Macaca fascicularis. J Comp Neurol 1987; 256:175–210
21. Giguere M, Goldman-Rakic PS: Mediodorsal nucleus: areal, laminar, and tangential distribution of afferents and efferents in the frontal lobe of rhesus monkeys. J Comp Neurol 1988; 277:195–213
22. Barbas H, Henion TH, Dermon CR: Diverse thalamic projections to the prefrontal cortex in the rhesus monkey. J Comp Neurol 1991; 313:65–94
23. Siwek DF, Pandya DN: Prefrontal projections to the mediodorsal nucleus of the thalamus in the rhesus monkey. J Comp Neurol 1991; 312:509–524
24. Ray JP, Price JL: The organization of projections from the mediodorsal nucleus of the thalamus to orbital and medial prefrontal cortex in macaque monkeys. J Comp Neurol 1993; 337:1–31
25. Bachevalier J, Meunier M, Lu MX, et al: Thalamic and temporal cortex input to medial prefrontal cortex in rhesus monkeys. Exp Brain Res 1997; 115:430–444
26. Selemon LD, Goldman-Rakic PS: Common cortical and subcortical targets of the dorsolateral prefrontal and posterior parietal cortices in the rhesus monkey: evidence for a distributed neural network subserving spatially guided behavior. J Neurosci 1988; 8:4049–4068
27. Vogt BA, Rosene DL, Pandya DN: Thalamic and cortical afferents differentiate anterior from posterior cingulate cortex in the monkey. Science 1979; 204:205–207
28. Baleydier C, Mauguiere F: The duality of the cingulate gyrus in monkey. Neuroanatomical study and functional hypothesis. Brain 1980; 103:525–554
29. Hatanaka N, Tokuno H, Hamada I, et al: Thalamocortical and intracortical connections of monkey congulate motor areas. J Comp Neurol 2003; 462:121–138
30. Cavada C, Company T, Tejedor J, et al: The anatomical connections of the macaque monkey orbitofrontal cortex. A review. Cereb Cortex 2000; 10:220–242
31. Yeterian EH, Pandya DN: Corticothalamic connections of the superior temporal sulcus in rhesus monkeys. Exp Brain Res 1991; 83:268–284
32. Gower EC: Efferent projections from limbic cortex of the temporal pole to the magnocellular medial dorsal nucleus in the rhesus monkey. J Comp Neurol 1989; 280:343–358
33. Markowitsch HJ, Emmans D, Irle E, et al: Cortical and subcortical afferent connections of the primate's temporal pole: a study of rhesus monkeys, squirrel monkeys, and marmosets. J Comp Neurol 1985; 242:425–458
34. Aggleton JP, Desimone R, Mishkin M: The origin, course, and termination of the hippocampothalamic projections in the macaque. J Comp Neurol 1986; 243:409–421
35. Russchen FT, Amaral DG, Price JL: The afferent connections of the substantia innominata in the monkey, Macaca fascicularis. J Comp Neurol 1985; 242:1–27
36. Hreib KK, Rosene DL, Moss MB: Basal forebrain efferent to the medial dorsal thalamic nucleus in the rhesus monkey. J Comp Neurol 1988; 277:365–390
37. Haber SN, Lynd-Balta E, Mitchell SJ: The organization of the descending ventral pallidal projections in the monkey. J Comp Neurol 1993; 329:111–128
38. Parent A, Pare D, Smith Y, et al: Basal forebrain cholinergic and noncholinergic projections to the thalamus and brainstem in cats and monkeys. J Comp Neurol 1988; 277:281–301
39. Middleton FA, Strick PL: Cerebellar projections to the prefrontal cortex of the primate. J Neurosci 2001; 21:700–712
40. Kelly RM, Strick PL: Cerebellar loops with motor cortex and prefrontal cortex of a nonhuman primate. J Neurosci 2003; 23:8432–8444
41. Price JL: Subcortical projections from the amygdaloid complex. Adv Exp Med Biol 1986; 203:19–33
42. Aggleton JP, Mishkin M: Projections of the amygdala to the thalamus in the cynomolgus monkey. J Comp Neurol 1984; 222:56–68
43. Mega MS, Cummings JL: Frontal-subcortical circuits and neuropsychiatric disorders [see comments]. J Neuropsychiatry Clin Neurosci 1994; 6:358–370
44. Mufson EJ, Pandya DN: Some observations on the course and composition of the cingulum bundle in the rhesus monkey. J Comp Neurol 1984; 225:31–43
45. Carmichael ST, Price JL: Limbic connections of the orbital and medial prefrontal cortex in macaque monkeys. J Comp Neurol 1995; 363:615–641

46. Amaral DG, Cowan WM: Subcortical afferents to the hippocampal formation in the monkey. J Comp Neurol 1980; 189:573–591
47. DeVito JL: Subcortical projections to the hippocampal formation in squirrel monkey (Saimira sciureus). Brain Res Bull 1980; 5:285–289
48. Shibata H, Yukie M: Differential thalamic connections of the posteroventral and dorsal posterior cingulate gyrus in the monkey. Eur J Neurosci 2003; 18:1615–1626
49. Morris R, Petrides M, Pandya DN: Architecture and connections of retrosplenial area 30 in the rhesus monkey (Macaca mulatta). Eur J Neurosci 1999; 11:2506–2518
50. Veazey RB, Amaral DG, Cowan WM: The morphology and connections of the posterior hypothalamus in the cynomolgus monkey (Macaca fascicularis). II. Efferent connections. J Comp Neurol 1982; 207:135–156
51. Yeterian EH, Pandya DN: Corticothalamic connections of the posterior parietal cortex in the rhesus monkey. J Comp Neurol 1985; 237:408–426
52. Yeterian EH, Pandya DN: Corticothalamic connections of extrastriate visual areas in rhesus monkeys. J Comp Neurol 1997; 378:562–585
53. Asanuma C, Anderson RA, Cowan WM: The thalamic relations of the cauda inferior parietal lobule and the lateral prefrontal cortex in monkeys: Divergent cortical projections from cell clusters in the medial pulvinar nucleus. J Comp Neurol 1985; 241:357–381
54. Castaigne P, Lhermitte F, Buge A, et al: Paramedian thalamic and midbrain infarct: clinical and neuropathological study. Ann Neurol 1981; 10:127–148
55. Graff-Radford NR, Damasio H, Yamada T, et al: Nonhaemorrhagic thalamic infarction. Clinical, neuropsychological and electrophysiological findings in four anatomical groups defined by computerized tomography. Brain 1985; 108:485–516
56. Bogousslavsky J, Regli F, Uske A: Thalamic infarcts: clinical syndromes, etiology, and prognosis [published erratum appears in Neurology 1988 Aug; 38(8):1335]. Neurology 1988; 38:837–848
57. Chung CS, Caplan LR, Han W, et al: Thalamic haemorrhage. Brain 1996; 119:1873–1886
58. Trzepacz PT, Meagher DJ, Wise MG: Neuropsychiatric aspects of delirium, in The American Psychiatric Publishing Textbook of Neuropsychiatry and Clinical Neurosciences. Edited by Yudofsky SC, Hales RE. Washington, DC, American Psychiatric Publishing, 2002, pp 525–564
59. Bassetti C, Mathis J, Gugger M, et al: Hypersomnia following paramedian thalamic stroke: a report of 12 patients. Ann Neurol 1996; 39:471–480
60. Lovblad KO, Bassetti C, Mathis J, et al: MRI of paramedian thalamic stroke with sleep disturbance. Neuroradiology 1997; 39:693–698
61. Kopelman MD: The Korsakoff syndrome. Br J Psychiatry 1995; 166:154–173
62. Belzunegui T, Insausti R, Ibanez J, et al: Effect of chronic alcoholism on neuronal nuclear size and neuronal population in the mammillary body and the anterior thalamic complex of man. Histol Histopathol 1995; 10:633–638
63. Zubaran C, Fernandes JG, Rodnight R:Wernicke-Korsakoff syndrome. Postgrad Med J 1997; 73:27–31
64. Lugaresi E, Medori R, Montagna P, et al: Fatal familial insomnia and dysautonomia with selective degeneration of thalamic nuclei. N Engl J Med 1986; 315:997–1003
65. Perani D, Cortelli P, Lucignani G, et al: [18F] FDG PET in fatal familial insomnia: the functional effects of thalamic lesions. Neurology 1993; 43:2565–2569
66. Cortelli P, Perani D, Parchi P, et al: Cerebral metabolism in fatal familial insomnia: Relation to duration, neuropathology, and distribution of protease-resistant prion protein. Neurology 1997; 49:126–133
67. Fiorino AS: Sleep, genes and death: fatal familial insomnia. Brain Res Rev 1996; 22:258–264
68. Benarroch EE, Stotz-Potter EH: Dysautonomia in fatal familial insomnia as an indicator of the potential role of the thalamus in autonomic control. Brain Pathol 1998; 8:527–530
69. Sandson TA, Daffner KR, Carvalho PA, et al: Frontal lobe dysfunction following infarction of the left-sided medial thalamus. Arch Neurol 1991; 48:1300–1303
70. Lim JS, Ryu YH, Kim BM, et al: Crossed cerebellar diachisis due to intracranial hematoma in basal ganglia or thalamus. J Nucl Med 1998; 39:2044–2047
71. Muller A, Baumgartner RW, Rohrenbach C, et al: Persistent Klüver-Bucy syndrome after bilateral thalamic infarction. Neuropsychiatry Neuropsychol Behav Neurol 1999; 12:136–139
72. Clarke S, Assal G, Bogousslavsky J, et al: Pure amnesia after unilateral left polar thalamic infarct: topographic and sequential neuropsychological and metabolic (PET) correlations [see comments]. J Neurol Neurosurg Psychiatry 1994; 57:27–34
73. Bogousslavsky J, Regli F, Delaloye B, et al: Loss of psychic self-activation with bithalamic infarction. Neurobehavioural, CT, MRI and SPECT correlates. Acta Neurol Scand 1991; 83:309–316
74. Pepin EP, Auray-Pepin L: Selective dorsolateral frontal lobe dysfunction associated with diencephalic amnesia. Neurology 1993; 43:733–741
75. Levasseur M, Baron JC, Sette G, et al: Brain energy metabolism in bilateral paramedian thalamic infarcts. A positron emission tomography study. Brain 1992; 115:795–807
76. Henselmans JM, de Jong BM, Pruim J, et al: Acute effects of thalamotomy and pallidotomy on regional cerebral metabolism, evalutated by PET. Clin Neurol Neurosurg 2000; 102:84–90
77. Tamura A, Tahira Y, Nagashima H, et al: Thalamic atrophy following cerebral infarction in the territory of the middle cerebral artery. Stroke 1991; 22:615–618
78. Ogawa T, Yoshida Y, Okudera T, et al: Secondary thalamic degeneration after cerebral infarction in the middle cerebral artery distribution: evaluation with MR imaging. Radiology 1997; 204:255–262
79. Sakashita Y, Matsuda H, Kakuda K, et al: Hypoperfusion and vasoreactivity in the thalamus and cerebellum after stroke. Stroke 1993; 24:84–87
80. De Reuck J, Decoo D, Lemahieu I, et al: Ipsilateral thalamic diaschisis after middle cerebral artery infarction. J Neurol Sci 1995; 134:130–135

Recent Publications of Interest

Cortelli P, Perani D, Montagna P, et al: Pre-symptomatic diagnosis in fatal familial insomnia: serial neurophysiological and ^{18}FDG-PET studies. Brain 2006; 129:668–675
Assessed cerebral glucose metabolism and clinical and electrophysiological measures in asymptomatic carriers of the mutation for fatal familial insomnia at multiple time points prior to and following symptom onset. Their data indicate that the degenerative process begins in thalamus 13–21 months prior to the advent of clinical symptoms.

Sanches-Gonzales MA, Garcia-Cabezas MA, Rico B, et al: The primate thalamus is a key target for brain dopamine. J Neurosci 2005; 25:6076–6083
Presents results from both macaque and human studies that support the existence of substantial dopaminergic innervation of thalamus, particularly in specific association, limbic, and motor nuclei. The origins of this innervation include dopaminergic neurons in hypothalamus, periaqueductal gray matter, ventral mesencephalon, and the lateral parabrachial nucleus.

Reprinted from Taber KH, Wen C, Khan A, et al: "The Limbic Thalamus." *Journal of Neuropsychiatry and Clinical Neurosciences* 16:127–132, 2004. Used with permission.

This study was supported by a grant from the Mike Hogg Fund to Dr. Taber. The authors thank Archibald J. Fobbs, Jr., B.S., curator of the National Museum of Health and Medicine, Armed Forces Institute of Pathology, Washington, D.C., for providing the myelin-stained coronal brain slices. This work was presented at the 15th Annual Meeting of the American Neuropsychiatric Association, February 21–24, 2004, Bal Harbour, Florida.

Chapter 27

UNDERSTANDING EMOTION REGULATION IN BORDERLINE PERSONALITY DISORDER

Contributions of Neuroimaging

PETER A. JOHNSON, B.A.
ROBIN A. HURLEY, M.D.
CHAWKI BENKELFAT, M.D., D.E.R.B.H.
SABINE C. HERPERTZ, M.D.
KATHERINE H. TABER, PH.D.

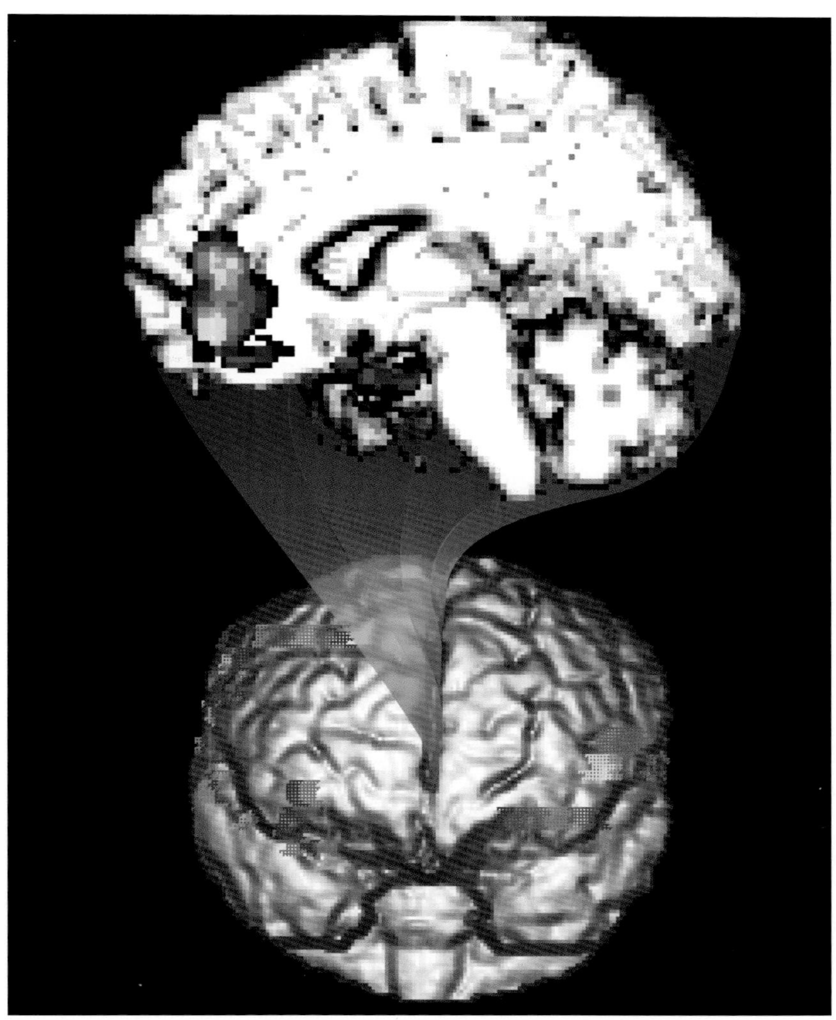

Magnetic resonance surface renderings of brain showing statistical probability mapping in patients with borderline personality disorder. (Top) PET scans demonstrate reduced accumulation of AMT in medial prefrontal, orbital prefrontal, and anterior cingulate cortices in patients relative to controls. Reprinted with permission from Leyton et al.[1] (Bottom) PET scans demonstrate reduced uptake of fluorodeoxyglucose in response to *d,l*-fenfluramine in similar regions of patients relative to controls. Reprinted with permission from Macmillan Publishers Ltd.[2]

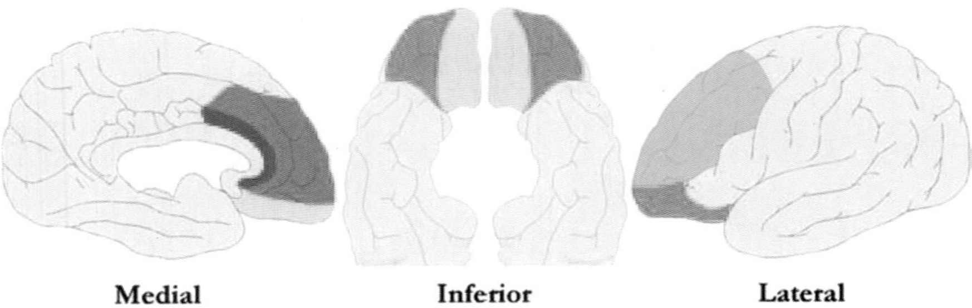

FIGURE 27–1. Regions of importance in emotion regulation. Anterior cingulate cortex (*dark pink*), adjacent medial prefrontal cortex (*light pink*), ventromedial prefrontal cortex (*yellow*), orbital prefrontal cortex (*orange*), and dorsolateral prefrontal cortex (*blue*) are illustrated on diagrams of the brain. These interconnected structures work together to generate, process, and control emotions. Pathology in any of these regions or in the pathways connecting them may result in dysregulation of emotions.

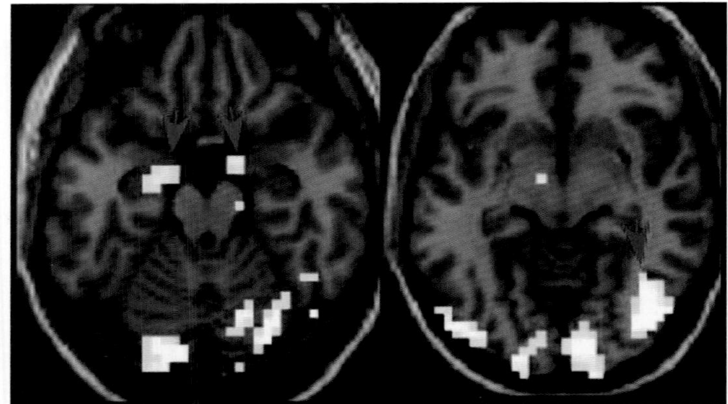

FIGURE 27–2. fMRI of regional cerebral hemodynamic changes in patients with borderline personality disorder after viewing emotionally aversive slides. Subtracting the difference in changes after viewing aversive versus neutral slides in seven female patients from the difference in seven female controls revealed activation of the amygdala (arrows, left image) and fusiform gyrus (arrow, right image) in the patients, as indicated on axial magnetic resonance images (threshold=5.2, extent threshold=7, $P<0.001$ uncorrected).

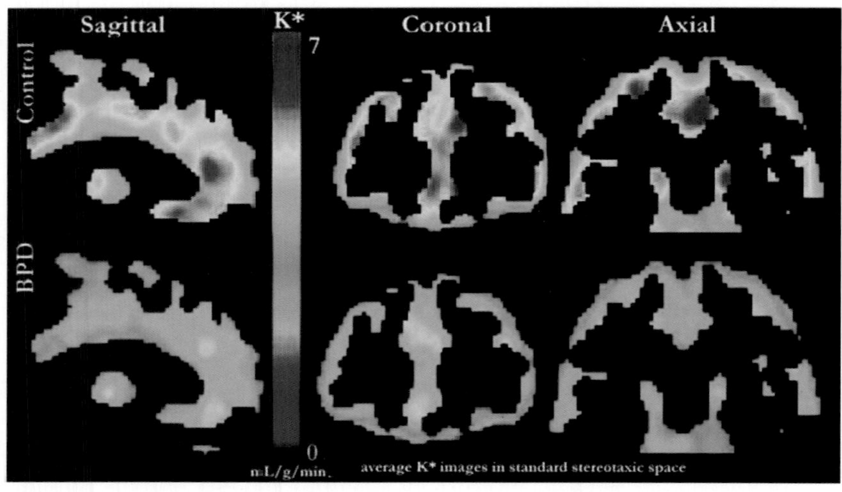

FIGURE 27–3. Positron emission tomography scans of AMT trapping in normal subjects (top row) compared to subjects with BPD (bottom row) indicate lower serotonin synthesis capacity in many regions, including medial, lateral, and orbital prefrontal cortex in BPD.

Borderline personality disorder (BPD) is a multidimensional, heterogeneous condition. Several maladaptive traits characterize patients with this "cluster B" personality disorder, including impulsive aggression, affective lability, self-injury, and identity diffusion. They often maintain volatile relationships. This volatility causes significant social and occupational impairment and yields a lifetime suicide mortality rate of almost 10%—a rate 50 times higher than in the general population.[3] Several recent publications review the diagnosis, prognosis, pathophysiology, and current treatment strategies for this debilitating condition.[3–5] BPD afflicts 1%–2% of the general population, up to 10% of psychiatric outpatients, and up to 20% of psychiatric inpatients. Clinicians diagnose it more often in women. A recent study of more than 40 twin pairs with BPD reported a concordance rate of 35% for monozygotic twins and almost 7% for dizygotic twins.[6]

Many patients with BPD suffer from comorbid psychiatric conditions. A study that included 59 patients with BPD found that all but one had a concurrent axis I disorder, and almost 70% had three or more.[7] Sixty-one percent of the patients met criteria for major depressive disorder (MDD), 35% for posttraumatic stress disorder (PTSD), 29% for panic disorder with agoraphobia, 20% for a somatoform disorder, and 13% for a substance use disorder. Another study found that of 240 patients with BPD, almost 40% were diagnosed with at least one mood disorder.[8] Specifically, 31% met criteria for MDD, 16% for dysthymia, 9% for bipolar I, and 4% for bipolar II.

Neural Circuitry of Emotion Regulation

One common denominator to the various clinical phenotypes of BPD appears to be dysfunctional regulation of emotions. According to Linehan,[9] individuals with BPD are characterized by high sensitivity to emotional stimuli, high emotional intensity, and slow return of emotional arousal to baseline. This theory is supported by a number of studies that indicate higher affective lability and higher affective intensity in subjects with BPD, as compared to individuals with other personality disorders.[10,11] Emotion regulation involves the processing, amplification, maintenance, and attenuation of emotions generated from internal and/or environmental stimuli. Davidson et al.[12] give an excellent overview of the present understanding of dysfunction in the neural circuitry of emotion regulation as it relates to impulsive aggression, a common feature of BPD. Evidence suggests that threatening or aversive stimuli activate the amygdala, which in turn activates the anterior cingulate and prefrontal cortices. While the anterior cingulate may play a role in the cognitive evaluation/processing of mood and affect regulation, it has also been implicated in responses to conflict. The orbital prefrontal cortex appears to inhibit impulsive aggression by regulating the amygdala. Related prefrontal regions include the dorsolateral prefrontal cortex (Figure 27–1, *blue*), which may integrate emotions with cognition, and the ventromedial prefrontal cortex (Figure 27–1, *yellow*), which may involve general processing of emotions. Of note is that while some consider the ventromedial and orbital prefrontal cortices to be distinct regions (Figure 27–1, *yellow* and *orange*), they are often grouped as orbital prefrontal cortex in the psychiatric literature.[13] In the psychiatric literature the anterior cingulate region includes not only the gyrus (Figure 27–1, *dark pink*) but also the adjacent medial prefrontal cortex (Figure 27–1, *light pink*).

Prefrontal serotonergic neurotransmission may play a role in modulating amygdala-driven emotional behavior.[12] A variety of data suggest that dysfunctional serotonergic regulation predisposes individuals to the emotional disinhibition and impulsive aggression responsible for many of the volatile behaviors seen in BPD. Recent studies investigating the neurophysiological and neuroanatomical components of emotion regulation in BPD have used a number of electrophysiological, structural, and functional modalities. While these studies have been few in number and mostly unreplicated, they suggest that dysfunction in the neural circuitry of emotion regulation plays an integral role in BPD.

Electrophysiological Studies

A recent focus for electrophysiological work in BPD has involved exploration of the relationship between BPD and MDD using sleep electroencephalography (EEG). While many of the initial sleep EEG studies did not differentiate between patients with and without comorbid MDD, more recent studies have taken this factor into account. These studies have evaluated several sleep parameters, including those of sleep continuity, non-REM sleep duration, and REM duration and latency. Both patients with BPD alone and those with MDD alone exhibited increased sleep latency and decreased total sleep time in three studies but not in a fourth.[14–17] Two studies found decreased REM latency in both groups.[14,16] Increased REM density may also be present,[16,18] and the differences from normal may be greater in MDD than BPD.[16] The relationship between BPD and MDD therefore remains unclear. It has been suggested that some of these parameters may serve as markers of predilection to mood disorders.[14,16] Whether there is a common biological origin for these two disorders is an open question.

EEG has also been used to study the electrophysiological mechanisms of self-injurious behavior in BPD. Interestingly, it has been reported that about one-half of these patients deny feeling pain during self-inflicted injury.[19] Some patients with depression also report decreased pain sensitivity. Given the high comorbidity between MDD and BPD, pain perception and mood regulation may be neurophysiologically correlated. To test this hypothesis, Russ et al.[20] compared power spectrum analysis of EEG in patients with BPD who did not feel pain during self-injury ($n = 19$) and those who did ($n = 22$), as well as in patients with MDD ($n = 15$) and controls. Participants were asked to place one hand in a 10°C water bath and verbally rate their level of pain every 15 seconds for 4 minutes. The study found that in patients with BPD who denied feeling pain, theta power significantly and inversely correlated with reported pain both at baseline and during the cold water bath. There was a similar trend for patients with BPD who did report pain, though this was not statistically significant. The authors commented that in other studies, some theta activity localizes to the anterior cingulate cortex, a region that has been associated with depersonalization.[19] They suggested that this association may correlate with decreased pain sensitivity, which in turn may play a role in mitigating noxious stimuli. The study also found that theta power directly correlated with the number of dissociative experiences resulting from the stimuli, providing further evidence that pain perception and mood regulation could be neuroanatomically and neurochemically related.

Structural Imaging Studies

Initial structural imaging studies using computed tomography (CT) revealed no volumetric or asymmetric abnormalities in patients with BPD,[21,22] other than a narrower third ventricle in healthy women and in those with BPD.[23] The authors questioned the significance of this finding, however, as it could be attributable to females in general.

Subsequent structural studies have used magnetic resonance imaging (MRI) to evaluate BPD. Lyoo et al.[24] measured cortical and ventricular volumes in patients with BPD ($n = 25$) and found 6.2% smaller frontal lobe volumes compared to control individuals. This study excluded patients with additional axis I or II diagnoses, which may render the results unrepresentative of BPD as a whole, given the high prevalence of comorbid disorders. Further, the study did not control for brain size.

Subcortical structures have also been studied in patients with BPD. Driessen et al.[25] measured hippocampal and amygdala volumes in patients with BPD reporting childhood physical or sexual abuse ($n = 21$), which are common in this disorder. While the study found no difference in whole brain volume between patients with BPD and controls, the patients had 16% smaller hippocampal volumes. A similar trend was found in the amygdala (8%), though this reduction was not statistically significant. These results concur with data from patients with PTSD from childhood abuse, suggesting that this decrease may correlate with traumatic experience rather than with BPD per se.[26] Driessen et al.[25] found no volume differences when they separated their patients with BPD by presence of PTSD. Of note is that the authors did not differentiate between patients who had an abusive background versus those who did not, nor did they consider comorbid MDD, which has also been associated with reductions in hippocampal volume.[27]

Functional Imaging Studies

In the following discussion, locations within the prefrontal cortex have been translated into three divisions most familiar to the psychiatric community (Figure 27–1).[13] In some instances, the description used within the study is included for completeness.

Functional MRI (fMRI) is a technique that localizes brain activity by imaging the influence of blood concentrations of deoxyhemoglobin, which alters signal through magnetic field changes. A recent fMRI study evaluated affective processing of women with BPD ($n = 6$) and no comorbid psychiatric illness or substance abuse while they viewed slides of emotionally aversive or neutral scenes.[28] Increased activity in the amygdala (6/6), fusiform gyrus (6/6), orbital prefrontal region (4/6), and anterior cingulate region (3/6, referred to as the medial prefrontal gyrus) was found in the patients compared to controls (Figure 27–2). Both patients and controls showed activation of the temporo-occipital cortex. The authors noted that increased activation of the amygdala has also been reported in PTSD and obsessive-compulsive disorder (OCD) and may reflect the intense and prolonged emotions seen in BPD. Increased activation of the fusiform gyrus, which processes complex visual features such as facial expression, may be attributable to influence from the amygdala. The orbital prefrontal region directly connects to the amygdala and may modulate amygdala-driven emotional behavior.[12] Enhanced prefrontal activation may therefore reflect cortical processing of the increased amygdala activity.

Proton magnetic resonance spectroscopy (^1H MRS) provides a measure of neuronal function. This technique generates signal by quantifying specified metabolites and plotting them on a spectrum. These metabolites include *N*-acetylaspartate (NAA, a marker of neuronal viability), choline (Cho, a neuronal membrane constituent), and creatine (Cr, used as a standard due to its stable level). Signal may be expressed as a ratio of NAA or Cho to Cr or as an absolute quantification of metabolite concentration.

A pilot ^{1}H MRS study in patients with BPD ($n=12$) and no comorbid psychiatric illness assessed NAA concentration in the left dorsolateral prefrontal cortex and left striatum.[29] Compared with controls, patients with BPD showed a significant (19%) reduction in absolute NAA concentration in the dorsolateral prefrontal region. Striatal levels were also decreased, but the difference was not significant, and ratios of NAA/Cr and Cho/Cr were not significantly changed, emphasizing the value of obtaining absolute quantification of metabolites.

Among the most widely used imaging techniques to measure brain activity is positron emission tomography (PET). This technique measures the signal of a radioactive tracer, such as [^{18}F]-fluorodeoxyglucose (FDG), and represents it on a tomographic map. FDG is a glucose analogue that is taken up into cells, including neurons, in the same manner as glucose. FDG cannot be metabolized, so it is trapped and thereby provides a measure of regional glucose metabolism. Various axis I disorders have demonstrated metabolic abnormalities, notably in the frontal lobes.[30] In some studies, patients with OCD or panic disorder have demonstrated hypermetabolism compared to controls. In others, patients with mood disorders, alcoholism, or schizophrenia have shown hypometabolism.

At least six studies have reported data on resting FDG uptake in patients with BPD. Among the first was De la Fuente et al.,[31] who studied FDG uptake specifically in the temporal lobes of patients with BPD ($n=10$). This region was selected to evaluate the theory that BPD may involve underlying epileptiform activity, as both patients with BPD and those with complex partial seizures share some common symptoms such as impulsivity. The study revealed no focal regions of asymmetry that would indicate an epileptic etiology, arguing against this theory.

Five studies measured resting FDG uptake throughout the brain in patients with BPD. Siever et al.[2] found no difference in uptake between patients with BPD and controls. Three studies reported decreased uptake relative to controls in the dorsolateral prefrontal region.[30,32,33] Both increased and decreased uptake have been reported in the medial and ventrolateral prefrontal regions.[30,32–34] One study reported decreased uptake in the orbital prefrontal region.[32,33] Another found that decreased FDG uptake in this area correlated with a greater history of aggression.[30] These findings support the theory that the orbital prefrontal region may modulate aggression through the inhibition of limbic regions (i.e., orbital prefrontal dysfunction results in limbic disinhibition).

Two studies reported differences in subcortical areas. De la Fuente et al.[32] found decreased uptake in the basal ganglia (caudate, lenticular nuclei, and ventral striatum) and thalamus. The anterior cingulate relays projections from higher-order sensory areas to other regions of the prefrontal cortex and basal ganglia, which is thought to enable emotions to affect motor planning. The basal ganglia are involved in the control of motor and emotional behavior, and the thalamus connects these nuclei to the cerebral cortex. The authors noted that hypometabolism of the thalamus has also been shown in bipolar depression, OCD, and schizophrenia. Hypometabolism of the basal ganglia has been shown in unipolar and bipolar depression, generalized anxiety disorder, OCD, schizophrenia, and alcohol abuse. One limitation of this study is that it included patients with BPD who had past comorbid MDD and/or past substance abuse. Juengling et al.,[34] using statistical parametric mapping rather than regions-of-interest, found decreased uptake in the hippocampus but not the basal ganglia or thalamus. The authors noted that this might be due to decreased hippocampal volume, a possibility that requires further study.

A variety of studies have linked reduced serotonergic activity with impulsivity and depressive symptoms, which are common in BPD (see review in Soloff et al.[33]). Two preliminary studies used *d,l*-fenfluramine (FEN)–activated FDG to investigate possible serotonergic dysfunction in BPD.[2,33] FEN is a serotonin-releasing agent, so a blunted response compared to placebo suggests reduced serotonergic activity. Both studies found an attenuated response to FEN in the orbital prefrontal region in patients relative to controls, supporting previous findings of dysfunction in this area. Siever et al.[2] reported a blunted response in the dorsolateral prefrontal region, though Soloff et al. did not. Siever et al. found a blunted response in the anterior cingulate region and right superior parietal lobe. Soloff et al. found a similar response in the left temporal lobe, left parietal lobe, and left caudate. Of note is that while Soloff et al. studied only patients with BPD ($n=5$), Siever et al. included patients ($n=6$) who had overlapping diagnoses of borderline, paranoid, and histrionic personality disorders.

Recent studies have used α-[^{11}C]methyl-L-tryptophan (AMT) with PET to more directly evaluate serotonin synthesis capacity. AMT is converted to α-methylserotonin, which is not a substrate for monoamine oxidase and thus accumulates in the brain. This, in turn, may provide a more direct index of serotonin synthesis than previous techniques.[35] Leyton et al.[1] studied AMT accumulation in patients with BPD ($n=13$) in conjunction with a test of behavioral disinhibition. They found that the patients made more errors than controls on a Go/No-Go task, and AMT accumulation inversely correlated with impulsivity scores.

Affected regions included the orbital prefrontal region, anterior cingulate region (including the medial prefrontal gyrus), temporal cortex, and caudate (Figure 27–3). The authors concluded that low serotonin synthesis capacity in the corticostriatal pathways may contribute to impulsivity in BPD. While none of the patients had MDD or substance abuse at the time of evaluation, several had additional cluster B personality disorders and/or a history of mood disorders or substance abuse.

Conclusion

The studies discussed in this paper are consistent in revealing dysfunction of interconnected prefrontal, limbic, and corticostriatal pathways that work together to process emotions and modulate behavior. They support the theory that reduced serotonin neurotransmission among these structures lowers the threshold for behavioral disinhibition, possibly involving downstream neurotransmitters such as γ-aminobutyric acid or dopamine.[2] They further suggest a multifaceted etiology that accounts not only for the impulsivity of BPD but also for affective lability, dissociation, and comorbid mood disorders.

While many of the individual findings from these studies do not appear to be unique to BPD, the combination may be, thereby producing its characteristic symptomatology. Differences in specific locations, boundaries, and laterality remain unclear but may relate to the few numbers of patients studied and myriad variations in approach and technique, making cross-comparisons challenging. Moreover, most of these studies have yet to be independently replicated and should therefore be considered exploratory. While not easily avoidable in BPD, many of these studies included patients with comorbid psychiatric disorders and substance abuse.

Despite these limitations, however, the findings are provocative and encouraging. They require further research to replicate these results and clarify implications. Neuroimaging promises to play an integral role in solving the mystery of emotion regulation in BPD, which in turn may guide future treatment strategies.

References

1. Leyton M, Okazawa H, et al: Brain regional alpha-[11C]methyl-L-tryptophan trapping in impulsive subjects with borderline personality disorder. Am J Psychiatry 2001; 158:775–782
2. Siever LJ, Buchsbaum MS, et al: *d,l*-fenfluramine response in impulsive personality disorder assessed with [18F]fluorodeoxyglucose positron emission tomography. Neuropsychopharmacology 1999; 20:413–423
3. Skodol AE, Gunderson JG, et al: The borderline diagnosis I: psychopathology, comorbidity, and personality structure. Biol Psychiatry 2002; 51:936–950
4. Skodol AE, Siever LJ, et al: The borderline diagnosis II: biology, genetics, and clinical course. Biol Psychiatry 2002; 51:951–963
5. Tyrer P: Practice guidelines for the treatment of borderline personality disorder: a bridge too far. J Personal Disord 2002; 16:113–118
6. Torgersen S, Lygren S, et al: A twin study of personality disorders. Compr Psychiatry 2000; 41:416–425
7. Zimmerman M, Mattia JI: Axis I diagnostic comorbidity and borderline personality disorder. Compr Psychiatry 1999; 40:245–252
8. Skodol AE, Stout RL, et al: Co-occurrence of mood and personality disorders: a report from the Collaborative Longitudinal Personality Disorders Study (CLPS). Depress Anxiety 1999; 10:175–182
9. Linehan M: Cognitive-Behavioral Treatment of Borderline Personality Disorder. New York, Guilford Press, 1993
10. Herpertz SC, Gretzer A, et al: Affective instability and impulsivity in personality disorder. Results of an experimental study. J Affect Disord 1997; 44:31–37
11. Henry C, Mitropoulou V, et al: Affective instability and impulsivity in borderline personality and bipolar II disorders: similarities and differences. J Psychiatr Res 2001; 35:307–312
12. Davidson RJ, Putnam KM, Larson CL: Dysfunction in the neural circuitry of emotion regulation—a possible prelude to violence. Science 2000; 289:591–594
13. Royall DR, Lauterbach EC, et al: Executive control function: a review of its promise and challenges for clinical research. J Neuropsychiatry Clin Neurosci 2002; 14:377–405
14. Battaglia M, Ferini-Strambi L, et al: Ambulatory polysomnography of never-depressed borderline subjects: A high-risk approach to rapid eye movement latency. Biol Psychiatry 1993; 33:326–334
15. De la Fuente JM, Bobes J, et al: Sleep-EEG in borderline patients without comorbid depression: a comparison with major depressives and normal control subjects. Psychiatry Res 2001; 105:87–95
16. Asaad T, Okasha T, Okasha A: Sleep EEG findings in ICD-10 borderline personality disorder in Egypt. J Affect Disord 2002; 71:11–18
17. Benson KL, King R, et al: Sleep patterns in borderline personality disorder. J Affect Disord 1990; 18:267–273
18. Battaglia M, Ferini-Strambi L, et al: First-cycle REM density in never-depressed subjects with borderline personality disorder. Biol Psychiatry 1999; 45:1056–1058
19. Leibenluft E, Gardner DL, Cowdry RW: The inner experience of the borderline self-mutilator. J Personal Disord 1987; 1:317–324
20. Russ MJ, Campbell SS, et al: EEG theta activity and pain insensitivity in self-injurious borderline patients. Psychiatry Res 1999; 89:201–214
21. Snyder S, Pitts WM, Gustin Q: CT scans of patients with borderline personality disorder (letter). Am J Psychiatry 1983; 140:272
22. Schulz SC, Koller MM, et al: Ventricular enlargement in teenage patients with schizophrenia spectrum disorder. Am J Psychiatry 1983; 140:1592–1595
23. Lucas PB, Gardner DL, et al: Cerebral structure in borderline personality disorder. Psychiatry Res 1989; 27:111–115

24. Lyoo IK, Han MH, Cho DY: A brain MRI study in subjects with borderline personality disorder. J Affect Disord 1998; 50:235–243
25. Driessen M, Herrmann J, et al: Magnetic resonance imaging volumes of the hippocampus and the amygdala in women with borderline personality disorder and early traumatization. Arch Gen Psychiatry 2000; 57:1115–1122
26. Bremner JD, Randall P, et al: Magnetic resonance imaging–based measurement of hippocampal volume in posttraumatic stress disorder related to childhood physical and sexual abuse—a preliminary report. Biol Psychiatry 1997; 41:23–32
27. Bremner JD, Narayan M, et al: Hippocampal volume reduction in major depression. Am J Psychiatry 2000; 157:115–117
28. Herpertz SC, Dietrich TM, et al: Evidence of abnormal amygdala functioning in borderline personality disorder: a functional MRI study. Biol Psychiatry 2001; 50:292–298
29. Tebartz van Elst L, Thiel T, et al: Subtle prefrontal neuropathology in a pilot magnetic resonance spectroscopy study in patients with borderline personality disorder. J Neuropsychiatry Clin Neurosci 2001; 13:511–514
30. Goyer PF, Andreason PJ, et al: Positron-emission tomography and personality disorders. Neuropsychopharmacology 1994; 10:21–28
31. De la Fuente JM, Lotstra F, et al: Temporal glucose metabolism in borderline personality disorder. Psychiatry Res 1994; 55:237–245
32. De la Fuente JM, Goldman S, et al: Brain glucose metabolism in borderline personality disorder. J Psychiatr Res 1997; 31:531–541
33. Soloff PH, Meltzer CC, et al: A fenfluramine-activated FDG-PET study of borderline personality disorder. Biol Psychiatry 2000; 47:540–547
34. Juengling FD, Schmahl C, et al: Positron emission tomography in female patients with borderline personality disorder. J Psychiatr Res 2003; 37:109–115
35. Young SN, Leyton M, Benkelfat C: PET studies of serotonin synthesis in the human brain, in Tryptophan, Serotonin, and Melatonin: Basic Aspects and Applications. Edited by Huether G. Kluwer Academic/Plenum Publishers, New York, 1999

Recent Publications of Interest

Binks CA, Fenton M, McCarthy L, et al: Pharmacological interventions for people with borderline personality disorder. Cochrane Database Syst Rev 2006; 25:CD005653

Comprehensively reviewed the literature on pharmacologic treatment of borderline personality disorder, and found that, although there is little good evidence available, antidepressants may have some positive effect.

Zanarini MC, Frankenburg FR, Hennen J, et al: The McLean Study of Adult Development (MSAD): overview and implications of the first six years of prospective follow-up. J Personal Disord 2005; 19:505–523

Prospectively studied the course and outcome in a cohort of adults with borderline personality disorder. The main findings for the first 6 years are presented, which together indicate that the prognosis is more favorable than previously thought.

Ruocco AC: The neuropsychology of borderline personality disorder: a meta-analysis and review. Psychiatry Res 2005; 137:191–202

Presents the combined results of 10 neuropsychological studies comparing subjects with borderline personality disorder to healthy comparison groups, and concludes that performance deficits are present in multiple neuropsychological domains.

Meares R, Melkonian D, Gordon E, et al: Distinct pattern of P3a event-related potential in borderline personality disorder. Neuroreport 2005; 16:289–293

Compared auditory event-related potentials in subjects with borderline personality disorder to a healthy comparison group, and concluded that the findings of abnormally enhanced amplitude, failure to habituate, and loss of temporal locking were consistent with a failure of frontal maturation.

Reeves RR, Struve FA, Patrick G: Auditory and visual P300 evoked potentials do not predict response to valproate treatment of aggression in patients with borderline and antisocial personality disorders. Clin EEG Neurosci 2005; 36:49–51

Compared auditory and visual evoked potentials in subjects hospitalized for aggressive behavior (borderline personality disorder, antisocial personality disorder) prior to treatment with valproate, and found no correlation between treatment responsiveness and evoked potential measures.

Reprinted from Johnson PA, Hurley RA, Benkelfat C, et al: "Understanding Emotion Regulation in Borderline Personality Disorder: Contributions of Neuroimaging." *Journal of Neuropsychiatry and Clinical Neurosciences* 15:397–402, 2003. Used with permission.

Chapter 28

FUNCTIONAL ANATOMY OF CENTRAL PAIN

KATHERINE H. TABER, PH.D.
ANIS RASHID, M.D.
ROBIN A. HURLEY, M.D.

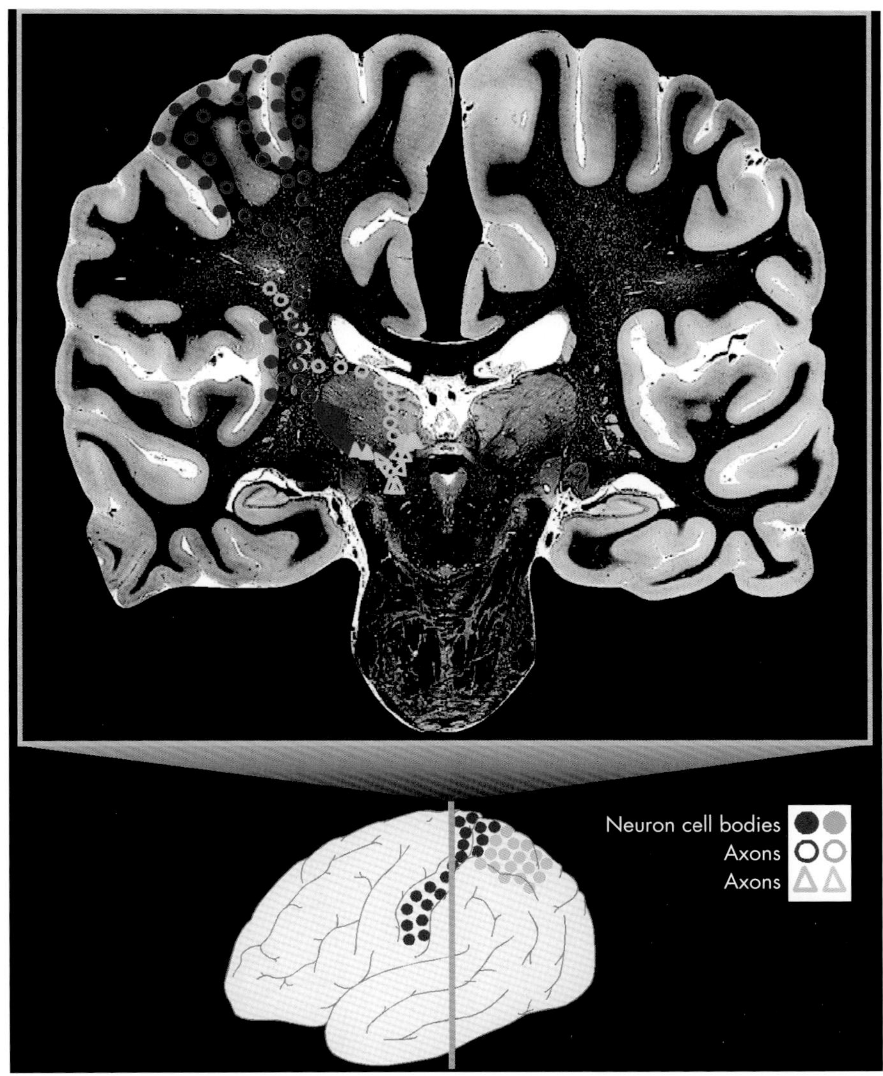

The approximate locations of the primary somatosensory nucleus (*pink*, perception of pain) and the midline and intralaminar nuclei (*blue*, emotional aspects of pain) of the thalamus are shown in the appropriate color on a myelin-stained coronal human brain section. Some of their cortical connections are illustrated on the lateral brain drawing. Color-coded circles indicate reciprocal connections between thalamus and cortical areas. Color-coded triangles indicate ascending inputs to thalamus from the spinothalamic tract (*green*) and dorsal raphe nucleus (*orange*). The approximate location of the coronal brain slice is indicated on the lateral brain drawing (*gold line*).

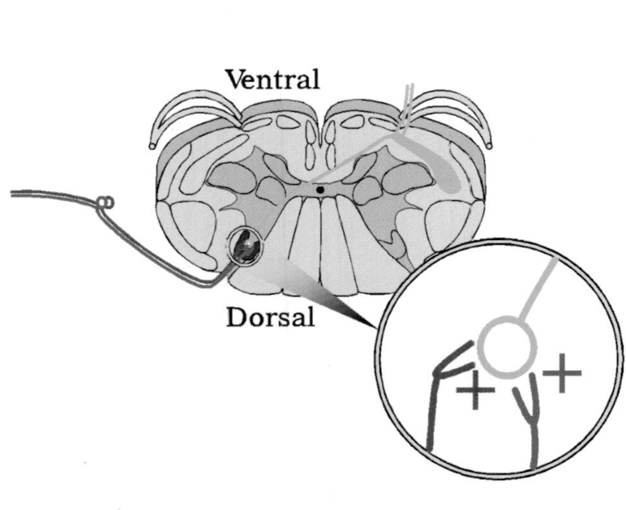

FIGURE 28–1. In the periphery, release of inflammatory substances following tissue injury activates C and A delta nociceptive endings (*red*) and increases their sensitivity. This decrease in the response threshold results in increased firing of these afferents in the spinal cord (felt as ongoing pain). Both nociceptive (*red*) and touch (*purple*) afferents activate the second-order spinal cord neurons (*green*), which send projections to the brain via the spinothalamic tract.

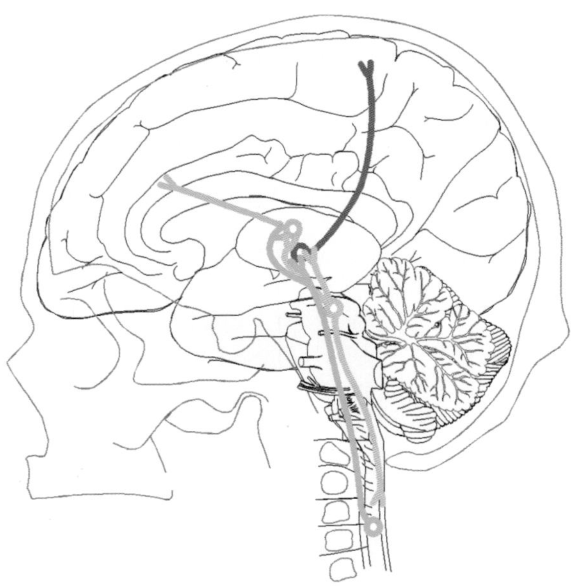

FIGURE 28–2. The spinothalamic tract (*green*, STT) projects to the primary somatosensory nucleus (*pink*) of the thalamus. This in turn projects to primary somatosensory cortex for perception of pain. The STT also projects to other thalamic nuclei. It is likely that the emotional aspects of pain are modulated in part by the influence of the midline and intralaminar nuclei (*blue*) on the anterior cingulate cortex. These higher centers also modulate perception of pain via brainstem structures. In particular, the dorsal raphe nucleus (*orange*) projects to both thalamus and spinal cord to modulate the intensity of pain.

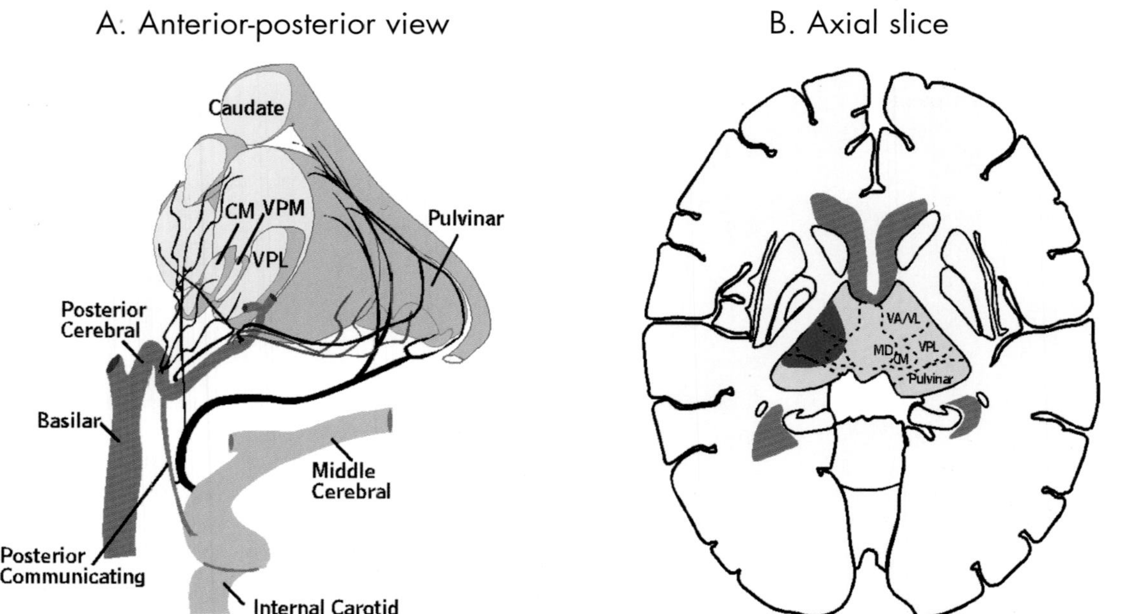

FIGURE 28–3. Thalamic pain is often associated with a lesion of the posterolateral thalamus (Dejerine and Roussy syndrome) involving the primary somatosensory nucleus (ventroposterior lateral [VPL] and ventroposterior medial [VPM] nuclei), centromedian [CM], and pulvinar. The arterial supply to this area of thalamus is the thalamogeniculate branches (*red*, A) of the posterior thalamoperforating arteries (also called geniculothalamic, inferolateral, or infero-external optic). The area commonly served by these branches is illustrated on an axial brain section (*red*, B). More than half of thalamic hemorrhages and infarctions occur in this arterial group.

Chronic pain is one of the most common and challenging problems facing our society. It is the second leading cause of work loss in the United States and the third greatest health care problem after cardiac disease and cancer. It has widespread impact on patients, their families, friends, and the workplace. Its influence extends to businesses, industry, and health care systems throughout the United States. Approximately 30% of the U.S. population (75 million Americans) suffer from chronic pain, with approximately $65 billion spent annually to treat and manage this problem.[1] Pain management has become an issue as studies have shown that only 40% of patients respond to current treatment regimens. Nursing organizations are proactively working to include pain as one of the basic vital signs, along with pulse, temperature, blood pressure, and respiration. Pain has already been included as the fifth vital sign by the Department of Veterans Affairs.[2] In many hospitals, nurses are using pain rating scales as an initial assessment and evaluation tool. Nurses are teaching patients to use a pain scale in which zero is the minimum and ten the maximum.[3] In 1999 the Joint Commission on Accreditation of Healthcare Organizations (JCAHO) approved revised standards for pain management and aggressive treatment. This has institutionalized pain nationwide as a vital sign for patient management. Currently a common strategy is to take an interdisciplinary approach that would help to recognize, document, and treat pain promptly and effectively.[4] The recommended JCAHO standards are given in the Patient Rights Section One of their official handbook, *The Comprehensive Accreditation Manual for Hospitals*. These standards can be used for both staff and patient education.[5]

The most difficult type of chronic pain to manage effectively is central pain. This type of pain results from injury to the ascending pain pathways and associated structures. Even quite small lesions to these areas can be clinically significant. Central pain has been reported following 3%–8% of strokes, occurs in 20%–44% of multiple sclerosis patients, and is recognized with increasing frequency in Parkinson's disease.[6,7] Commonly, patients are referred to psychiatry for evaluation when central pain has gone unrecognized or misdiagnosed as "drug-seeking," mood disorder, or somatoform disorder. The purpose of this paper is to summarize the complex functional anatomy of central pain and briefly note the therapeutic options for its treatment.

Functional Anatomy of Pain

Normal pain (nociceptive pain) results from activation of free nerve endings in peripheral tissues. These nociceptive primary afferents have little or no activity under normal circumstances. Release of inflammatory substances following tissue injury activates A delta nerve endings (small-diameter myelinated fibers that carry pinprick or primary pain) and C nerve endings (small-diameter unmyelinated fibers that carry slow-burning or secondary pain), increasing their sensitivity. This decrease in the response threshold results in increased firing of these afferents in the spinal cord (felt as ongoing pain). Both nociceptive and touch afferents converge on and activate second-order spinal cord neurons, which send projections to the brain via the spinothalamic tract (Figure 28–1). This convergent input (and co-release of substance P, which activates neurokinin receptors) causes hyperexcitability in the second-order neurons in the spinal cord. Responses are increased both to nociceptive input (hyperalgesia) and to touch. Light touch in and around the area of injury evokes pain (allodynia). Peripheral tenderness spreads beyond the actual area of injury as a result of this sensitization (secondary hyperalgesia).

From the spinal cord, pain sensation is relayed to thalamus and brainstem via the spinothalamic and spinomesencephalic tracts (Figure 28–2). From the thalamus, the pain system is believed to separate into a lateral system involved in perception of pain (sensory and discriminative) and a medial system involved in emotional coloring of pain (affect and motivation).[7–12] The projection to the primary somatosensory nucleus of the thalamus (ventral posterior complex, VP) is important for perception of pain.[13] VP in turn projects to primary (SI) and secondary (SII) somatosensory cortices as well as the dorsal portion of middle-posterior insular and posterior parietal cortices (see image at opening of chapter and Figure 28–2).[14] The spinothalamic tract also projects to other thalamic nuclei. It is likely that the emotional aspects of pain are modulated in part by the influence of the midline and intralaminar nuclei on the anterior cingulate cortex (Brodmann's area 24) as well as anterior insular and orbitofrontal cortex (see image at opening of chapter and Figure 28–2).[14]

Higher centers also modulate pain via brainstem structures. In particular, the dorsal raphe nucleus in the brainstem projects to both the thalamus and spinal cord to modulate the intensity of pain.[15] The periaqueductal gray receives projections from many limbic, sensory, and autonomic structures. Among other actions, it modulates the activity level of the dorsal raphe nucleus.[16] Functional brain imaging studies using positron emission tomography and functional magnetic resonance imaging have shown activation in somatosensory, prefrontal, cingulate, insular, and parietal cortices, thalamus, midbrain, and basal ganglia in response to painful stimuli.[11,17,18] Receptor mapping and binding studies indicate that many areas included in the medial pain system are also part of the endogenous opiate system.[19] Opiate binding is decreased in some of these structures in patients with central pain, perhaps indicating maximal activation of the endogenous pain control system.[20] This may be why opiates are generally not effective in patients with central pain.[11]

Central pain is neuropathic pain resulting from damage to portions of the central nervous system involved in perception of pain. Central pain arises most commonly from injury to the ascending spinothalamic tract or VP of the thalamus. It is frequently referred to as thalamic pain (Dejerine and Roussy syndrome; Figure 28–3).[21–23] However, because injury to other areas can give rise to central pain, the more general term *central poststroke pain* (CPSP) has also been used. This term is also too narrow. Although stroke is the most common etiology, central pain can follow injury from many other conditions, such as subarachnoid hemorrhage, compression, traumatic brain injury, abscess, and demyelinating or degenerative processes.

Central pain develops within a week after injury in 35%–40% of patients. However, its appearance may be delayed by more than a year in as many as 11% of patients.[6,22,24] If the pain is late in onset, its relationship to the initial injury may not be obvious. Thus a detailed clinical history and appropriate neuroimaging are vital. The pain is frequently perceived as arising from the peripheral area affected by the central injury and is felt to be diffuse rather than deep or superficial. It is exacerbated by any stimulus or movement of the affected area of the body. Once established, it tends to spread. There is no inflammation in the affected area. A common aspect of central pain is allodynia, in which the sensation of pain is experienced from a nonpainful stimulus. Even brief movement of clothing, for example, can cause severe burning pain.

Therapeutic Options for Central Pain

Treatment of central pain can be difficult. To manage these patients effectively, it is very important to recognize and diagnose central pain early, because the longer it goes untreated, the harder it is to control.[25] In the last two decades many different approaches have been tried. There is no single method that will reliably and effectively work in all patients.

Medications are successful in some patients, but only a few double-blind studies have been done. Systemic narcotic analgesics are occasionally effective.[26] Tricyclic antidepressants are reported to relieve central pain in more than one-half of patients.[25,27] Addition of mexiletine to amitriptyline may provide pain relief in previously unresponsive patients.[25] Tricyclic antidepressants, however, come with significant drawbacks due to their anticholinergic and sedative properties as well as the small safety margin (lethal in overdose). Carbamazepine may also be useful. Other medications, such as lamotrigine, gabapentin, and nefazodone, also show promise for the treatment of central pain, but at present the evidence is limited to case studies and anecdotal reports.[25,28,29] Initial double-blind studies indicate that the newer generation antidepressants that are specific serotonin reuptake inhibitors are probably not effective.[6]

Electrical brain stimulation has been tried in patients in whom medications have failed. Common targets are VP of the thalamus, posterior limb of the internal capsule, and motor cortex, although brainstem stimulation is used in some instances. Deep brain stimulation is reported to be successful in more than half of chronic pain patients overall, but it provides relief to only 20%–24% of patients experiencing central pain.[30,31] Surface stimulation of motor cortex, in which electrodes are placed in the epidural space over the portion of motor cortex serving the body area where the pain is experienced, is reported to provide relief in 46%–77% of central pain patients.[26,32]

Brain lesioning is the last resort for the treatment of central pain patients. It is seldom used because of the high risk of developing iatrogenic central pain.[33,34] The main targets for this type of treatment are thalamic (VP, medial thalamus, intralaminar nuclei).[33,34] Success rates are difficult to determine, although one series reported 60% of patients (3/5) benefited from lesion of the centromedian nucleus (one of the intralaminar nuclei).[34]

Summary

Central pain is the most difficult type of chronic pain to manage. It results from injury to the ascending pain pathways and associated structures, and may be seen in a wide range of conditions, including stroke, multiple sclerosis, and Parkinson's disease. To manage these patients effectively, it is very important to diagnose central pain promptly. A better understanding of the basic pain mechanisms and pathways will aid the clinician in recognizing central pain and help in choosing treatments customized to specific patients. Aggressive treatment of central pain also complies with the recent recommendations made by the JCAHO.

References

1. Tollison CD: Pain and its magnitude, in Pain Management: A Practical Guide for Clinicians. Edited by Weiner RS. Boca Raton, FL, St. Lucie Press, 1998, pp 3–6
2. Newman BY: Pain as the fifth vital sign. J Am Optom Assoc 1999; 70:619–620

3. Pasero CL, McCaffery M: Pain ratings: the fifth vital sign. Am J Nurs 1997; 97:15–16
4. Pasero CL, McCaffery M, Gordon DB: Build institutional commitment to improving pain management. Nurs Manage 1999; 30:27–33
5. Williams-Lee P: Managing pain by the book. Nurs Manage 1999; 30:9
6. Andersen G, Vestergaard K, Ingeman-Nielsen M, et al: Incidence of central post-stroke pain. Pain 1995; 61:187–193
7. Casey KL: The imaging of pain: background and rationale, in Pain Imaging: Progress in Pain Research and Management, vol 18. Edited by Casey KL, Bushnell MC. Seattle, WA, IASP Press, 2000, pp 1–29
8. Applebaum AE, Leonard RB, Kenshalo DR, et al: Nuclei in which functionally identified spinothalamic tract neurons terminate. J Comp Neurol 1979; 188:575–586
9. Bushnell MC, Duncan GH: Sensory and affective aspects of pain perception: is medial thalamus restricted to emotional issues? Exp Brain Res 1989; 78:415–418
10. Price DD: Psychological and neural mechanisms of the affective dimension of pain. Science 2000; 288:1769–1772
11. Rainville P, Bushnell MC, Duncan GH: PET studies of the subjective experience of pain, in Pain Imaging: Progress in Pain Research and Management, vol 18. Edited by Casey KL, Bushnell MC. Seattle, WA, IASP Press, 2000, pp 123–156
12. Vogt BA, Sikes RW: The medial pain system, cingulate cortex, and parallel processing of nociceptive information. Prog Brain Res 2000; 122:223–235
13. Craig AD, Bushnell MC, Zhang ET, et al: A thalamic nucleus specific for pain and temperature sensation. Nature 1994; 372:770–773
14. Craig AD, Chen K, Bandy D, et al: Thermosensory activation of insular cortex. Nature 2000; 3:184–190
15. Wang QP, Nakai Y: The dorsal raphe: an important nucleus in pain modulation. Brain Res Bull 1994; 34:575–585
16. Behbehani MM: Functional characteristics of the midbrain periaqueductal gray. Prog Neurobiol 1995; 46:575–605
17. Coghill RC, Sang CN, Maisog JM, et al: Pain intensity processing within the human brain: a bilateral, distributed mechanism. J Neurophysiol 1999; 82:1934–1943
18. Davis KD: The neural circuitry of pain as explored with functional MRI. Neurol Res 2000; 22:313–317
19. Jones AKP, Qi LY, Fujirawa T, et al: In vivo distribution of opioid receptors in man in relation to the cortical projections of the medial and lateral pain systems measured with positron emission tomography. Neurosci Lett 1991; 126:25–28
20. Willoch F, Tolle TR, Wester HJ, et al: Central pain after pontine infarction is associated with changes in opioid receptor binding: a PET study with ^{11}C-diprenorphine. AJNR Am J Neuroradiol 1999; 20:686–690
21. Martin JJ: Thalamic syndromes, in Handbook of Clinical Neurology, edited by Vinken PJ, Bruyn GW. Amsterdam, North-Holland, 1969, pp 469–496
22. Bowsher D: Central pain: clinical and physiological characteristics. J Neurol Neurosurg Psychiatry 1996; 61:62–69
23. Bowsher D, Leijon G, Thuomas KA: Central poststroke pain: correlation of MRI with clinical pain characteristics and sensory abnormalities. Neurology 1998; 51:1352–1358
24. Nasreddine ZS, Saver JL: Pain after thalamic stroke: right diencephalic predominance and clinical features in 180 patients. Neurology 1997; 48:1196–1199
25. Bowsher D: Central pain following spinal and supraspinal lesions. Spinal Cord 1999; 37:235–238
26. Yamamoto T, Katayama Y, Hirayama T, et al: Pharmacological classification of central post-stroke pain: comparison with the results of chronic motor cortex stimulation therapy. Pain 1997; 72:5–12
27. Leijon G, Boivie J: Central post-stroke pain: a controlled trial of amitriptyline and carbamazepine. Pain 1989; 36:27–36
28. Canavero S, Bonicalzi V: Lamotrigine control of central pain. Pain 1996; 68:179–181
29. Sindrup SH, Jensen TS: Efficacy of pharmacological treatments of neuropathic pain: an update and effect related to mechanism of drug action. Pain 1999; 83:389–400
30. Levy RM, Lamb S, Adams JE: Treatment of chronic pain by deep brain stimulation: long term follow-up and review of the literature. Neurosurgery 1987; 21:885–893
31. Kumar K, Toth C, Nath RK: Deep brain stimulation for intractable pain: a 15-year experience. Neurosurgery 1997; 40:736–746
32. Nguyen JP, Lefaucheur JP, Decq P, et al: Chronic motor stimulation in the treatment of central and neuropathic pain: correlations between clinical, electrophysiological and anatomical data. Pain 1999; 82:245–251
33. Tasker RR, Kiss ZHT: The role of the thalamus in functional neurosurgery. Neurosurg Clin N Am 1995; 6:73–104
34. Hariz MI, Bergenheim AT: Thalamic stereotaxis for chronic pain: ablative lesion or stimulation? Stereotact Funct Neurosurg 1995; 64:47–55

Recent Publications of Interest

Frese A, Husstedt IW, Ringelstein EB, et al: Pharmacologic treatment of central post-stroke pain. Clin J Pain 2006; 22:252–260

Comprehensively reviewed the literature on pharmacologic treatment of central poststroke pain to derive evidence-based recommendations for treatment.

Brooks J, Tracey I: From nociception to pain perception: imaging the spinal and supraspinal pathways. J Anat 2005; 207:19–33

Provides an overview of pain research employing structural and functional neuroimaging.

Weigel R, Krauss JK: Center median-parafascicular complex and pain control. Review from a neurosurgical perspective. Stereotact Funct Neurosurg 2004; 82:115–126
Summarizes the current understanding of the anatomy and connectivity of the center median-parafascicular complex, which in humans is the major portion of the intralaminar thalamus and important for pain processing.

Craig AD: Pain mechanisms: labeled lines versus convergence in central processing. Annu Rev Neurosci 2003; 26:1–30
Presents the evidence for a different view of pain processing that is specific to humans and higher primates, that of pain as a homeostatic emotion, part of the representation of the physiological condition of the body (interoception).

Reprinted from Taber KH, Rashid A, Hurley RA: "Functional Anatomy of Central Pain." *Journal of Neuropsychiatry and Clinical Neurosciences* 13:437–440, 2001. Used with permission.

Work on this article was supported by a grant from the Mike Hogg Fund, Houston, TX.

Chapter 29

An Update on Estrogen

Higher Cognitive Function, Receptor Mapping, Neurotrophic Effects

Katherine H. Taber, Ph.D.
Diane D. Murphy, Ph.D.
Mathew M. Blurton-Jones, M.S.
Robin A. Hurley, M.D.

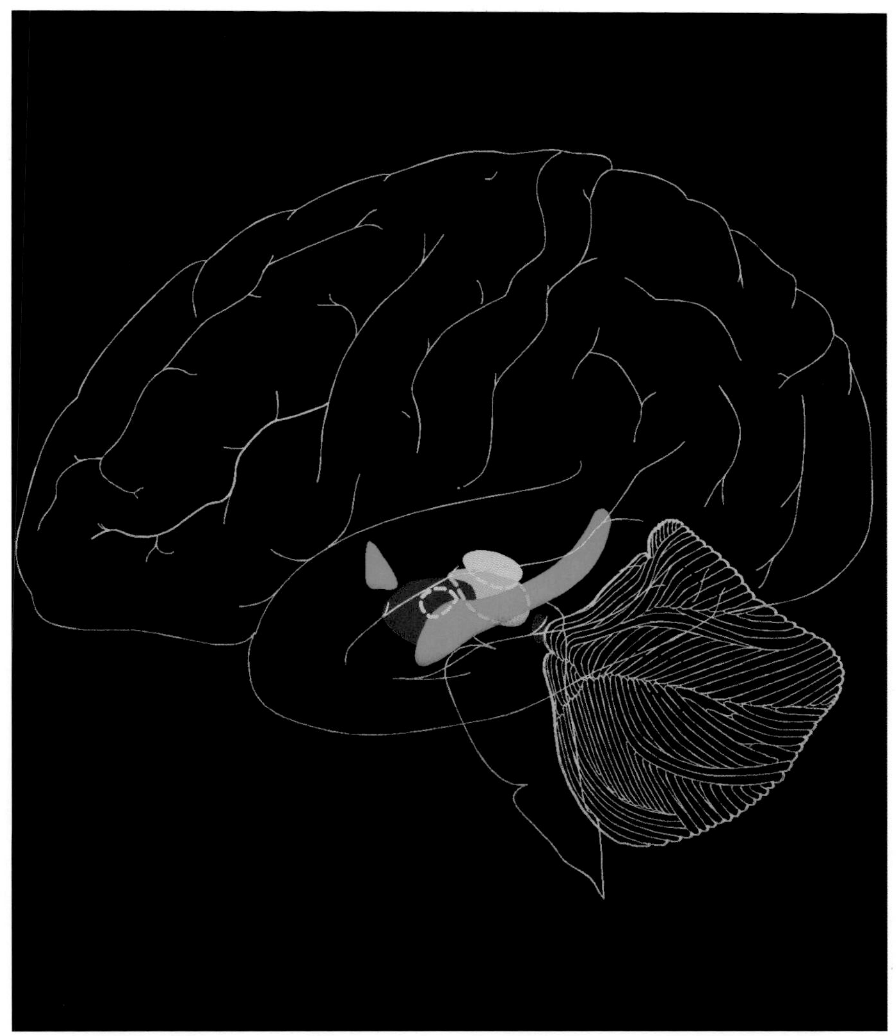

New areas in which estrogen receptors have been confirmed in primates are illustrated on a sagittal drawing of the human brain. Structures are color-coded by function: memory (*blue:* basal forebrain, hippocampal formation, mammillary body); emotion (*pink:* amygdala, dorsal raphe nucleus); movement (*green:* subthalamic nucleus, substantia nigra).

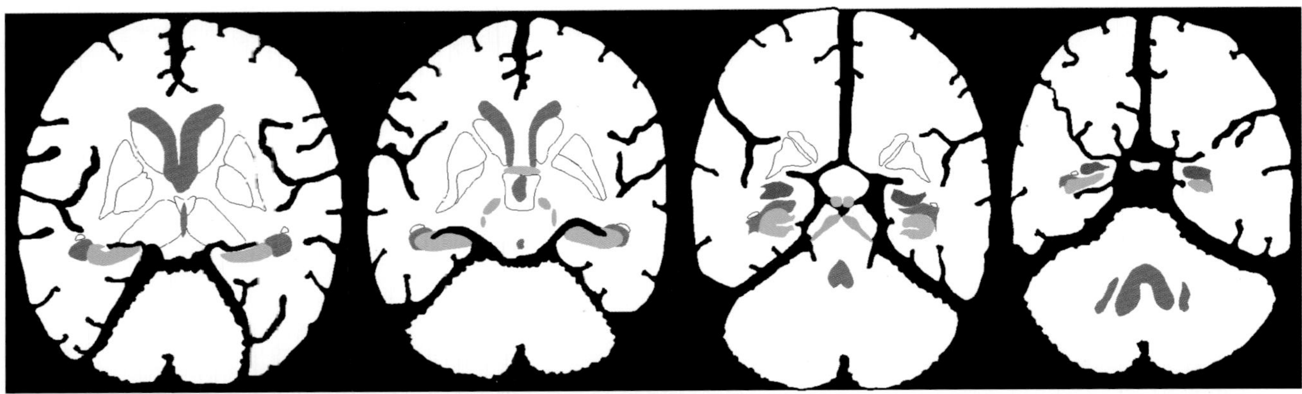

FIGURE 29–1. New areas in which estrogen receptors have been confirmed in primates are illustrated on drawings of axial human brain slices. Structures are color-coded by function: memory (*blue:* basal forebrain, hippocampal formation, mammillary body); emotion (*pink:* amygdala); movement (*green:* subthalamic nucleus, substantia nigra).

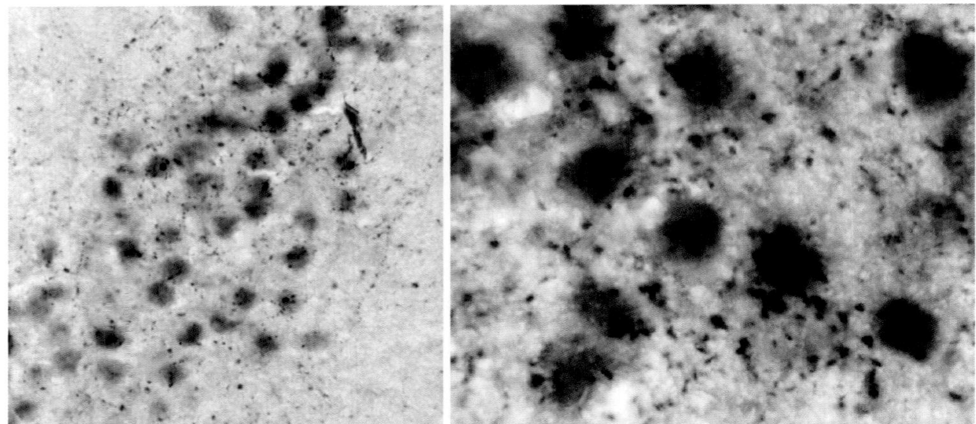

FIGURE 29–2. Immunchistochemical double labeling shows localization of the estrogen alpha receptor (*yellow-brown label* in neuronal nuclei) and choline acetyltransferase (*blue label* in cytoplasm) in the primate amygdala. Note that the co-association of cholinergic axon terminals with estrogen receptor–containing neuronal cell bodies is clear on the higher-magnification image (right).

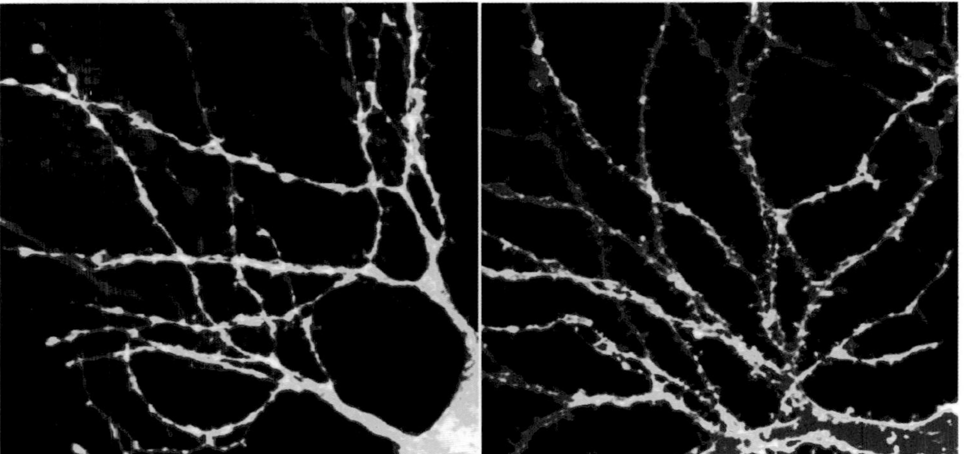

FIGURE 29–3. Photomicrographs of cultured hippocampal neurons immunohistochemically labeled with DiI (a plasma membrane dye) so that individual spine morphology could be visualized in the confocal microscope. The neurons on the right have been exposed to estradiol (0.1 μg/mL) for 48 hours; the ones on the left have not. Note the marked increase of the number of mature spines on the dendrites of neurons exposed to estradiol.

The sex steroids have been associated with brain development and global functioning directly or indirectly for thousands of years. Writings from the ancient Greeks and Egyptians linked emotional instability or any unacceptable behavior from a female with the uterus.[1] Modern medicine continues to be perplexed by the influence of reproductive steroids on behavior. For example, a PubMed search of "estrogen and brain" gives 10,846 references since 1963. As 21st-century neuropsychiatrists try to understand the brain circuits and neurotransmitters that underlie emotion and behavior, the influence of sex steroids begins to establish its importance. Estrogen and mood is a much-studied area. Recent evidence indicates that at least a subset of depressive disorders are influenced by estrogen's effects at many points, particularly the premenstrual and perimenopausal times. A recent issue of a neuropsychiatric journal was dedicated to summarizing the current literature on the effects of estrogen on mood throughout the female life cycle.[2] But what about estrogen's effects on other cortical functions? Cognition is an area of particular interest to the neuropsychiatrist. The current database and established truths for a relationship between cognition, neurodegeneration, and the sex steroids are much more limited. As our population ages and dementias become more prominent in our medical practices, it is vital that we more clearly understand any relationship between these steroids and neurodegeneration. The following discussion summarizes some of the most recent evidence linking one sex steroid, estrogen, with cognition and neurodegeneration.

Estrogen and Cognitive Function

There have been numerous reports of an association between estrogen and performance on specific measures of higher cognitive function. In particular, higher estrogen levels have been associated with improvements in verbal performance and decrements in visual-spatial performance.[3–5] However, a subsequent summary of the literature concluded that although there is observational evidence for estrogen enhancement of certain aspects of cognitive functioning, quantitative comparison across studies cannot be performed because of heterogeneity among subjects and variability in the cognitive measures used.[6] A comparison of two more recent studies illustrates this problem. Both were prospective studies in which performance on the Forward and Backward Digit Span test was compared in groups of postmenopausal females over time. In one, females receiving estrogen replacement therapy (ERT) performed better than females not receiving ERT at both study initiation and 18 months later.[7] In the other, there were no differences in performance on this task, either at initiation or 2 years later.[8] However, the second study matched participants for educational level. In general, females on ERT are better educated, have higher socioeconomic status, and are healthier than females who are not.[9] Mood is also a critical variable that is sometimes overlooked. In most studies circulating levels of hormones have not been measured, making comparisons difficult. The situation is further complicated by the report that cerebrospinal fluid levels of estradiol (presumably representing hormone levels in the brain) are very different from circulating levels and do not decrease as much following menopause.[10]

Estrogen Receptor Mapping

In addition to the well-known localization of estrogen receptors within hypothalamic nuclei, which are important for regulation of sexual and reproductive behaviors (not illustrated), estrogen receptors have now been found in other areas of the brain (see image at opening of chapter and Figure 29–1). There are at least two forms of the estrogen receptor (alpha and beta), and their distributions within the brain are different.[11–13] Receptor mapping studies do not all agree, perhaps because several different techniques (autoradiography, in situ hybridization, immunocytochemistry) and multiple species (mouse, rat, guinea pig, monkey, human) have been used. There are clear species differences, so the following summary is based only on studies of human and nonhuman primates (see image at opening of chapter and Figure 29–1). Several studies have found estrogen receptors in the hippocampal formation (hippocampus proper, dentate gyrus, subiculum, and entorhinal cortex), basal forebrain (septal nucleus, diagonal band of Broca, and nucleus basalis of Meynert), and mammillary bodies (see image at opening of chapter and Figure 29–1, *blue areas*).[11,13–19] These support an influence on declarative (autobiographical, explicit) memory. Presence in the amygdala and dorsal raphe nucleus may underlie some of the effects of estrogen on mood and emotion (see image at opening of chapter and Figure 29–1, *pink area*).[11,14–19] Estrogen receptors are present in movement-related areas including the substantia nigra and the subthalamic nucleus (see image at opening of chapter and Figure 29–1, *green areas*).[13,17–19] They may also be present in the cerebellum (not illustrated), but exact localization is still unclear.[11,13] Most studies have not found estrogen receptors in the basal ganglia (caudate, putamen, or globus pallidus).[11,13–16,18,19] Several studies have reported estrogen receptors in various areas of the cerebral cortex (not illustrated), but this is still controversial.[11,13,18] No obvious differences have been reported between females and males in regional distribution of the alpha estrogen receptor.[15,16] There may be gender differences in the distribution of the beta form of the receptor.[11] One study has reported similar distributions of estrogen receptors in intact and ovariectomized females.[15]

Estrogen has multiple modes of action within the central nervous system.[12,20–24] It binds to a nuclear receptor, acting intracellularly to alter gene expression. Estrogen actions via this genomic mechanism, which are necessarily slow, may include inhibition of apoptosis, suppression of inflammatory reactions, and modulation of neurotrophins and growth factors as well as neuronal structure and synapse formation. Estrogen also has rapid actions, occurring far too quickly for genomic mechanisms. These may include its antioxidant effects as well as enhancement of cerebral blood flow and cerebral glucose utilization. These nongenomic effects probably occur via both plasma membrane receptors and non-receptor-mediated pathways. Some actions, such as modulation of neurotransmitters, may occur by both genomic and nongenomic mechanisms.

Estrogen interacts with multiple neurotransmitter systems at multiple sites. For instance, it has been shown to modulate the levels of dopamine (upregulation), serotonin (downregulation), norepinephrine (downregulation), and acetylcholine (upregulation) in prefrontal cortex.[25] This may occur via direct actions within cortex, or indirectly via estrogen receptor–mediated changes in brainstem or basal forebrain areas. Estrogen co-localizes with some neurotransmitters. Estrogen receptors have been found in serotonergic neurons within the dorsal raphe nucleus, where estrogen appears to facilitate serotonergic transmission by several mechanisms.[26] Estrogen alpha receptor–containing neurons in the amygdala are heavily invested with cholinergic terminals projecting from the basal forebrain (Figure 29–2).[15] Estrogen modulates aspects of neuronal plasticity, including dendritic spine formation. In the hippocampus, for instance, estrogen receptors are localized in GABAergic interneurons. Estradiol exposure decreases the activity of these inhibitory interneurons (via an interaction with a neurotrophin), resulting in an increase in pyramidal cell excitability, which in turn promotes formation of new dendritic spines and synapses (Figure 29–3).[27–29]

Neurotrophic and Neuroprotective Effects of Estrogen

Estrogen has neuroprotective and neurotrophic actions that may be mediated by a variety of routes. Estrogen receptors (both alpha and beta forms) have been found in microglia and within reactive astrocytes.[30,31] In addition, there is evidence that estrogen suppresses activation of microglia and astrocytes and thereby the inflammatory cascade.[31,32] Circulating estrogen is critical to the health of some types of neurons. This has been clearly demonstrated for a subpopulation of dopaminergic neurons in the substantia nigra, suggesting the importance of estrogen in Parkinson's disease.[33] It is not yet clear whether this effect on dopaminergic neurons is mediated via the intracellular estrogen receptor or by a plasma membrane receptor for estradiol, although the antioxidant actions of estrogen have been implicated.[21]

Estrogen may also be important in other neurodegenerative diseases. Epidemiological studies generally support the view that ERT reduces the risk of developing Alzheimer's disease (AD),[22–24,34,35] which occurs more frequently and progresses more quickly in females.[23] It has been suggested that estrogen's anti-inflammatory action may be one important protective mechanism.[31] The process is not yet clear, since there is not a decrease in cortical estradiol or testosterone in AD.[36] The influence of ERT on the progression of neurodegeneration after onset is more controversial, as are ERT's effects on cognition. There was an absence of therapeutic effect on measures of cognition, mood, and cerebral blood flow in a recent double-blind, placebo-controlled study of ERT in AD,[37] suggesting that its therapeutic use needs further study.

The incidence of stroke is lower in premenopausal females than in other groups (males, postmenopausal females), perhaps a result of estrogen's influence on cerebral vasculature, its effect on circulating levels of cholesterol, and/or its antioxidant actions.[20,23,38] Although some reports indicate ERT lowers the risk of stroke after menopause, not all studies agree.[38] A recent large study actually found more clinically significant brain atrophy in postmenopausal females who were receiving ERT than in those who were not.[39] In that study, the prevalence of infarcts as demonstrated by magnetic resonance imaging was not different between ERT and non-ERT groups, and measures of cognitive functioning did not correlate with duration of estrogen treatment. Similarly, although some studies have reported that females fare better than males following traumatic brain injury, a recent meta-analysis of the few studies available reporting outcome by gender found that females fared worse than males on virtually every outcome measure, with the interesting exception of "return to work."[40,41] Thus, although the neuroprotective actions of estrogen have been convincingly demonstrated in animal models of ischemia, contusion, hypoxia, and drug-induced toxicity, its protective effects in humans are less clear.[20,23,24] There is a need for careful clinical studies in which potentially confounding factors such as premorbid conditions, severity of injury, and treatment differences can be assessed.

Implications

The influence of estrogen on such a wide range of brain functions has important implications for neuropsychiatry. It may be one reason why there are gender differences in both vulnerability to some mental illnesses and disease course. It suggests, as well, the potential for differences in response to therapeutics both across gender and as a function of life stage. The neuroprotective effects of estrogen raise the hope that it can be used to treat degenerative diseases of the central nervous system, such as Alzheimer's disease. It may also be helpful in salvaging tissue after stroke and traumatic brain injury. The existence of at least two forms of the estrogen receptor, and the differences in their distribution among brain areas, raises the possibility of designing pharmaceutical interventions that are targeted to specific aspects of estrogen's wide range of functions. It is clear, however, that estrogen has such widespread effects that it will be very difficult to predict what the effect of estrogen agonists and antagonists will be for particular aspects of cognitive function. Thus, new therapeutics will have to be very carefully evaluated.

References

1. Catonne JP: [Hippocratic concept of hysteria] (French). Ann Med Psychol (Paris) 1992; 150:705–719
2. Special Issue: Female-Specific Mood Disorders. CNS Spectrums: The International Journal of Neuropsychiatric Medicine 2001; 6:125–174
3. Sherwin BB: Estrogen effects on cognition in menopausal women. Neurology 1997; 48:S21–S26
4. Williams CL: Estrogen effects on cognition across the lifespan. Horm Behav 1998; 34:80–84
5. Drake EB, Henderson VW, Stanczyk FZ, et al: Associations between circulating sex steroid hormones and cognition in normal elderly women. Neurology 2000; 54:599–603
6. Haskell SG, Richardson ED, Horwitz RI: The effect of estrogen replacement therapy on cognitive function in women: a critical review of the literature. J Clin Epidemiol 1997; 50:1249–1264
7. Carlson LE, Sherwin BB: Higher levels of plasma estradiol and testosterone in healthy elderly men compared with age-matched women may protect aspects of explicit memory. Menopause 2000; 7:168–177
8. Maki PM, Resnick SM: Longitudinal effects of estrogen replacement therapy on PET cerebral blood flow and cognition. Neurobiol Aging 2000; 21:373–383
9. Yaffe K, Grady D, Pressman A, et al: Serum estrogen levels, cognitive performance, and risk of cognitive decline in older community women. J Am Geriatr Soc 1998; 46:816–821
10. Molnar G, Kassai-Bazsa Z: Gonadotropin, ACTH, prolactin, sexual steroid and cortisol levels in postmenopausal women's cerebrospinal fluid (CSF). Archives of Gerontology and Geriatrics 1997; 24:269–280
11. Pau CY, Pau KY, Spies HG: Putative estrogen receptor beta and alpha mRNA expression in male and female rhesus macaques. Mol Cell Endocrinol 1998; 146:59–68
12. McEwen BS: Clinical review 108: the molecular and neuroanatomical basis for estrogen effects in the central nervous system. J Clin Endocrinol Metab 1999; 84:1790–1797
13. Taylor AH, Al-Azzawi F: Immunolocalisation of oestrogen receptor beta in human tissues. J Mol Endocrinol 2000; 24:145–155
14. Register TC, Shively CA, Lewis CE: Expression of estrogen receptor alpha and beta transcripts in female monkey hippocampus and hypothalamus. Brain Res 1998; 788:320–322
15. Blurton-Jones MM, Roberts JA, Tuszynski MH: Estrogen receptor immunoreactivity in the adult primate brain: neuronal distribution and association with p75, trkA, and choline acetyltransferase. J Comp Neurol 1999; 405:529–542
16. Donahue JE, Stopa EG, Chorsky RL, et al: Cells containing immunoreactive estrogen receptor-alpha in the human basal forebrain. Brain Res 2000; 856:142–151
17. Gundlah C, Kohama SG, Mirkes SJ, et al: Distribution of estrogen receptor beta (ERbeta) mRNA in hypothalamus, midbrain and temporal lobe of spayed macaque: continued expression with hormone replacement. Brain Res Mol Brain Res 2000; 76:191–204
18. Osterlund MK, Keller E, Hurd YL: The human forebrain has discrete estrogen receptor alpha messenger RNA expression: high levels in the amygdaloid complex. Neuroscience 2000; 95:333–342
19. Osterlund MK, Grandien K, Keller E, et al: The human brain has distinct regional expression patterns of estrogen receptor alpha mRNA isoforms derived from alternative promoters. J Neurochem 2000; 75:1390–1397
20. Roof RL, Hall ED: Gender differences in acute CNS trauma and stroke: neuroprotective effects of estrogen and progesterone. J Neurotrauma 2000; 17:367–388
21. Sawada H, Shimohama S: Neuroprotective effects of estradiol in mesencephalic dopaminergic neurons. Neurosci Biobehav Rev 2000; 24:143–147
22. Birkhauser MH, Strnad J, Kampf C, et al: Oestrogens and Alzheimer's disease. Int J Geriatr Psychiatry 2000; 15:600–609
23. Garcia-Segura LM, Azcoitia I, DonCarlos LL: Neuroprotection by estradiol. Prog Neurobiol 2001; 63:29–60
24. Wise PM, Dubal DB, Wilson ME, et al: Estrogens: trophic and protective factors in the adult brain. Front Neuroendocrinol 2001; 22:33–66
25. Kritzer MF, Kohama SG: Ovarian hormones differentially influence immunoreactivity for dopamine beta-hydroxylase, choline acetyltransferase, and serotonin in the dorsolateral prefrontal cortex of adult rhesus monkeys. J Comp Neurol 1999; 409:438–451
26. Bethea CL, Pecins-Thompson M, Schutzer WE, et al: Ovarian steroids and serotonin neural function. Mol Neurobiol 1998; 18:87–123
27. Woolley CS, Weiland NG, McEwen BS, et al: Estradiol increases the sensitivity of hippocampal CA1 pyramidal cells to NMDA receptor–mediated synaptic input: correlation with dendritic spine density. J Neurosci 1997; 17:1848–1859
28. Murphy DD, Cole NB, Greenberger V, et al: Estradiol increases dendritic spine density by reducing GABA neurotransmission in hippocampal neurons. J Neurosci 1998; 18:2550–2559

29. Murphy DD, Cole NB, Segal M: Brain-derived neurotrophic factor mediates estradiol-induced dendritic spine formation in hippocampal neurons. Proc Natl Acad Sci USA 1998; 95:11412–11417
30. Blurton-Jones M, Tuszynski MH: Reactive astrocytes express estrogen receptors in the injured primate brain. J Comp Neurol 2000; 433:115–123
31. Vegeto E, Bonincontro C, Pollio G, et al: Estrogen prevents the lipopolysaccharide-induced inflammatory response in microglia. J Neurosci 2001; 21:1809–1818
32. Garcia-Estrada J, Del Rio JA, Luquin S, et al: Gonadal hormones down-regulate reactive gliosis and astrocyte proliferation after a penetrating brain injury. Brain Res 1993; 628:271–278
33. Leranth C, Roth RH, Elsworth JD, et al: Estrogen is essential for maintaining nigrostriatal dopamine neurons in primates: implications for Parkinson's disease and memory. J Neurosci 2000; 20:8604–8609
34. Tang MX, Jacobs D, Stern Y, et al: Effect of oestrogen during menopause on risk and age at onset of Alzheimer's disease. Lancet 1996; 348:429–432
35. Kawas C, Resnick S, Morrison A, et al: A prospective study of estrogen replacement therapy and the risk of developing Alzheimer's disease: the Baltimore Longitudinal Study of Aging. Neurology 1997; 48:1517–1521
36. Twist SJ, Taylor GA, Weddell A, et al: Brain oestradiol and testosterone levels in Alzheimer's disease. Neurosci Lett 2000; 286:1–4
37. Wang PN, Liao SQ, Liu RS, et al: Effects of estrogen on cognition, mood, and cerebral blood flow in AD: a controlled study. Neurology 2000; 54:2061–2066
38. Hurn PD, Macrae IM: Estrogen as a neuroprotectant in stroke. J Cereb Blood Flow Metab 2000; 20:631–652
39. Luoto R, Manolio T, Meilahn E, et al: Estrogen replacement therapy and MRI-demonstrated cerebral infarcts, white matter changes, and brain atrophy in older women: the Cardiovascular Health Study. J Am Geriatr Soc 2000; 48:467–472
40. Groswasser Z, Cohen M, Keren O: Female TBI patients recover better than males. Brain Inj 1998; 12:805–808
41. Farace E, Alves WM: Do women fare worse: a metaanalysis of gender differences in traumatic brain injury outcome. J Neurosurg 2000; 93:539–545

Recent Publications of Interest

Maki PM: Hormone therapy and cognitive function: is there a critical period for benefit? Neuroscience 2006; 138:1027–1030
Reviews the evidence that, while hormone therapy appears to be detrimental when started later in life, early hormone replacement may be beneficial.

Deroo BJ, Korach KS: Estrogen receptors and human disease. J Clin Invest 2006; 116:561–570
Summarizes the influence of estrogen on multiple physiologic processes and its involvement in the development or progression of many diseases, including cancer, osteoporosis, lupus, and neurodegenerative and cardiovascular diseases.

Dykens JA, Moos WH, Howell N: Development of 17alpha-estradiol as a neuroprotective therapeutic agent: rationale and results from a phase I clinical study. Ann N Y Acad Sci 2005; 1052:116–135
Provides an overview of the therapeutic potential of isomers of estradiol that have potent neuroprotective activity coupled with greatly reduced hormonal activity.

Reprinted from Taber KH, Murphy DD, Blurton-Jones MM, et al: "An Update on Estrogen: Higher Cognitive Function, Receptor Mapping, Neurotrophic Effects." *Journal of Neuropsychiatry and Clinical Neurosciences* 13:313–317, 2001. Used with permission.

Part 4

TREATMENT

In the last 10 years, great strides have been made in the application of technology to medicine. Procedures that previously were inconceivable have become possible with the help of computers. Diagnostics have certainly taken advantage of the technological revolution. Although treatment of psychiatric disease has improved, it has been at a significantly slower pace. This is probably due to many factors, including the great complexity of the brain and the circuits that underlie behavior and cognition.

In this section of the text, applications of imaging to the treatment of neuropsychiatric disease are presented. This section is the briefest. However, treatment-related applications of imaging may have the most life-changing impact for our patients in the near future. As neuroreceptor-specific ligands become more widely available, imaging may help to identify which medications or nonmedication treatments will help the patient the most, identify treatments to avoid, and be useful in the prevention of functional decline. The reader should be mindful that this area of study is very new and many advances are yet to be made. The papers can be read in sequence or individually for a particular area of interest. At the conclusion of this section, the reader should have a basic understanding of how imaging helps to explain why particular treatment strategies did not work in history or may be useful in future therapeutics.

Chapter 30

PREDICTING TREATMENT RESPONSE IN OBSESSIVE-COMPULSIVE DISORDER

ROBIN A. HURLEY, M.D.
SANJAYA SAXENA, M.D.
SCOTT L. RAUCH, M.D.
RUDOLF HOEHN-SARIC, M.D.
KATHERINE H. TABER, PH.D.

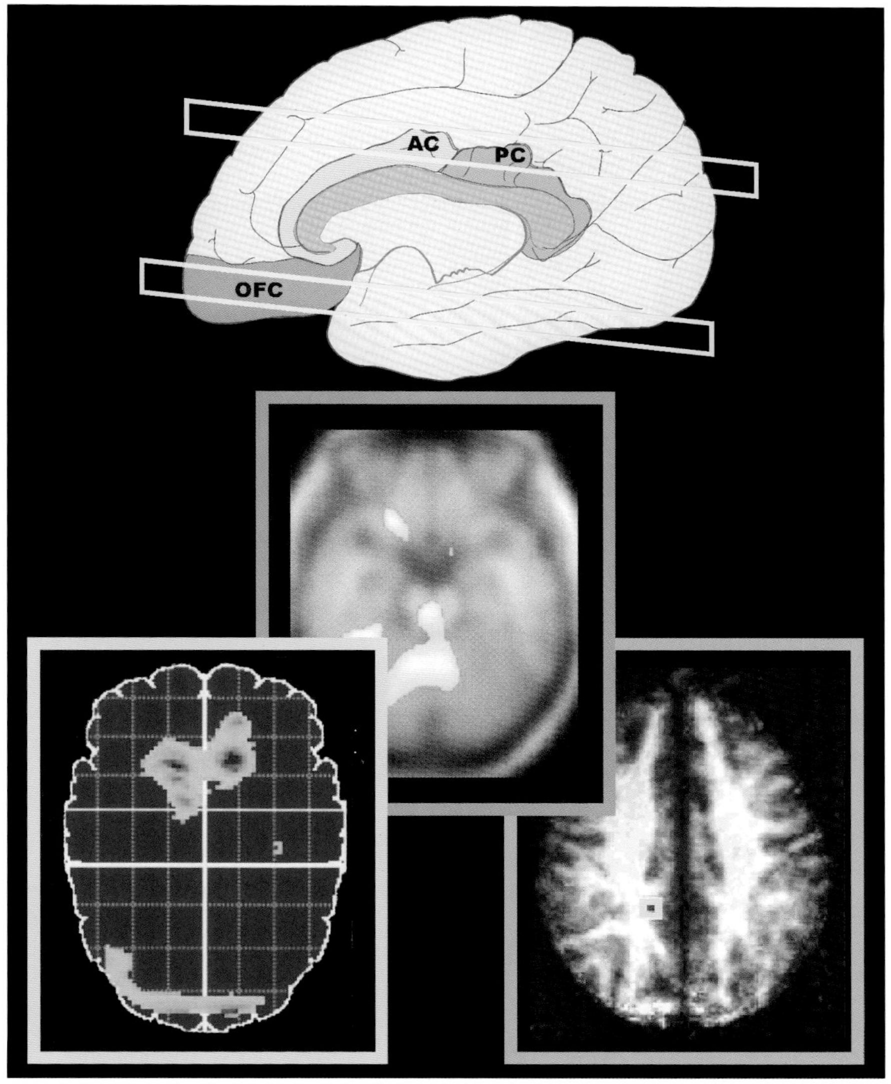

Axial sections show areas of importance in obsessive-compulsive disorder as revealed by different functional imaging techniques (see Figures 30–1 through 30–3 for details). Each panel is color-coded to the relevant brain region shown on the sagittal illustration of midline cortex (top): orbitofrontal cortex (OFC, *orange*), anterior cingulate cortex (AC, *green*), and posterior cingulate cortex (PC, *blue*). The approximate axial cuts are indicated in yellow on the sagittal illustration.

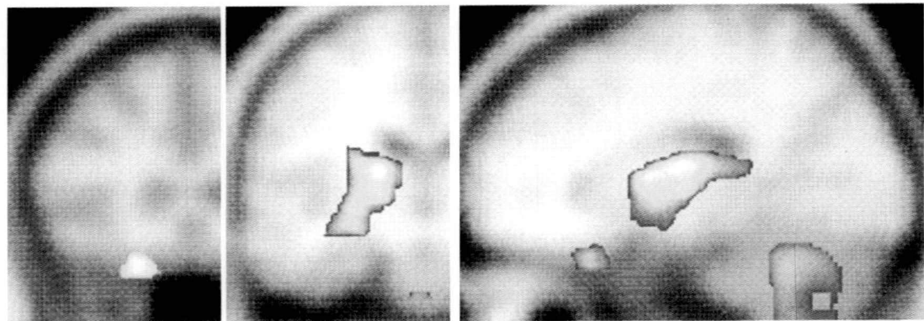

FIGURE 30–1. Retrospective analysis of pretreatment PET regional cerebral glucose uptake (rCMRglu) scans in OCD patients. Response of OCD to paroxetine was associated with higher pretreatment rCMRglu in the right caudate, whereas response to adjunctive risperidone in refractory patients was associated with higher pretreatment rCMRglu in right orbitofrontal cortex and bilateral thalamus, as indicated in color (*light yellow* is highest level of significance) on coronal (left, middle) and sagittal (right) magnetic resonance images.

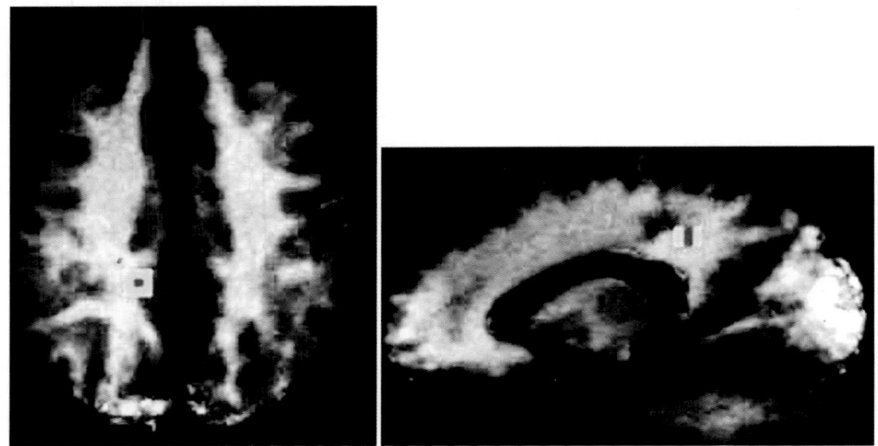

FIGURE 30–2. Retrospective analysis of preoperative PET regional cerebral glucose uptake (rCMRglu) scans in OCD patients prior to cingulotomy. A correlation analysis was performed between preoperative rCMRglu and improvement in postoperative Yale-Brown Obsessive Compulsive Scale score. The only area that was statistically significant was the posterior cingulate, in which higher preoperative rCMRglu was associated with greater postoperative improvement. This area is indicated on axial (left) and sagittal (right) magnetic resonance images. Reprinted with permission from Rauch et al.[21]

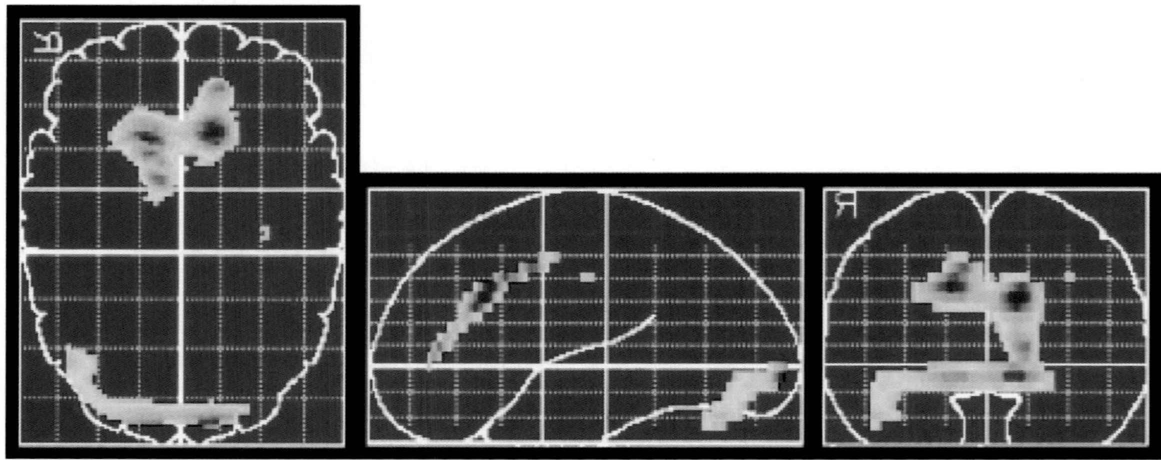

FIGURE 30–3. Retrospective analysis of pretreatment SPECT regional cerebral blood flow (rCBF) scans in OCD patients. Higher rCBF in anterior cingulate prior to treatment was found in medication responders, as indicated in color (*red* indicates highest level of difference) on axial (left), sagittal (middle), and coronal (right) brain templates. Reprinted with permission from Hoehn-Saric et al.[22]

"Possession" by evil spirits was once the diagnosis for those who were having obsessive ruminations about religion, sex, or other subjects that were intrusive or distressing. Although the concept of "possession" was dismissed long ago, modern medicine still does not have a complete understanding of what is now termed *obsessive-compulsive disorder* (OCD). This anxiety disorder is characterized by intrusive reoccurring thoughts or images that have such themes as danger, contamination, religion, sex, or symmetry. These thoughts are distressing to the sufferer and are recognized as irrational. To relieve anxiety associated with the thoughts, the obsessor often engages in compulsions or ritualistic actions. These include counting, checking, hand washing, and repetition of words, phrases, or other actions. Many good reviews of this disorder have been published to update clinicians on the latest theories of pathologic development, diagnosis, prognosis, and treatment strategies.[1–3] OCD has a worldwide prevalence of 2%–3% and a mean age at onset in the twenties to thirties, although it often arises in childhood.[4] It is a chronic disorder with many comorbid conditions. For example, two-thirds of OCD patients have major depressive disorder.

Many studies have been done to identify the neuroanatomical substrate of OCD. Much of this work has involved neuroimaging. Initial structural studies with computed tomography (CT) and magnetic resonance imaging (MRI) revealed a variety of volumetric or asymmetric changes in cortical and subcortical structures of OCD patients. The consistent theme was abnormalities in the circuits that include the orbitofrontal and anterior cingulate cortices, basal ganglia, and thalamus. Additional work with functional imaging has allowed a further refinement in the proposed abnormal circuitry, including increased activity in the excitatory or direct pathways as compared with the indirect or inhibitory pathways through the basal ganglia. Saxena et al.[5] have published an excellent review describing these pathways and the neuroimaging studies that led to the current neuroanatomical theory of OCD. They not only review the circuitry, but also update the four areas of imaging studies in OCD: studies comparing OCD patients and control subjects; studies of patients before and after treatment; studies provoking symptoms; and studies of cognitive activation. Theories to explain these circuit abnormalities include absence of normal developmental "pruning" during neuronal maturation, streptococcal infection, hypoxia to the striosomes of the striatum, and genetic abnormalities in enzyme and monoamine functions.[5,6]

Treatment is presently unpredictable, with most patients achieving only a partial response. The current standard of care is to offer behavioral psychotherapy and medication. The medications of choice are selective serotonin reuptake inhibitors (SSRIs), which allow 65%–70% of patients to attain a moderate (30%–60%) improvement in symptoms.[7] Psychosurgery (cingulotomy or capsulotomy) is done very infrequently to help the most severe nonresponders to all other therapeutic options. This treatment also provides only modest improvements.[3] It would clearly be immensely valuable to separate patients into more homogeneous groups in order to target treatment strategies. The literature relevant to prediction of treatment response is both promising and sparse. The varied approaches can be grouped into those focused on pretreatment symptoms, electrophysiological parameters, and functional brain imaging.

Prediction Based on Symptoms: Dimensional Model of OCD

An obvious hypothesis, given the extensive range of symptoms that may be present in OCD, is that the predominant symptoms displayed can be used to group patients into treatment categories. Most studies have approached this by categorizing patients into subgroups based on presence/absence of specific OCD symptoms, such as compulsions or cleaning rituals. This approach has not been particularly successful (see reviews[8,9]). A more promising approach applies factor analysis techniques to identify symptoms that are highly intercorrelated, thus collapsing many symptoms into a few symptom dimensions.[8–10] In the initial study, the many items in the Yale-Brown Obsessive Compulsive Scale symptom checklist were subsumed into three major dimensions: aggressive/sexual/religious; contamination; and symmetry/hoarding.[10] The symmetry/hoarding dimension correlated with comorbid Tourette's syndrome or chronic tic disorder, suggesting that this subgroup would benefit from neuroleptic medication. In the larger follow-up study, the number of dimensions was expanded to five: symmetry/ordering; hoarding; contamination/cleaning; aggressive/checking; and sexual/religious obsessions.[9] Not surprisingly, overall severity of symptoms prior to treatment was related to post-treatment severity of symptoms. In addition, higher scores on the hoarding dimension correlated with poorer response to SSRIs.

Prediction Based on Electrophysiological Measures

Both quantitative electroencephalography (qEEG) and event-related potential (ERP) studies have been done in the context of predicting treatment response in OCD.

In qEEG analyses, a mathematical method (the fast Fourier transform) is used to convert a block of EEG into a power spectrum so that concrete measures can be made. The power spectrum is split into standard frequency bands (delta, 1.5–3.5 Hz; theta, 3.5–7.5 Hz; alpha, 7.5–12.5 Hz; beta, 12.5–25 Hz) prior to measurement of absolute and relative power, mean frequency, and inter/intrahemispheric coherence/symmetry. In a pilot study, baseline (pretreatment) measures were compared for responders and nonresponders to medication (clomipramine or fluoxetine).[11] Responders showed increased power in the alpha and beta bands, particularly in frontal regions. Nonresponders showed decreased power in the delta band, particularly in the posterior regions. In a follow-up study, cluster analysis was used to identify subgroups.[12] Decreased power in the delta band was present in both subgroups of patients. Increased power in the theta band, particularly in anterior regions, defined patient group 1. Increased power in the alpha and beta bands, particularly in the anterior and central regions, defined patient group 2. Group 1 contained mostly nonresponders (71%), group 2 mostly responders (88%). These results were replicated in a larger study from the same group.[13] The authors note that SSRIs have been shown to decrease alpha activity. Thus, SSRIs may help normalize brain activity in responsive patients. On the basis of these findings, they suggest that OCD may include pathophysiologically different subgroups with a similar clinical expression.

ERPs are the summed electrical activity recorded from scalp electrodes following a stimulus presentation. A variety of situations or tasks are used in this type of study, and the ERP has a characteristic shape for each. A very simple task commonly used requires monitoring of a series of sounds (e.g., tones, words) and responding in some manner (e.g., pushing a button, keeping count) whenever a designated different sound is presented ("oddball" task). The different, rarely occurring, sound is the target. Early portions of the waveform are related to initial sensory reception and analysis of the stimulus. The subsequent N2 and P3 peaks relate to stimulus evaluation and perceptual synthesis.[14,15] In one set of studies, the latencies of the N2 and P3 peaks were shortened in patients who later responded well to SSRIs.[14,15] The amplitude of the N2 component may also be predictive of SSRI responsiveness, but in a complex manner. When simple sound stimuli (tones) were used, an increased N2 amplitude correlated with SSRI responsiveness.[16] When complex sound stimuli (words) were used, decreased N2 amplitude correlated with SSRI responsiveness.[14,15] Thus, both accelerated processing and abnormal stimulus evaluation in this task may identify OCD patients likely to respond well to SSRIs The authors note that these findings are consistent with the cortical hyperarousal model of OCD. These are promising results, but relatively few patients were studied, and the robustness and generalizability of the findings have not yet been demonstrated.

Prediction Based on Functional Brain Imaging

Two types of functional brain imaging have been used to study prediction of treatment response in OCD patients: positron emission tomography (PET) and single-photon emission computed tomography (SPECT). Functional imaging uses radioactive tracers followed by imaging to measure brain activity. All of the PET studies mentioned below used glucose utilization ([^{18}F]-fluorodeoxyglucose; FDG-PET) as their tool for examining brain function. The published SPECT study involved measurements of regional cerebral blood flow (rCBF) using [^{99m}Tc]HMPAO. In comparison with SPECT, PET has better spatial resolution, but it is more expensive and not widely available. Although together these studies are very few in number, complex, and expensive to undertake, the concepts studied are exciting and the results are encouraging.

PET Imaging

One of the first studies to look for predictors of treatment response used FDG-PET scans in 18 adults with childhood-onset OCD.[17] Patients who had pretreatment lower metabolic rates in the right orbitofrontal and right anterior cingulate cortices responded better initially to clomipramine (2 months of treatment). However, these measures were not predictive of good therapeutic response at 1 year.[18] Interestingly, good therapeutic response at 1 year correlated with pretreatment normalized rate of metabolism (region of interest divided by whole hemisphere) in the left caudate. However, on later follow-up scans, responders and nonresponders had similar left caudate metabolic rates. The authors noted uncertainty as to how this finding should be interpreted.

Brody et al.[19] performed FDG-PET before and after treatment in 27 patients diagnosed with OCD. Eighteen of the patients had chosen behavioral therapy, and nine had chosen fluoxetine treatment. Results were surprising. In the behavioral therapy group, patients with *higher* pretreatment normalized metabolism in left orbitofrontal cortex had a better response. In the medication group, patients with *lower* pretreatment normalized metabolism in left orbitofrontal cortex had a better response. The authors propose that the behavioral therapy results may be related to the orbitofrontal cortex function of mediating responses to situations where the "affective value" changes.

Behavioral therapy targets that assignment of value. Results for the fluoxetine group were similar to previous work in which higher orbitofrontal metabolism (although on the right rather than left) was associated with more severe illness and less robust response to medication.[18] One possible source of bias in this study is that the patients self-selected their therapy. A patient's biology may be associated with choice of treatment.

A follow-up study by the same group[20] examined changes in brain metabolism before and after paroxetine treatment. A secondary finding in this study is important to prediction of treatment response. Patients with lower normalized metabolism bilaterally in orbitofrontal cortex prior to treatment responded better to paroxetine. More specifically, the left posterior medial orbitofrontal cortex had the "strongest relationship" with better response. As noted by the authors, further work with large groups and placebo controls is needed. This group has also studied SSRI-refractory patients treated with adjunctive risperidone (S. Saxena, personal communication). Risperidone responders had higher pretreatment glucose metabolism in right posteromedial orbitofrontal cortex and bilateral thalamus (Figure 30–1). Lower pretreatment glucose metabolism in left parietal and bilateral dorsolateral prefrontal cortices, however, was also associated with better response. Thus, there may be different, and perhaps opposite, neurochemistries among patients who respond to atypical antipsychotics.

Another SSRI, fluvoxamine, has been used in a PET study to predict treatment response. Results are in press, but the authors refer to the outcome in another published article. In this work, an inverse correlation was found between rCBF in the orbitofrontal cortex and treatment response, as well as a direct relationship between rCBF in the posterior cingulate cortex and treatment response.[21]

One other area of PET prediction of treatment response has had a first examination. It is prediction of response to anterior cingulotomy. Rauch et al.[21] retrospectively examined the presurgical PET scans of 11 patients who underwent anterior cingulotomies for refractory severe OCD. Higher presurgical regional cerebral metabolic rates for glucose utilization within posterior cingulate cortex were associated with better postoperative improvement in symptoms (Figure 30–2). The authors suggest that this finding may be related to a direct influence of the posterior cingulate on orbitofrontal cortex and caudate, in addition to its influence on the anterior cingulate. As noted with other pretreatment studies, this one had limitations including small numbers, scans done during a resting state, and reliance on a linear model of evaluation that did not account for variables such as comorbid conditions and medication effects.

SPECT Imaging

In a recent double-blind trial of sertraline versus desipramine for patients with OCD and comorbid major depression, 11 of 16 participants were classified as OCD treatment responders.[22] In a retrospective examination of pretreatment scans, responders had higher rCBF in the orbitofrontal cortex (left>right), cingulate cortex, and basal ganglia than did nonresponders, irrespective of the medication used (Figure 30–3). The authors propose that "changes in cerebral activity correspond with changes in psychopathology rather than reflecting response-independent effects of treatment modalities." The study, however, had small numbers and all patients had comorbid major depression.

Although the data are not available in a PubMed-indexed journal, a recent SPECT study of 37 OCD patients was reported at the Seventh World Congress of Biological Psychiatry.[23] In this report, the presenter noted that the SSRI responders had greater pretreatment rCBF in the right caudate and lower rCBF in the anterior cingulate with symptom provocation.

Conclusion

Unlike many other neuropsychiatric disorders, OCD has reasonably well established circuitry. However, a substantial subset of OCD patients remain treatment refractory. As with most psychiatric conditions, there are no robust predictive tests to guide sequencing of treatment trials. Although traditionally considered a single diagnostic entity, OCD is now thought to be an etiologically and phenotypically diverse condition.[8] The heterogeneous nature of this severely disabling condition creates a substantial challenge. Pretreatment indicators of likely treatment response would therefore be immensely valuable.

Previous studies of treatment prediction have not separated patients according to subtypes of OCD. Many have not included patients with comorbid disorders, although these are common. The meaning and interpretation of these studies might be different if more homogeneous subgroups of patients were compared. The great variety of approaches that has been used creates another challenge, making comparisons across studies difficult. Most studies have used relatively small groups and most have not been independently replicated. All studies to date were retrospective rather than prospective. Functional imaging studies have not all measured the same areas of brain, further complicating comparisons across studies.

Even with these problems, the reported results suggest that particular patterns of pretreatment regional brain activity in OCD differentially predict treatment response (to behavioral therapy, SSRIs, adjunctive atypical antipsychotics, and neurosurgery). Prediction of treatment response based on pretreatment brain activity could become increasingly important in the future for understanding the mechanisms of treatment response. This opens the door to an exciting new prospect of being able to use functional testing to help guide treatment.

References

1. Allen A, Hollander E (eds): Obsessive-Compulsive Spectrum Disorders (special issue). Psychiatr Clin North Am 2000; 23:xv, 469–687
2. Neel JL, Stevens VM, Stewart JE: Obsessive-compulsive disorder: identification, neurobiology, and treatment. J Am Osteopath Assoc 2002; 102:81–86
3. Jenike MA: An update on obsessive-compulsive disorder. Bull Menninger Clin 2001; 65:4–25
4. Horwath E, Weissman MM: The epidemiology and cross-national presentation of obsessive-compulsive disorder. Psychiatr Clin North Am 2000; 23:493–507
5. Saxena S, Bota RG, Brody AL: Brain–behavior relationships in obsessive-compulsive disorder. Semin Clin Neuropsychiatry 2001; 6:82–101
6. Stein DJ: Advances in the neurobiology of obsessive-compulsive disorder: implications for conceptualizing putative obsessive-compulsive and spectrum disorders. Psychiatr Clin North Am 2000; 23:545–562
7. Hollander E, Kaplan A, Allen A, et al: Pharmacotherapy for obsessive-compulsive disorder. Psychiatr Clin North Am 2000; 23:643–656
8. Leckman JF, Grice DE, Boardman J, et al: Symptoms of obsessive-compulsive disorder. Am J Psychiatry 1997; 154:911–917
9. Mataix-Cols D, Rauch SL, Manzo PA, et al: Use of factor-analyzed symptom dimensions to predict outcome with serotonin reuptake inhibitors and placebo in the treatment of obsessive-compulsive disorder. Am J Psychiatry 1999; 156:1409–1416
10. Baer L: Factor analysis of symptom subtypes of obsessive compulsive disorder and their relation to personality and tic disorders. J Clin Psychiatry 1994; 55(suppl):18–23
11. Prichep LS, Mas F, John ER, et al: Neurometric subtyping of obsessive compulsive disorders in psychiatry: a world perspective, in Proceedings of the VIII World Congress of Psychiatry, Athens, October 12–19, 1989. Edited by Stefanis CN, Rabavilas AD, Soldatos CR. New York, Elsevier, 1989, pp 557–562
12. Mas F, Prichep LS, John ER, et al: Neurometric quantitative electroencephalogram subtyping of obsessive compulsive disorders, in Imaging of the Brain in Psychiatry and Related Fields, edited by Maurer K. Berlin-Heidelberg, Springer-Verlag, 1993, pp 277–280
13. Prichep LS, Mas F, Hollander E, et al: Quantitative electroencephalographic subtyping of obsessive-compulsive disorder. Psychiatry Research: Neuroimaging 1993; 50:25–32
14. Morault PM, Bourgeois M, Laville J, et al: Psychophysiological and clinical value of event-related potentials in obsessive-compulsive disorder. Biol Psychiatry 1997; 42:46–56
15. Morault P, Guillem F, Bourgeois M, et al: Improvement predictors in obsessive-compulsive disorder: an event-related potential study. Psychiatry Res 1998; 81:87–96
16. Towey J, Bruder G, Tenke C, et al: Event-related potential and clinical correlates of neurodysfunction in obsessive-compulsive disorder. Psychiatry Res 1993; 49:167–181
17. Swedo SE, Schapiro MB, Grady CL, et al: Cerebral glucose metabolism in childhood-onset obsessive-compulsive disorder. Arch Gen Psychiatry 1989; 46:518–523
18. Swedo SE, Pietrini P, Leonard HL, et al: Cerebral glucose metabolism in childhood-onset obsessive-compulsive disorder: revisualization during pharmacotherapy. Arch Gen Psychiatry 1992; 49:690–694
19. Brody AL, Saxena S, Schwartz JM, et al: FDG-PET predictors of response to behavioral therapy and pharmacotherapy in obsessive compulsive disorder. Psychiatry Research: Neuroimaging 1998; 84:1–6
20. Saxena S, Brody AL, Maidment KM, et al: Localized orbitofrontal and subcortical metabolic changes and predictors of response to paroxetine treatment in obsessive-compulsive disorder. Neuropsychopharmacology 1999; 21:683–693
21. Rauch SL, Dougherty DD, Cosgrove GR, et al: Cerebral metabolic correlates as potential predictors of response to anterior cingulotomy for obsessive compulsive disorder. Biol Psychiatry 2001; 50:659–667
22. Hoehn-Saric R, Schlaepfer TE, Greenberg BD, et al: Cerebral blood flow in obsessive-compulsive patients with major depression: effect of treatment with sertraline or desipramine on treatment responders and non-responders. Psychiatry Research: Neuroimaging 2001; 108:89–100
23. Sherman C: Brain studies predict OCD treatment response. Clinical Psychiatry News, Sept 2001, p 12. www.imng.com/IMNG/psyche/

Recent Publications of Interest

Evans KC, Dougherty DD, Pollack MH, et al: Using neuroimaging to predict treatment response in mood and anxiety disorders. Ann Clin Psychiatry 2006; 18:33–42

Provides an overview of the factors that must be considered when designing studies of treatment response, then summarizes the functional neuroimaging literature related to treatment prediction in depressive and anxiety disorders.

Mataix-Cols D: Deconstructing obsessive-compulsive disorder: a multidimensional perspective. Curr Opin Psychiatry 2006; 19:84–89

Summarizes the various approaches to dividing obsessive-compulsive disorder into more homogeneous groups based upon clinical characteristics and symptom clusters. A multidimensional model is suggested in which multiple overlapping syndromes may be present.

Denys D, de Geus F: Predictors of pharmacotherapy response in anxiety disorders. Curr Psychiatry Rep 2005; 7:252–257

Briefly summarizes the recent literature on predictors of response to pharmacotherapy in anxiety disorders (obsessive-compulsive disorder, social anxiety disorder, panic disorder, posttraumatic stress disorder).

Hollander E, Kaplan A, Schmeidler J, et al. Neurological soft signs as predictors of treatment response to selective serotonin reuptake inhibitors in obsessive-compulsive disorder. J Neuropsychiatry Clin Neurosci 2005; 17:472–477
Presents evidence of an association between neurological soft signs and treatment response to fluvoxamine in OCD patients.

Mergl R, Mavrogiorgou P, Juckel G, et al: Can a subgroup of OCD patients with motor abnormalities and poor therapeutic response be identified? Psychopharmacology (Berl) 2005; 179:826–837
Found that kinematical analysis of handwriting movements shows potential for the prediction of poor response to treatments in OCD patients.

Denys D, Burger H, van Megen H, et al: A score for predicting response to pharmacotherapy in obsessive-compulsive disorder. Int Clin Psychopharmacol 2003; 18:315–322
Summarized the literature on predictors of good and poor treatment response in OCD, and used the identified variables to prospectively identify independent predictors of response. A model is presented that can estimate the probability of treatment response to antidepressants.

Reprinted from Hurley RA, Saxena S, Rauch SL, et al: "Predicting Treatment Response in Obsessive-Compulsive Disorder." *Journal of Neuropsychiatry and Clinical Neurosciences* 14:249–253, 2002. Used with permission.

Chapter 31

SCHIZOPHRENIA

What's Under the Microscope?

KATHERINE H. TABER, PH.D.
DAVID A. LEWIS, M.D.
ROBIN A. HURLEY, M.D.

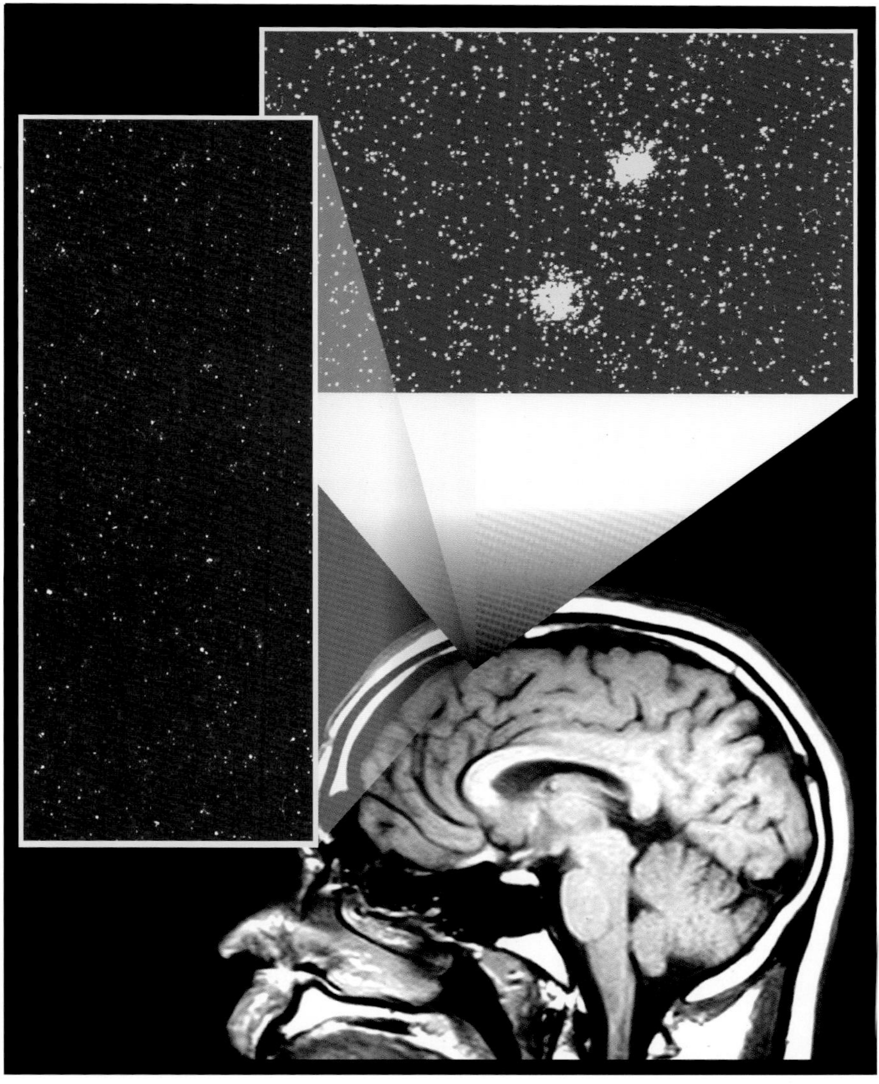

A sagittal magnetic resonance image of patient with chronic schizophrenia is overlaid with photomicrographs of dopamine transporter–labeled axons (left) and glutamic acid decarboxylase–positive neurons (top).

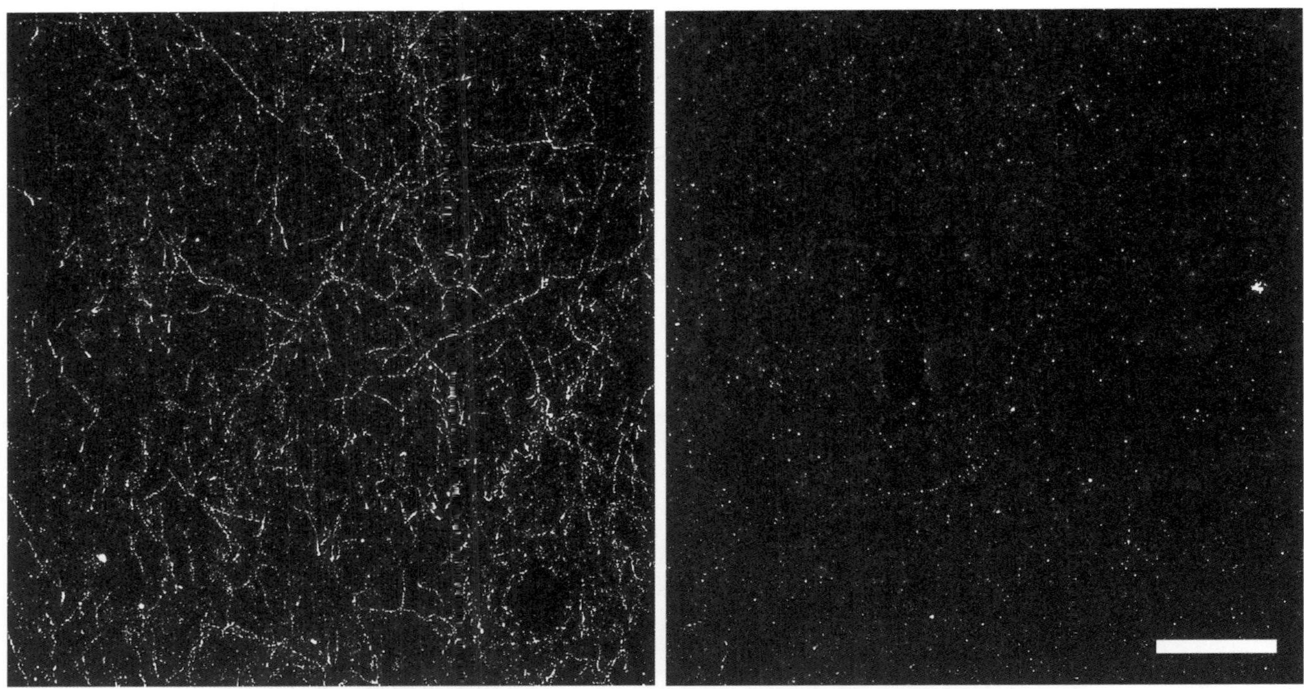

FIGURE 31–1. Darkfield photomicrograph of dopamine transporter–labeled axons in layer 6 of prefrontal cortex (area 9) from control (left) and schizophrenic (right) subjects (calibration bar=200 μm). Note the clearly diminished density of dopamine axons in the schizophrenic subject. Adapted from Akil et al.[1] Copyright © 1999, American Psychiatric Association.

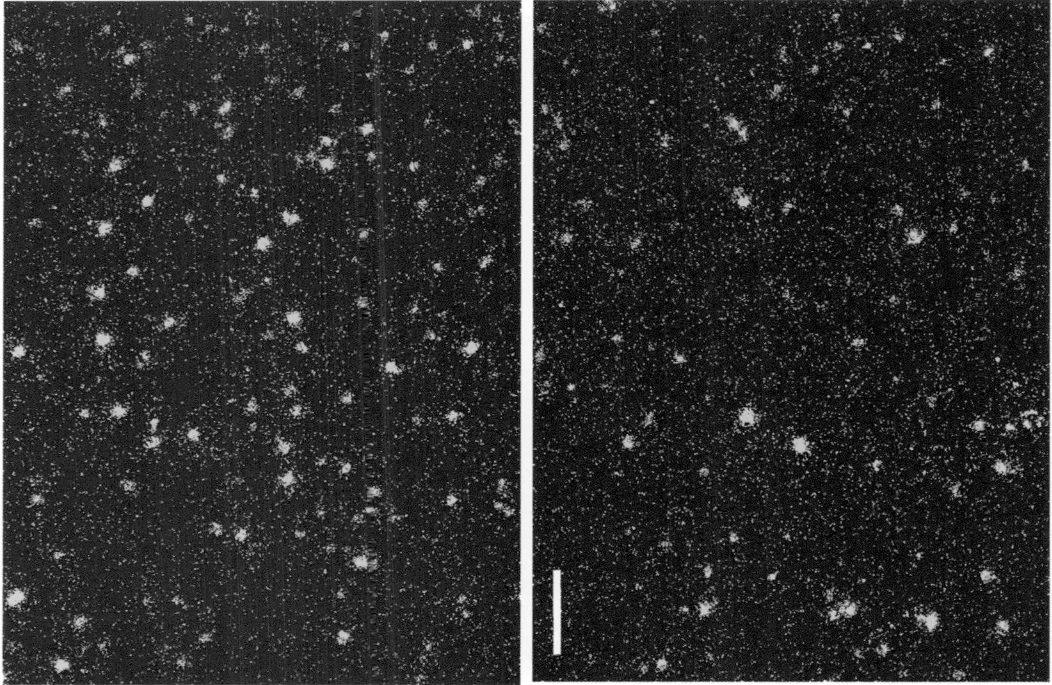

FIGURE 31–2. Darkfield photomicrographs of the glutamic acid decarboxylase (GAD) mRNA-positive neurons in deep layer 3 of prefrontal cortex (area 9) from control (left) and schizophrenic (right) subjects (calibration bar=150 μm). Note the reduction in labeled GABAergic neurons in the schizophrenic subject. Adapted from Volk et al.[2] Copyright © 2000, American Medical Association. All rights reserved.

Dementia praecox, as formally described by Emil Kraepelin in 1898, is a devastating illness affecting every aspect of life for the patient and the patient's family. Over the past century, theories of the cause of schizophrenia have ranged from original sin to in utero viral infection. Heritability patterns support a strong genetic component, yet other factors are clearly involved. Schizophrenia, as this illness is now known, affects 1% of the population worldwide. In 1990, the socioeconomic impact of schizophrenia in the United States alone was $32.5 billion. These patients accounted for 25% of all hospital admissions and occupied 40% of all long-term care beds.[3,4]

A vital part of fully understanding an illness is identification of the underlying pathology. Initially the search for the biologic basis of schizophrenia focused on changes in gross brain structure (macroscopic neuropathology). Volumetric studies undertaken in recent decades comparing normal subjects and individuals with schizophrenia have shown considerable variability in results.[5,6] There is a consensus that the ventricles are commonly enlarged. More subtle abnormalities have been reported for many areas, including prefrontal cortex, basal ganglia, thalamus, and hippocampus, but specific claims are controversial. No single brain region is consistently abnormal in schizophrenia, and no pattern of gross brain abnormalities has been identified that is diagnostic of schizophrenia (see image at opening to this chapter for a sagittal T_1-weighted magnetic resonance image of a 31-year-old male with chronic paranoid schizophrenia). It may well be, as suggested recently, that schizophrenia results from "the cumulative effect of deviant brain structure."[7] Thus, schizophrenia may be the functional end result of various combinations of brain abnormalities. More recently the focus has shifted to seeking the abnormal brain circuits that could account for the symptoms of schizophrenia. This approach requires measures that can be related to how brain regions function together as parts of the circuits that support complex cognitive functions. Widespread functional circuits can be studied by detailed examination of individual areas and by global examination of entire networks.

Many studies focus on the fine structure (microscopic neuropathology) of brain areas implicated in schizophrenia. Significant decreases in neuronal numbers have been found in the medial dorsal and anterior nuclei of the thalamus (parts of the thalamus with intimate connections to prefrontal and limbic areas) and in the nucleus accumbens (part of the basal forebrain).[8] In the anterior nucleus of the thalamus, the reductions are in projection neurons rather than interneurons, suggesting a decrease in thalamocortical transmission.[9] Some studies have also reported decreased neuronal numbers in the cingulate cortex, which is reciprocally connected to these thalamic nuclei.[10] Most studies have not found decreased numbers of projection neurons (pyramidal cells) in the other major connection area considered important in schizophrenia, prefrontal cortex.[11] More subtle differences may exist between individuals with schizophrenia and normal subjects in this area. For instance, several lines of evidence, including those involving increased neuronal density and decreased presynaptic proteins (i.e., synaptophysin), are consistent with a decrease in the density of synapses in prefrontal cortex.[12]

Alterations have been reported in several neurotransmitter systems in this illness. Immunoreactivity for tyrosine hydroxylase—which is known to mark dopamine (DA)-containing axons—and immunoreactivity for the DA membrane transporter are both decreased in prefrontal cortex (see Figure 31–1).[1] Several measures of the γ-aminobutyric acid (GABA) system are altered in prefrontal cortex, as well. There may be a decrease in inhibitory (GABAergic) interneurons.[11,13] The tissue content of GABA and the cellular expression of the mRNA for the GABA transporter and for glutamic acid decarboxylase (synthetic enzyme for GABA; see Figure 31–2) are all decreased.[2,14] In contrast, cellular expression of the mRNA for the $GABA_A$ receptor is increased.[14] These changes may be concentrated in a specific subgroup of GABAergic interneurons (chandelier neurons) that provide inhibitory input to the axon initial segment of pyramidal cells, thus exerting control over the excitatory output of the prefrontal cortex.[15] Studies of the serotonin (5-HT) system have mixed findings. Postmortem studies have found increased 5-HT receptor density in several cortical areas, including prefrontal and temporal.[16] On the other hand, labeling of axons immunoreactive to the serotonin transporter was unchanged in prefrontal cortex.[1] The glutamate system has been studied less than other neurotransmitters, but there is evidence for altered expression of some receptor subtypes in hippocampus and some areas of cortex.[17]

Functional brain imaging is another way of examining neurochemistry. Initial studies focused on imaging DA receptors because the first successful pharmacologic treatment for schizophrenia acted by blockade of DA D_2 receptors.[16] In addition, amphetamines, which can produce a state similar to paranoid schizophrenia, act by increasing presynaptic DA release and inhibiting uptake.[18] These findings led to the development of the "dopamine hypothesis" of schizophrenia, in which the symptoms were attributed to excessive DA activity. Many, but not all, patients with schizophrenia have increased D_2 receptor density in the striatum. Synaptic concentrations of DA may also be greater in schizophrenia. Dopaminergic responsiveness may also be increased, as indicated by a greater amphetamine-induced release of DA in the striatum. Studies have concentrated on striatum because of its high concentration of DA receptors. The low density of D_2 receptors in other areas of brain has precluded their study in vivo, although newly developed ligands may change this in the future.[16]

The atypical antipsychotics act powerfully on other neurotransmitter systems in addition to DA. In particular, they are potent 5-HT receptor antagonists.[19] The balance between 5-HT and DA antagonism may be critical to the lower rate of side effects with these agents.[20] Although changes in 5-HT receptor density have been found in postmortem studies of brains from individuals with schizophrenia, two in vivo studies (measuring fluorine-18-labeled setoperone binding) did not find any difference.[16] Similarly, in vivo studies of GABA receptor density have not found any abnormalities in individuals with schizophrenia, although alterations have been reported in postmortem studies.[16] The basis for this divergence of findings has not yet been established.

Functional imaging can also indirectly observe summed synaptic activity, as mirrored in the metabolic demand of an area. There is sufficient anatomic resolution to observe functional subregions of the brain and thus gain insight into interacting circuits. Many studies have found a decrease in resting metabolism (as measured by regional cerebral blood flow or glucose metabolism) in areas of prefrontal cortex in schizophrenia.[21,22] This hypofrontality is most closely associated with the negative symptoms of schizophrenia. Prefrontal cortex is made up of many functional areas, and it is clear that areas of increased and decreased metabolism coexist within individuals, indicating the importance of looking at subregions rather than prefrontal cortex in totality.[22] Many other brain regions also show altered resting metabolism, including portions of anterior cingulate, temporal and parietal cortices, striatum, thalamus, and cerebellum.[21,22] Correlation analysis has been used to examine functional relationships among many of these areas. The strength of correlation between frontal cortex and related regions is decreased in schizophrenia, suggesting changes in functional connectivity.[21] Alterations in neuronal numbers, in the density of synaptic proteins (and therefore of synapses), in the density of transporters for neurotransmitters, and in their synthetic enzymes, found with micropathological studies, all may underlie the findings of changes in connectivity from functional brain imaging studies.

Even more informative, from the perspective of treatment, are the studies examining the effects of antipsychotic agents on regional brain metabolism. Medication-related increases in striatal metabolism have been found by several groups. It has been suggested that this is a "normalization" of function. A low resting striatal metabolic rate may even be predictive of good medication response.[21] Similarly, medication-induced increased metabolic rate in striatal areas (caudate, globus pallidus) may predict development of tardive dyskinesia. Regional patterns of antipsychotic-induced metabolic changes vary with the agent. It is possible that careful systematic studies relating these differences to individual patients' medication response may provide a means of predicting responders and nonresponders in future.

In recent years the original DA hypothesis of schizophrenia has been transformed as understanding of interactions among neurotransmitter systems has evolved. It has become evident that considering the DA system in isolation does not provide a full picture of schizophrenia. Many new formulations have been suggested that incorporate other neurotransmitter systems in a wide variety of ways.[15,20,23–26] Some emphasize the interactions between DA and 5-HT, others the interactions between DA and glutamate. GABA is central in some theories, glutamate in others. Most of these theories involve multiple brain areas, although not necessarily the same areas.

A core similarity among these diverse approaches to understanding schizophrenia is an incorporation of the very complex interactions that exist among neurotransmitter systems at the level of individual synapses and at the level of interconnected brain regions. As a result of this wider view, new medications are being developed that target more neurotransmitter systems and different receptor subtypes than previously. Their success or failure will provide valuable insight into the pathophysiology of schizophrenia, as well as a source for new therapeutic agents.

References

1. Akil M, Pierri JN, Whitehead RE, et al: Lamina-specific alterations in the dopamine innervation of the prefrontal cortex in schizophrenic subjects. Am J Psychiatry 1999; 156:1580–1589
2. Volk DW, Austin MC, Pierri JN, et al: Decreased glutamic acid decarboxylase$_{67}$ messenger RNA expression in a subset of prefrontal cortical gamma-aminobutyric acid neurons in subjects with schizophrenia. Arch Gen Psychiatry 2000; 57:237–245
3. Pickar D: Prospects for pharmacotherapy of schizophrenia. Lancet 1995; 345:557–562
4. Rice DP: The economic impact of schizophrenia. J Clin Psychiatry 1999; 60 (suppl 1):4–6; discussion 28–30
5. McCarley RW, Wible CG, Frumin M, et al: MRI anatomy of schizophrenia. Biol Psychiatry 1999; 45:1099–1119
6. Pearlson GD, Marsh L: Structural brain imaging in schizophrenia: a selective review. Biol Psychiatry 1999; 46:627–649
7. Leonard CM, Kuldau JM, Breier JI, et al: Cumulative effect of anatomical risk factors for schizophrenia: an MRI study. Biol Psychiatry 1999; 46:374–382

8. Danos P, Baumann B, Bernstein HG, et al: Schizophrenia and anteroventral thalamic nucleus: selective decrease of parvalbumin-immunoreactive thalamocortical projection neurons. Psychiatry Res 1998; 82:1–10
9. Dixon G, Dissanaike S, Harper CG: Parvalbumin-immunoreactive neurons in the human anteroventral thalamic nucleus. Neuroreport 2000; 11:97–101
10. Benes FM: Emerging principles of altered neural circuitry in schizophrenia. Brain Res Brain Res Rev 2000; 31:251–269
11. Thune JJ, Pakkenberg B: Stereological studies of the schizophrenic brain. Brain Res Brain Res Rev 2000; 31:200–204
12. Honer WG, Falkai P, Chen C, et al: Synaptic and plasticity-associated proteins in anterior frontal cortex in severe mental illness. Neuroscience 1999; 91:1247–1255
13. Beasley CL, Reynolds GP: Parvalbumin-immunoreactive neurons are reduced in the prefrontal cortex of schizophrenics. Schizophr Res 1997; 24:349–355
14. Ohnuma T, Augood SJ, Arai H, et al: Measurement of GABAergic parameters in the prefrontal cortex in schizophrenia: focus on GABA content, GABA(A) receptor alpha-1 subunit messenger RNA and human GABA transporter-1 (HGAT-1) messenger RNA expression. Neuroscience 1999; 93:441–448
15. Pierri JN, Chaudry AS, Woo TU, et al: Alterations in chandelier neuron axon terminals in the prefrontal cortex of schizophrenic subjects. Am J Psychiatry 1999; 156:1709–1719
16. Soares JC, Innis RB: Neurochemical brain imaging investigations of schizophrenia. Biol Psychiatry 1999; 46:600–615
17. Meador-Woodruff JH, Healy DJ: Glutamate receptor expression in schizophrenic brain. Brain Res Brain Res Rev 2000; 31:288–294
18. Vollenweider FX: Advances and pathophysiological models of hallucinogenic drug actions in humans: a preamble to schizophrenia research. Pharmacopsychiatry 1998; 31(suppl):92–103
19. Ichikawa J, Meltzer HY: Relationship between dopaminergic and serotonergic neuronal activity in the frontal cortex and the action of typical and atypical antipsychotic drugs. Eur Arch Psychiatry Clin Neurosci 1999; 249(suppl):90–98
20. Kasper S, Tauscher J, Kufferle B, et al: Dopamine- and serotonin-receptors in schizophrenia: results of imaging-studies and implications for pharmacotherapy in schizophrenia. Eur Arch Psychiatry Clin Neurosci 1999; 249(suppl):83–89
21. Buchsbaum MS, Hazlett EA: Positron emission tomography studies of abnormal glucose metabolism in schizophrenia. Schizophr Bull 1998; 24:343–364
22. Kim JJ, Mohamed S, Andreasen NC, et al: Regional neural dysfunctions in chronic schizophrenia studied with positron emission tomography. Am J Psychiatry 2000; 157:542–548
23. Carlsson A, Waters N, Carlsson ML: Neurotransmitter interactions in schizophrenia—therapeutic implications. Eur Arch Psychiatry Clin Neurosci 1999; 249(suppl):37–43
24. Moore H, West AR, Grace AA: The regulation of forebrain dopamine transmission: relevance to the pathophysiology and psychopathology of schizophrenia. Biol Psychiatry 1999; 46:40–55
25. Olney JW, Newcomer JW, Farber NB: NMDA receptor hypofunction model of schizophrenia. J Psychiatr Res 1999; 33: 523–533
26. Aghajanian GK, Marek GJ: Serotonin model of schizophrenia: emerging role of glutamate mechanisms. Brain Res Brain Res Rev 2000; 31:302–312

Recent Publications of Interest

Carlsson A: The neurochemical circuitry of schizophrenia. Pharmacopsychiatry 2006; 39:S10–S14
Describes the basic neuronal circuits that are thought to underlie the generation of symptoms in schizophrenia, and the roles of various neurotransmitters. The importance of the balance between inhibition and excitation is emphasized.

Winterer G: Cortical microcircuits in schizophrenia—the dopamine hypotheses revisited. Pharmacopsychiatry 2006; 39:S68–S71
Presents the evidence from recent studies that supports a critical role for cortical dopamine circuits in the pathophysiology of schizophrenia.

Scherk H, Falkai P: Effects of antipsychotics on brain structure. Curr Opin Psychiatry 2006; 19:145–150
Summarizes recent studies on the effects of typical and atypical antipsychotics on brain structure, which suggest that atypical antipsychotics may ameliorate structural changes in the brain caused by the disease process underlying schizophrenia.

Abbott C, Bustillo J: What have we learned from proton magnetic resonance spectroscopy about schizophrenia? A critical update. Curr Opin Psychiatry 2006; 19:135–139
Provides an overview of studies utilizing proton magnetic resonance spectroscopy to investigate schizophrenia.

Lewis DA, Hashimoto T, Volk DW: Cortical inhibitory neurons and schizophrenia. Nat Rev Neurosci 2005; 6:312–324
Reviews the evidence that specific cognitive deficits in schizophrenia may reflect alterations in cortical inhibitory circuits arising from specific pathogenetic processes that have implications for therapeutic interventions.

Reprinted from Taber KH, Lewis DA, Hurley RA: "Schizophrenia: What's Under the Microscope?" *Journal of Neuropsychiatry and Clinical Neurosciences* 13:1–4, 2001. Used with permission.

Chapter 32

Surgical Treatment of Mental Illness

Impact of Imaging

Robin A. Hurley, M.D.
Deborah N. Black, M.D.
Emmanuel Stip, M.D.
Katherine H. Taber, Ph.D.

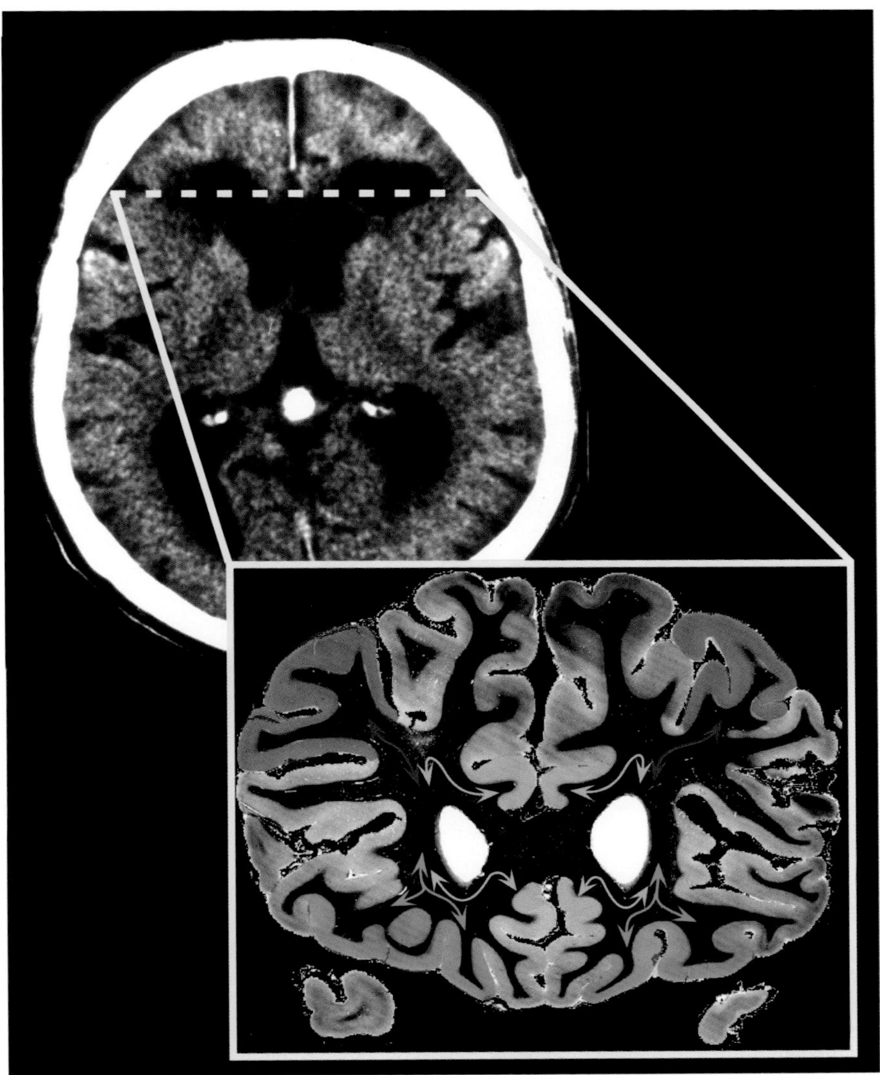

An axial (CT) scan from a patient who underwent frontal leukotomy (top left) shows massive damage to the anterior parts of the brain. A coronal myelin-stained brain section from a normal individual is color-coded with the locations for the three major prefrontal cortical circuits: orbitofrontal (*blue*); dorsolateral (*pink*); anterior cingulate (*green*). The approximate anterior-posterior location of the coronal section is indicated by the dashed line on the axial section. Note that connections from all three circuits may have been damaged in this patient.

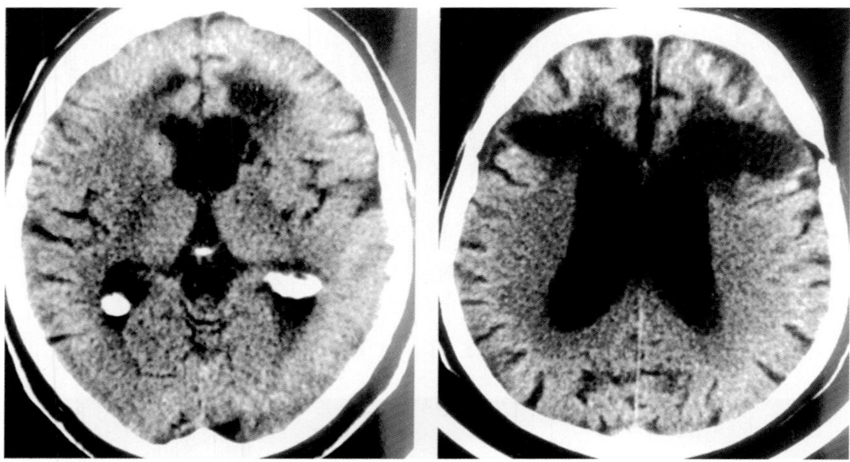

FIGURE 32–1. Axial CT scans from two patients who underwent frontal leukotomy (transection of the fiber tracts leading from the frontal gray matter) are shown (a third case is shown in the image at the opening of this chapter). Early surgeries were necessarily performed freehand, resulting in considerable variability in actual lesion location and size. Note the dramatic differences among these three cases.

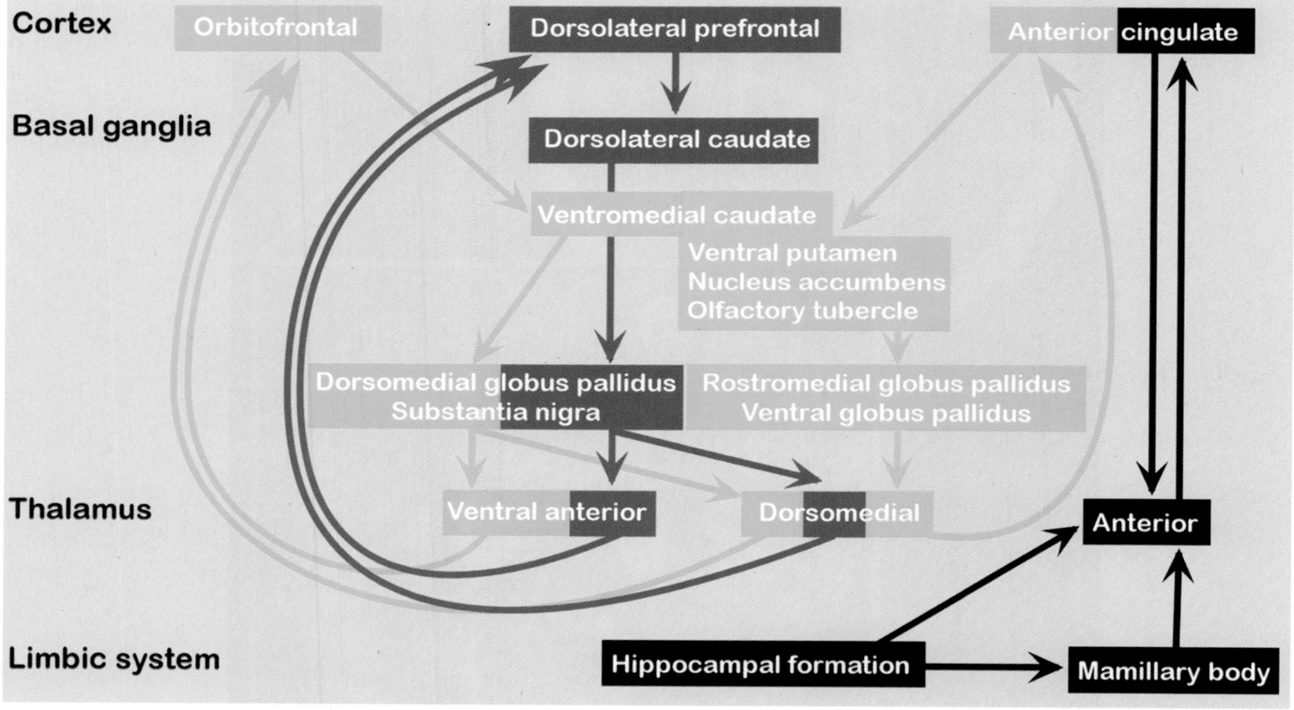

FIGURE 32–2. The original emotion and memory circuit proposed by Papez is diagrammed above in *black*. Current theories emphasize the presence of parallel processing of different aspects of behavior. The orbitofrontal circuit is thought to mediate socially appropriate behavior, impulse control, and empathy (*blue*). The dorsolateral circuit is thought to accomplish organization, planning, and attention (*pink*). The anterior cingulate circuit is thought to produce motivation by balancing the inhibitory input of the supplemental motor area with its own stimulus that supports wakefulness and arousal (*green*). The three circuits are color-coded at the level of the leukotomy on a coronal myelin-stained brain slice in the image at the opening to this chapter. Note that these pathways run close together. Subcortical injury is likely to affect more than one.

The accidental brain injury suffered by Phineas Gage in 1848 planted the seeds for a later formulation of the influence of the frontal lobes on personality and behavior. In the late 19th century, personality changes were also seen in patients following resection of frontal lobe tumors. Early studies correlating frontal lobe lesions (resulting from head wounds sustained in World War I) and changes in personality, affect, and behavior added to the preliminary theories of frontal lobe function. This knowledge was expanded with experimental studies in primates.[1,2] Since then, intensive study of both brain-injured patients and animals has broadened and deepened our understanding of the brain circuits that underlie many aspects of normal cognition and personality, as well as mental illnesses.

The application of the neurosurgical approach to treatment of mental illness began in earnest with Moniz in 1936. He was convinced that lesions in the frontal lobes, by interrupting the fibers connecting the frontal lobes with other brain regions, would provide relief from the devastating symptoms of severe mental illness. His work came at a time in which the only treatments available for mental illness (other than heavy sedation or physical restraint) were hydrotherapy or convulsive treatment (by induction of hypoglycemic coma or metrazol seizures). Although these somatic therapies were sometimes effective, the remission of symptoms was usually transitory. The possibility of a treatment approach that could provide more permanent relief was thus of great interest, although it was recognized early on that there was a high likelihood of unwanted personality changes.

Surgical treatment of mental illness was prevalent prior to the development of antipsychotic medications in the 1950s. The white matter connecting the orbitofrontal and/or cingulate cortices with other cortical and subcortical structures was a common surgical target. The choice of this target was not primarily based on knowledge of the underlying brain circuits, but rather was based on symptom relief and better surgical outcome. Thus, surgical treatment brought passivity and apathy in many cases where before there were agony and aggression. It was also recognized from tumor surgeries that white matter lesions bled less than gray matter and had fewer postoperative complications.

During this early period, surgery was necessarily performed freehand, resulting in considerable variability in actual lesion location and size (see Figure 32–1) as well as surgical complications. Although therapeutic improvements were reported in many patients, there were also clear changes in personality and drive. Little was done to correlate lesion size and/or location with therapeutic effect. Such studies were difficult because the areas affected could only be assessed postmortem. Limited autopsy studies from 1947 to 1950 documented great differences in the lesions.[2] The refinement of lesion size and placement was then attempted, based on experimental studies in primates, in an effort to diminish the occurrence of personality changes (still without a cohesive knowledge of circuitry). For a more complete account of the history of neurosurgical treatment of mental illness in the early years, see Dorman[1] or Swayze.[2]

Parallel to this era, a better understanding of brain circuitry was taking form. Near the turn of the century, Eduard Hitzig had proposed the concept of cortical localization and the motor cortex from his work with voltage studies in canine brains. After getting no motor response from frontal lobe stimulation, Hitzig deduced that "the frontal lobes have abstract thought."[1] Papez formally introduced the idea of the limbic circuit in 1937, naming specific brain structures associated with emotion and memory (see Figure 32–2). This initial circuit was expanded by McLean in 1952 to include, notably, the frontal and temporal lobes.[3] The concept of specific brain circuits mediating cognition, emotion, and memory gained wide acceptance in neuropsychiatry. As the 20th century passed, knowledge of these circuits greatly expanded—as did their clinical applications. Later refinements emphasized the presence of parallel processing of different aspects of behavior (see Figure 32–2).

Development of pathophysiologic models of psychiatric disease has been greatly enhanced by the explosive increase in the techniques available to study the living brain that has occurred during the past three decades. Improvements in our understanding of the functional circuitry underlying both normal cognitive functions and mental illness have benefited enormously from the availability of methods for probing, in vivo, both structure (computed tomography [CT], magnetic resonance imaging [MRI]) and function (positron emission tomography [PET], single-photon emission computed tomography [SPECT], functional magnetic resonance imaging [fMRI], magnetoencephalography [MEG], tomographic electroencephalography [tEEG]).

Just as these imaging techniques expanded the knowledge of normal circuitry and pathophysiology, so did they influence treatment of disease.

Surgical treatment of mental illness is critically dependent upon a solid understanding of these circuits and the locations of the pathways connecting them.[4–7] Currently neurosurgery for mental illnesses is done, very infrequently, in expert centers for intractable mood or anxiety disorders. However, all stages of this treatment have benefited from these new imaging techniques. Imaging now allows preoperative localization of target areas at high resolution and has improved the placement of lesions significantly.[8,9]

Although primarily used for treatment of "neurological" conditions (e.g., intractable Parkinson's disease, central pain, uncontrollable seizures), stereotactic planning with MRI or CT is done to localize the exact target for radiofrequency lesions with electrodes in cingulctomies (accurate within 1–3 mm).[5] Oblique coronal T_1-weighted magnetic resonance images currently are done, as well as the traditional sagittal T_1-weighted images.[10] MRI localization is also used for anterior capsulotomy for intractable obsessive-compulsive disorder.[11]

There are reports that now address the three-dimensional differences in target localization between CT and MRI, as well as which MRI sequence is best for visualizing small anatomical landmarks needed for stereotactic planning.[8,9,12] CT is less prone to image distortion but has lower anatomic resolution. MRI provides much better visualization of anatomy, although image distortion may be present, which is highly dependent on scanner and pulse sequence. Overall, the accuracy of stereotactic localizations with CT and MRI appears to be equivalent.[12,13] The greater anatomic resolution of MRI is now being exploited to provide direct visualization of target structures. For example, a heavily T_1-weighted fast spin echo inversion recovery MRI sequence (FSE-IR) has been used to directly localize the internal globus pallidus.[9] This approach allows individual variations in anatomy to be taken into account in surgical planning, something not possible with the previously used gradient echo sequence—thus allowing more accurate ablation of the internal globus pallidus in intractable Parkinson's disease. The FSE-IR images are acquired in both the axial and coronal planes of section, providing localization of the target in all three dimensions.[8,9]

Postoperatively, imaging has an important role in many arenas. The gross extent and location of ablation can be easily evaluated by using CT or (preferably) MRI. Studies correlating lesion location and size with differential outcome are beginning to provide valuable insights. For instance, there is an ongoing controversy as to whether cingulotomy or anterior capsulotomy provides better symptom resolution in obsessive-compulsive disorder patients.[10,14,15] In the immediate postoperative period (first few months), fatigue and loss of initiative and mental drive have been correlated with MRI-based visualization of edema surrounding the lesion site.[11] In addition, imaging allows postoperative comparison of different surgical techniques (e.g., thermocapsulotomy with electrodes versus gamma capsulotomy with irradiation; thermocontrolled electrocoagulation versus radioactive yttrium-induced lesions).[11,16]

Remote changes and degeneration of major pathways subsequent to surgical intervention can also be studied by using standard clinical MRI.[17–19] In addition, newer MRI techniques such as magnetization transfer (MT) and diffusion tensor imaging (DTI) may provide more sensitive ways to study these changes, allowing a more accurate delineation of the pathways disrupted by the lesion.[20–22] MT imaging is sensitive to interactions between free protons (unbound water in tissue) and bound protons (water bound to macromolecules such as those in myelin membranes). The amount of MT correlates with the degree of myelination. Thus, MT imaging is a promising method for studying both normal development and injury-induced pathway degeneration.[20,23,24] DTI is a more complicated version of diffusion-weighted (DW) MRI. DW MRI is sensitive to the speed of water diffusion. In DTI, a set of at least six DW images is collected, each sensitized to a different anatomic direction. From this set of images several measures can be derived, including the principal direction of diffusion within each voxel of the image. Diffusion within white matter occurs much faster along the length of axons than transaxonally, so the principal direction of diffusion within white matter reflects the average direction of the fibers and may be useful in tracing pathways.[21] In areas of pathway degeneration this directionality is diminished or lost.[22] The greater sensitivity of these methods to injury-related changes may well provide a better correlation with differential outcome.[23,24]

Metabolic imaging provides a way to ascertain functional alterations remote from the lesion site. Only a few studies have been done comparing metabolic measures before and after surgery.[25,26] A case report of bifrontal leukotomy for refractory obsessive-compulsive disorder found that regional glucose metabolism (as measured by PET) was decreased toward normal in the orbital frontal cortex in concert with clinical improvement. Another study reported a correlation between symptom reduction and decreased cerebral blood flow (as measured by SPECT) in anterior frontal and cingulate cortex following subcaudate tractotomy for refractory depression. These findings are consistent with the present understanding of the brain circuits involved.

Imaging has changed the face of neurosurgical interventions for psychiatric diseases. It has made possible refined and carefully controlled procedures. The future holds yet more promise with the applications of functional MRI and other techniques such as three-dimensional spiral CT and intraoperative MRI.[27–29] Ultimately these should lead to better treatments for severe and intractable mood and anxiety disorders.

References

1. Dorman J: The history of psychosurgery. Tex Med 1995; 91:54–61
2. Swayze VW: Frontal leukotomy and related psychosurgical procedures in the era before antipsychotics (1935–1954): a historical overview. Am J Psychiatry 1995; 152:505–515
3. Cosgrove GR, Rauch SL: Psychosurgery. Neurosurg Clin N Am 1995; 6:167–176
4. Trivedi MH: Functional neuroanatomy of obsessive-compulsive disorder. J Clin Psychiatry 1996; 57(suppl):26–35
5. Marino R Jr, Cosgrove GR: Neurosurgical treatment of neuropsychiatric illness. Psychiatr Clin North Am 1997; 20:933–943
6. Trimble MR, Mendez MF, Cummings JL: Neuropsychiatric symptoms from the temporolimbic lobes. J Neuropsychiatry Clin Neurosci 1997; 9:429–438
7. Burruss JW, Hurley RA, Taber KH, et al: Functional neuroanatomy of the frontal lobe circuits. Radiology 2000; 214:227–230
8. Starr PA, Vitek JL, DeLong M, et al: Magnetic resonance imaging-based stereotactic localization of the globus pallidus and subthalamic nucleus. Neurosurgery 1999; 44:303–313
9. Reich CA, Hudgins PA, Sheppard SK, et al: A high-resolution fast spin-echo inversion-recovery sequence for preoperative localization of the internal globus pallidus. AJNR Am J Neuroradiol 2000; 21:928–931
10. Spangler WJ, Cosgrove GR, Ballantine HT Jr, et al: Magnetic resonance image–guided stereotactic cingulotomy for intractable psychiatric disease. Neurosurgery 1996; 38:1071–1076
11. Mindus P, Rasmussen SA, Lindquist C: Neurosurgical treatment for refractory obsessive-compulsive disorder: implications for understanding frontal lobe function. J Neuropsychiatry Clin Neurosci 1994; 6:467–477
12. Holtzheimer PE, Roberts DW, Darcey TM: Magnetic resonance imaging versus computed tomography for target localization in functional stereotactic neurosurgery. Neurosurgery 1999; 45:290–297
13. Bednarz G, Downes MB, Corn BW, et al: Evaluation of the spatial accuracy of magnetic resonance imaging–based stereotactic target localization for gamma knife radiosurgery of functional disorders. Neurosurgery 1999; 45:1156–1161
14. Sachdev P, Hay P: Site and size of lesion and psychosurgical outcome in obsessive-compulsive disorder: a magnetic resonance imaging study. Biol Psychiatry 1996; 39:739–742
15. Irle E, Exner C, Thielen K, et al: Obsessive-compulsive disorder and ventromedial frontal lesions: clinical and neuropsychological findings. Am J Psychiatry 1998; 155:255–263
16. Malhi GS, Bartlett JR: A new lesion for the psychosurgical operation of stereotactic subcaudate tractotomy (SST). Br J Neurosurg 1998; 12:335–339
17. Sawlani V, Gupta RK, Singh MK, et al: MRI demonstration of Wallerian degeneration in various intracranial lesions and its clinical implications. J Neurol Sci 1997; 146:103–108
18. Yamada K, Shrier DA, Rubio A, et al: MR imaging of the mamillothalamic tract. Radiology 1998; 207:593–598
19. Khurana DS, Strawsburg RH, Robertson RL, et al: MRI signal changes in the white matter after corpus callosotomy. Pediatr Neurol 1999; 21:691–695
20. Rademacher J, Engelbrecht V, Burgel U, et al: Measuring in vivo myelination of human white matter fiber tracts with magnetization transfer MR. Neuroimage 1999; 9:393–406
21. Jones DK, Simmons A, Williams SC, et al: Noninvasive assessment of axonal fiber connectivity in the human brain via diffusion tensor MRI. Magn Reson Med 1999; 42:37–41
22. Wieshmann UC, Symms MR, Clark CA, et al: Wallerian degeneration in the optic radiation after temporal lobectomy demonstrated in vivo with diffusion tensor imaging. Epilepsia 1999; 40:1155–1158
23. Bagley LJ, McGowan JC, Grossman RI, et al: Magnetization transfer imaging of traumatic brain injury. J Magn Reson Imaging 2000; 11:1–8
24. McGowan JC, Yang JH, Plotkin RC, et al: Magnetization transfer imaging in the detection of injury associated with mild head trauma. AJNR Am J Neuroradiol 2000; 21:875–880
25. Malizia AL, Allen SJ, Maisey MN, et al: Changes in low frontal cerebral blood flow correlate with outcome in stereotactic subcaudate tractotomy carried out for refractory depression, in Refractory Depression: Current Strategies and Future Directions, edited by Nolen W, et al. New York, Wiley, 1994, pp 163–167
26. Biver F, Goldman S, Francois A, et al: Changes in metabolism of cerebral glucose after stereotactic leukotomy for refractory obsessive-compulsive disorder: a case report. J Neurol Neurosurg Psychiatry 1995; 58:502–505
27. Moringlane JR, Bartylla K, Hagen T, et al: Stereotactic neurosurgery planning with 3-D spiral CT-angiography. Minim Invasive Neurosurg 1997; 40:83–86
28. Rubino GJ, Farahani K, McGill D, et al: Magnetic resonance imaging–guided neurosurgery in the magnetic fringe fields: the next step in neuronavigation. Neurosurgery 2000; 46:643–653
29. Hall WA, Liu H, Martin AJ, et al: Safety, efficacy, and functionality of high-field strength interventional magnetic resonance imaging for neurosurgery. Neurosurgery 2000; 46:632–641

Recent Publications of Interest

Hall W: Avoiding potential misuses of addiction brain science. Addiction 2006; 101:1529–1532

A cautionary editorial about the use of psychosurgery to treat opiate addiction in China and Russia and the potential danger that this unproven approach may be introduced into other nations.

Breit S, LeBas JF, Koudsie A, et al: Pretargeting for the implantation of stimulation electrodes into the subthalamic nucleus: a comparative study of magnetic resonance imaging and ventriculography. Neurosurgery 2006; 58:ONS83–ONS95

Compares the accuracy of preoperative magnetic resonance imaging and stereotactic ventriculography for targeting the subthalamic nucleus. They found that mismatches were present with both techniques, but indirect targeting by use of radiological landmarks (ventriculography) was more accurate than direct targeting by anatomic visualization. They note that regardless of the imaging methods used for targeting, electrophysiological exploration is mandatory to obtain optimal clinical results.

Mashour GA, Walker EE, Martuza RL: Psychosurgery: past, present, and future. Brain Res Brain Res Rev 2005; 48:409–419
Provides an overview of psychosurgery including the origins and history, the four major procedures used in current practice, and likely future developments.

Kotowicz Z: Gottlieb Burckhardt and Egas Moniz—two beginnings of psychosurgery. Gesnerus 2005; 62:77–101
Discusses the origins of psychosurgery and the factors that lead to its acceptance as a treatment procedure.

Rezai AR, Bajer KB, Tkach JA, et al: Is magnetic resonance imaging safe for patients with neurostimulation systems used for deep brain stimulation? Neurosurgery 2005; 57:1056–1062
A commentary on the known dangers of performing magnetic resonance imaging examinations in patients with implanted electrodes for deep brain stimulation and the importance of following manufacturers' exposure guidelines.

Sachdev PS, Sachdev J: Long-term outcome of neurosurgery for the treatment of resistant depression. J Neuropsychiatry Clin Neurosci 2005; 17:478–485
Presents the long-term outcomes of psychosurgery on patients with treatment-resistant depression at their center. Although significant improvement or remission was obtained in many cases, no prognostic indicators were identified.

Anderson CA, Arciniegas DB: Neurosurgical interventions for neuropsychiatric syndromes. Curr Psychiatry Rep 2004; 6:355–363
Reviews the history of and recent developments in psychosurgery for the treatment of mental illnesses.

Reprinted from Hurley RA, Black DN, Stip E, et al: "Surgical Treatment of Mental Illness: Impact of Imaging." *Journal of Neuropsychiatry and Clinical Neurosciences* 12:421–424, 2000. Used with permission.

INDEX

Page numbers printed in **boldface** *refer to figures.*